Praise for *Women of the 14th Moon*

"A valuable collection, practically a support group in a package."
— *Publishers Weekly*

"Thank goodness for the diversity of emotions and symptoms described in the stories and poems of *Women of the 14th Moon . . .* Women are finally speaking about menopause and sharing their stories . . ."
— *Women's Review of Books*

". . . unique first-person accounts . . . encourage women to consider menopause as a positive change bringing new freedom . . . The contributors discuss personal thoughts and urge women to use menopause as an opportunity to make creative changes in their lives."
— *Library Journal*

". . . one of the most informative, lively and woman-focused books on menopause I've ever seen."
— *Toronto Star*

". . . for any woman who has experienced menopause or who knows she one day will and doesn't quite know what to expect."
— *Sojourner*

"*Women of the 14th Moon* is an extraordinary impressionistic work, brilliantly presenting the immense diversity of aging and menopause experience."
— *Women Library Workers Journal*

"An incredible wealth of information is revealed in first-person accounts . . ."
— Judy Askew, *Menopause News*

"*Women of the 14th Moon* is a wonderful collection of personal accounts of the many different shapes our journeys through menopause may take. It provides what I looked for a decade ago and couldn't find . . ."
— Christine Downing, author *Journey Through Menopause*

WOMEN
of the 14th
MOON

writings on
menopause

Edited by
Dena Taylor and
Amber Coverdale Sumrall

Preface by Grace Paley
Foreword by Rosetta Reitz

The Crossing Press • Freedom, CA 95019

The "Hot Flash Fan" on the cover is by Ann Stewart Anderson in collaboration with 52 artists. It is in the collection of the Kentucky Foundation for Women in Louisville. The Hot Flash Fan is a visual description of the myths and facts about menopause. Based on academic research and responses from menopausal women, the Fan's twelve blades, in colors representing the spectrum, describe the many facets of this change in a woman's body. Beginning at the lower left, the fan depicts the myth that menopausal women are no longer interested in sex. It pictures the hag, the dried up woman with a permanent scar. This leads to several panels about aging, a general slowing and the specific phenomena of the dowager's hump, dried up mucus membranes, aching joints and obesity. At the top of the fan, the seventh panel represents freedom from pregnancy and birth control leading to the blue figure who leaps with spiritual joy at her new liberation. But society imposes on these women the myth of strangeness, hysteria and melancholia. Finally the woman is shown with post menopausal zest, enjoying her new sexual freedom.

The fan is 8' x 16' and constructed from fabric. It is embellished with applique, embroidery, couching, beading, trapunto, quilting, paint and photographs.

Library of Congress Cataloging-in-Publication Data

Women of the Fourteenth Moon: Writings on Menopause / edited by Dena
   Taylor and Amber Coverdale Sumrall.
                    p. cm.
   ISBN 0-89594-478-2   ISBN 0-89594-477-4 (pbk.)
   1. Menopause. I. Taylor, Dena. II. Sumrall, Amber Coverdale.
   III. Title: Women of the Fourteenth Moon.
RG186.W64 1991
612.6'65--dc20   91-20297
                                                  CIP

We dedicate this book
to our mothers and grandmothers
who made the journey through menopause
in silence and isolation.

The mind of a post-menopausal woman is virtually uncharted territory.
—Barbara G. Walker

I don't want to get around it. I want to live it. I don't want to "treat" it or "cure" it, though I do want to honor it with curiosity and with therapy (therapeia), attention of the kind one devotes to sacred mysteries. I want menopause to be a soul event, which means letting it be transformative.
—Christine Downing

TABLE OF CONTENTS

PREFACE
Grace Paley

About a year ago a friend, a woman, a writer, called long distance to ask, How come you've never written anything about menopause. I don't mean to be critical, she said, I'm just asking. I decided it was a critical statement and immediately added it to other important life facts and worries I hadn't written about yet. Life is complicated and so short, I thought, and I'm not getting anything done. But really, what about menopause?

The fact is I'm 68 and I seem to have forgotten those years or maybe that year. They happened, in my optimistic reconstruction, between my late 40s and early 50s. On medical forms I have written 49, 52, 50—whatever number was useful to that day's mindset. I *did* write a review of Rosetta Reitz's fine book on menopause when it came out and admired Paula Weideger's as well, so it must have been on my mind at some point.

I suspect that my menstrual periods simply ceased one month having grown lighter and easier. That probable easiness was accompanied by something I do remember: heat, the taking off and putting on of shirts and sweaters, my face reddening first into rosy health then a fierce faceful of fever. A crazy barometer, I'd explain to people who thought I was about to faint. Give that barometer two degrees and it takes twenty, I said. I was joking and it did have a certain comedy to it. Excess, when not dangerous, often does. I laughed. My friends laughed.

We could laugh because the kids were just about grown. Something else was coming. We could laugh because the years were lively, energetic, risky, hopeful, lots of politics, literature, friendship, love.

That was because of luck and the historical moment. This is what luck might have meant for some of us: fortunate family experience, maybe your mother and two aunts say *oh it was easy for me, that change of life*. Luck also makes itself known by inhabiting a gene or two. This is how good teeth appear in certain generally toothless families. But when luck is thickened with good food or bad, with early loving care or neglect, it becomes the historical moment. On the simplest level, when women's lives were measured by their reproductive years, menopause was the end. Poor women! That public and psychological description—quite frequent when I was young—enraged me, disgusted me.

But I want to take the historical moment a little past that ancient idea—well-trounced by the women's movement of the last couple of decades, sometimes called *the second wave.* All in lucky time for my aging generation.

The historical moments of my change of life occurred in the late 1960s to early 70s when those important communities of civil rights activists and anti-war workers began to break apart dramatically, the women of those movements reforming, reshaping into feminist organizers, thinkers, wild, delighted activists.

The women's movement, that world changer, had been scattering consciousness-raising groups all over the country. Concluding that the personal was political gave a way of speaking and writing and thinking—a way for all women to make art, educate themselves, find new work, rename time and themselves. A book like *Our Bodies Our Selves* was almost enough to air out the last few dusty centuries.

I have written this little bit of history because I believe that the high, anxious, but hopeful energy of the time, the general political atmosphere and the particular female moment had a lot to do with the fact that I can't quite remember my menopause, or remembering it, haven't thought to write much about it. Writing for me has always come from being bugged—agitated by a life, a speaking voice, an idea. I've asked some of my age-mates, old friends, and they feel pretty much the same way. We were busy, our lives heightened by opposition and hope.

Now I write this as the war in the Gulf, the Great American Gulf War, has ended and not ended. Hundreds of thousands have died by our high-flying hand. Our anti-war coalitions didn't have time to set out branches and roots. They did well, but the war was so swift, so vicious, that many of us are left with considerable sorrow/despair. I think of women entering their period of menopause now and I wonder will it be different for them. I think it must be. We live in this world which takes our children and sets terrible barriers before them: war—a new one just for their generation, a gift of their fathers—drugs, a narrow nationalism of hatred, poverty, absurdity. Our insides *do* know something about what is happening to our outsides. Our bodies live in this world and are picked up, shaken, and what is natural becomes difficult. What is difficult becomes painful and hopeless.

Still, I must remind myself, having said all this, that there is now a women's community, women's communities where women stand still, almost breathless, to talk to one another, or gather at homes or meeting places—or in a book like *Women of the Fourteenth Moon,* to listen, to tell, *This is where my trouble is, this is where it hurts.* And then someone answers, *Me too. This is what I did about it.*

FOREWORD

Rosetta Reitz

Menopause has had a poor press. The bad parts have been touted and the good parts have been kept secret. Hot flashes and mood swings are TV fare for talk shows but they don't give equal time to the pleasure of no longer being burdened with a monthly flow of blood which must be absorbed or the freedom of sex without birth control.

It's the same kind of thing that happened to the women who sang the blues. The negative side was emphasized as though every black woman who sang was moaning and groaning about lost love and being abandoned. As if every song was a variation of, "Daddy won't you please come home./ Mama's so all alone." Victims. We've been led to believe the blues, like menopause, is sad and sorry. It can be and is, some of the time, but that's only part of the picture.

What about the women who sang, "I bake the best jelly roll," or "I've got the sweetest cabbage in town"? Or those who gave sexual instructions:

> I may want love for one hour,
> then decide to make it two.
> Takes an hour before I get started,
> maybe three before I'm through.*

Those aren't victims, those are proud women with plenty of self-esteem and a big sense of humor.

Why, then, historically, have the negatives received so much publicity while the good stuff has been kept hidden? That was one of the questions I asked when I began to search for information about menopause twenty years ago.

It was a wasteland. There was so little. And what there was, was written mostly by male doctors who looked upon menopause as a deficiency disease. The books were patronizing, trying to make me feel worthless. Worst of all, they reduced women, around the age of 50, to only being in menopause; robbing

---

* From *One Hour Mama* by Ida Cox on the album *Mean Mothers*, Women's Independent Blues, Volume 1, Rosetta Records.

us of our personhood and our identities.

The only thing I could find 20 years ago which was literature was a deplorable book written by Thomas Mann toward the end of his life. A novel called *The Black Swan* was horrid enough to make you clutch at your ovaries. Hateful, that's what it was; women after menopause were worthless. They were good to no one and were merely taking up space on this planet. Could this travesty against women be written by the same person who moved me so much (before the Women's Movement) with *The Magic Mountain* and *Buddenbrooks*? Yes, it was. I have never had the courage to read those books again, but I hope to, one day.

I wanted to hear from women themselves, what they were feeling, not from men who distorted us and our feelings through their own biased filters.

That is why it is such a delight to know that a book like this exists, where menopause is celebrated in prose and poetry. I liked the poems most and wish there were more of them but I can imagine how hard it must be to find good poems, especially ones about menopause, not yet a common choice for a subject by poets.

When I started my search for information in the early seventies, I was in my mid-forties; I asked women who were older and had had the experience, as well as women my own age. My friends were as ignorant as I was and the older women weren't used to talking about such matters. I was fired up from consciousness raising in those days and was looking for the truth.

At that time, I was the director of the Classified section of the *Village Voice* and easily placed ads. MENOPAUSE in caps, "want to talk about it? Free! Call this number."

Women called and came to my house; they travelled from Westchester and New Jersey and Connecticut. They were like me, enthusiastic to talk to each other.

There was only one rule, one taboo word. *Should.* No one was to tell another person what she *should* do. Each woman came to her own conclusions for herself and no one was to reprimand herself for what she *should* have done. We were all searching together and what may work for one, might not for another.

To tell you those meetings were thrilling is only part of the story. They had historic reverberations of the pleasure of women meeting together at the river to wash clothes; in a sewing circle to make a quilt. There was such an honesty about it all. Nothing like the phoney stuff where people instantaneously love each other. Nothing like that at all.

To say I became addicted to these groups is perhaps an overstatement but they were feeding me, nurturing me in a way that was filling a place I hadn't fully understood. No matter, I was involved for five years, writing notes after each session so I wouldn't forget some of the nuances which were fascinating.

The range and scope of the "symptoms" were baffling. How much was aging and how much was menopause and how much was an individual's own baggage?

I became known, among women's groups, as a person who was seriously searching for information about menopause and was invited to speak and facilitate workshops. It wasn't long before I realized I'd have to put this material in a book. When I was hunting for information I wanted to find a book about "us," not "them." So I wrote the book I was searching for, using many women's voices in addition to my own.

I tried to sell it. A few publishers offered to consider it if I eliminated the word MENOPAUSE. This was the middle seventies when that word was still only whispered. They wanted euphemisms, like "mid-life crisis," or "middle years." But I refused. That idea violated everything I believed in. The whole point was to confront menopause, not hide from it or make it sound like anything other than it was.

I insisted on naming it *Menopause: A Positive Approach* and it was published in 1977, picked by The Book Of The Month Club in 1978 and issued in paperback by Penguin in 1979 and is still selling, including many foreign editions.

How lucky women are today who are searching for information. *Women of the 14th Moon* has an abundance of it, by women, first hand, who have lived the experience.

It is curious that the woman who is probably most read is Jane E. Brody, who writes about health for the *New York Times*. She seems eager to report on the various new uses of estrogen. Why, I still wonder, would women fool around with their endocrine systems by putting foreign hormones into themselves? Not only does it throw the system out of whack but adds the possibility of serious damage. It also creates a sluggishness in one's own ability to make estrogen. Our body's capacity to supply us with estrogen doesn't shut off the day we become 50 years old. And when the ovaries slow down, the adrenals pick up some of that work and so does our fatty tissue. What an irony it is that many nationally known women advisors on health matters look to be anorexic. They don't seem to know about nature's miraculous self-healing extraglandular estrogen in our own fatty tissue.

The myths we were fighting 20 years ago about estrogen enabling the user to be "feminine forever" are not as far behind us as I had hoped. The pharmaceutical companies keep pushing their products and when they lose sales from birth control pills because women are afraid of the side effects, they try PMS to sell their estrogen. When that doesn't catch on into the multi-million dollar industry they hoped for they go after older women. With promises, promises of estrogen being the cure for their complaints, including osteoporosis and maybe even heart disease. Without, of course, nearly enough warning about the detrimental effects. While other companies are trying to push anti-estrogens on healthy women to prevent breast cancer. Contradictions! Contradictions! The NATIONAL WOMEN'S HEALTH NETWORK in Washington, D.C. has effectively influenced National policies which have an impact on women's health. For example, the Network prevented the manufacturer of Premarin estrogen tablets from gaining FDA approval for routine use in all women over 50 with hysterectomies. The FDA's decision is still pending because of the Network's opposition. And further, they went on record as having told the FDA that, "The Network strongly opposes the proposed new indication for Premarin as a coronary heart disease preventative. Premarin has not been adequately studied." This statement influenced the FDA Advisory Committee from giving full support to Wyeth-Ayerest's request to add coronary heart disease prevention to the list of reasons why women should use ERT. Not a full victory by any means, but when you consider their lobbying opponents are the AMA and gargantuan drug companies, I take my hat off to them.

Women of the 14th Moon is a fascinating collection of poetry and prose which represents a variety of voices and viewpoints. In addition to being entertaining, it will go a long way toward enlightening and informing women about this very significant time of their lives.

INTRODUCTION

Dena Taylor & Amber Coverdale Sumrall

When we realized that we were on the brink of menopause, we went in search of women's stories describing in their own voices this time in their lives. We did not find them. Instead, we found medical texts by men, self-help books by women, anthropological reports on menopause in other cultures, and many articles on the pros and cons of various remedies. One exception was Rosetta Reitz' landmark book, *Menopause: A Positive Approach,* documenting the experiences of many women. Still, there was no literature telling women's stories, so we decided to collect them ourselves.

We expected to find common experiences of hot flashes, a sense of loss, and a general feeling of the blahs. Instead we found tremendous diversity and individuality in the women's accounts. Some had terrible hot flashes. Some had incredible dreams. Some went through a period of important self-discovery, often realizing a profound sense of spirituality. Some left long-standing relationships, and some found new ones. Some laughed about what was happening. For some, menopause lasted one year; for others, ten years. Some had very heavy bleeding. Some couldn't get by without taking estrogen, and others wouldn't hear of it. Many came through it much stronger. And some told us they had nothing to write because they hardly noticed their menopause.

Menopause is a natural event, not a deficiency disease or a signal that the end is near. Nor is it an end to vitality and sexuality. It has been, however, a taboo subject, shrouded in silence, negativity, denial and fear.

Nevertheless, when women themselves are asked about their menopause, it seems that for many it is not particularly negative. Sonja McKinlay, who has been studying menopause for years, collecting data on 2,500 women in the Boston area, found that often the women experience a year or two of irregular periods, some hot flashes and sleepless nights, and "that is that." Women in Newfoundland, in fact, are said to experience hot flashes as generally cleansing, and the heat is believed to purify the blood.

Medical information is constantly changing, with new and often conflicting studies being published every few weeks on the risks and benefits of hormone replacement therapy and other help for the symptoms of menopause.

We are told in the popular magazines that if we are lucky we will get through this stage as quickly and as effortlessly as possible. We are taught not to accept our aging and the wisdom of our lives, to discount our new selves, to ignore the phenomenon of menopause. It is what Germaine Greer calls "the invisible experience."

Perhaps there is a different attitude. Perhaps we could see menopause as a transformative process, and relish the possibilities contained therein. We need to claim this time as vital to our growth, as important as the changes of adolescence, which Kurt Vonnegut has termed "children's menopause."

Our mothers and grandmothers often "went crazy" and were even institutionalized during menopause. The subject was considered shameful and not openly discussed. It has only begun to come out of the closet. Women in the past had little support or information. They could only turn to their (male) doctors who, from what we can glean from old medical texts, believed menopausal women were fit for the garbage heap.

Until recently, historically speaking, women didn't live long past their child-bearing years, which is one of the reasons little research has been done on the subject of menopause. Also, the practice of medicine is largely a male-dominated one, and menopausal women are not taken seriously.

Hopefully with more women in fields of research and medicine, this aspect of women's lives will receive the thoughtful study it deserves. Hopefully too we will see menopause as a subject of literature.

A new generation of women is coming into menopause which views this time as an important process, challenging the myths and misogyny that exist today in our North American society. Ours is a culture which is not only sexist but ageist—factors which put menopausal women in a very low position. As Paula Weideger has said, "Our cultural inheritance has dictated that woman is valued and valuable *only* as long as she can reproduce."

Women in some non-Western cultures experience menopause quite differently, and often have a definite and positive place in society after this passage. Marcha Flint found that women in India, for instance, were rewarded for attaining menopause, and did not experience any negative menopausal symptoms.

Women of the 14th Moon presents a wide range of North American women's experiences with menopause: inspiring, painful, funny, informative, poetic. We see from these accounts what happens when a pattern of 35-40 years of cyclic bleeding is disrupted, with the inevitable accompanying physical and emotional changes.

As can be seen from the stories and poems in this book, women do emerge from menopause not simply older, but invariably changed in some way. For many this journey is a positive, empowering experience, full of discovery and excitement. For others it is difficult, but there always seems to be an end, a point where women say, "Yes, that's over now, and I feel very much alive again." Although we cannot know how menopause is going to affect us, we can prepare for it by informing ourselves and listening to those who have been there.

It is important to develop resources, talk to one another, and keep our sense of humor. This is a time to let go, to accept ourselves as we are, to listen to our inner voice.

This book will help demystify menopause for women in their late thirties and forties. It will educate and hopefully prepare them for this process. And for women going through menopause, we hope that by reading other women's stories, their journey will be enriched. We also think this is a book for partners of women in menopause, because it will provide some understanding of how menopause can be experienced.

In 1975, Paula Weideger wrote, "If menopause is to become an integrated part of life rather than the separate crisis it now is, women must define and share their own experiences." *Women of the Fourteenth Moon* is a beginning, the first wave of what we hope will be many more women's stories of menopause.

Our title is taken from Eleanor Piazza's piece in the book. She says, "...if there are thirteen full moons in a given year, a woman who has not had a period for a year will begin a new phase of her life upon the fourteenth full moon..."

A resource section is included at the end, listing periodicals, books, and organizations which provide information and support for women going through menopause.

We want to thank Elaine Goldman Gill of The Crossing Press for her enthusiasm and support for this project. We also gratefully acknowledge and thank the writers in this book who wrote so personally and genuinely. For us, the experience of putting these inspiring women's voices together in one place was exhilarating. It is with tremendous pride that we present these works so that all of us may learn from them and that as a society we may begin to claim this part of our lives as vital and important.

Dena Taylor
Amber Coverdale Sumrall
Santa Cruz, CA, 1991

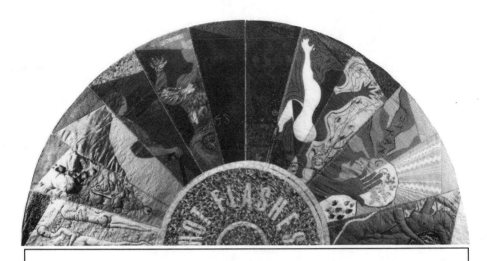

THE M-WORD

It makes me sad to know that if someone speaks of the myths of menopause, they mean the untruths, the fallacies, the misogynist distortions.

—Christine Downing

What I want to do is draw middle-aged women out of their purdah, make them really joyous. Menopause is the invisible experience. People don't want to hear about it. But this is the time when everything comes good for you—your humor, your style, your bad temper.

—Germaine Greer

I hope it gets here soon—I'm 22.

—from Mary Beth Edelson's Menstruation Stories

THE SPACE CRONE

Ursula K. Le Guin

The menopause is probably the least glamorous topic imaginable; and this is interesting, because it is one of the very few topics to which cling some shreds and remnants of taboo. A serious mention of menopause is usually met with uneasy silence; a sneering reference to it is usually met with relieved sniggers. Both the silence and the sniggering are pretty sure indications of taboo.

Most people would consider the old phrase "change of life" a euphemism for the medical term "menopause," but I, who am now going through the change, begin to wonder if it isn't the other way round. "Change of life" is too blunt a phrase, too factual. "Menopause," with its chime-suggestion of a mere pause after which things go on as before, is reassuringly trivial.

But the change is not trivial, and I begin to wonder how many women are brave enough to carry it out whole-heartedly. They give up their reproductive capacity with more or less of a struggle, and when it's gone they think that's all there is to it. Well, at least I don't get the Curse any more, they say, and the only reason I felt so depressed sometimes was hormones. Now I'm myself again. But this is to evade the real challenge, and to lose, not only the capacity to ovulate, but the opportunity to become a Crone.

In the old days women who survived long enough to attain the menopause more often accepted the challenge. They had, after all, had practice. They had already changed their life radically once before, when they ceased to be virgins and became mature women/wives/matrons/mothers/mistresses/whores/etc. This change involved not only the physiological alterations of puberty—the shift from barren childhood to fruitful maturity—but a socially recognized alteration of being: a change of condition from the sacred to the profane.

With the secularisation of virginity now complete, so that the once awesome term "virgin" is now a sneer or at best a slightly dated word for a person who hasn't copulated yet, the opportunity of gaining or regaining the dangerous/sacred condition-of-being at the Second Change has ceased to be apparent.

Virginity is now a mere preamble or waiting-room to be got out of as soon as possible; it is without significance. Old age is similarly a waiting-room, where you go after life's over and wait for cancer or a stroke. The years before and after the menstrual years are vestigial: the only meaningful condition left to women is that of fruitfulness. Curiously, this restriction of significance coincided with the development of chemicals and instruments which make fertility itself a meaningless or at least secondary characteristic of female maturity. The significance of maturity now is not the capacity to conceive but the mere ability to have sex. As this ability is shared by pubescents and by postclimacterics, the blurring of distinctions and elimination of opportunities is almost complete. There are no rites of passage, because there is no significant change. The Triple Goddess has only one face: Marilyn Monroe's, maybe. The entire life of a woman from 10 or 12 through 70 or 80 has become secular, uniform, changeless. As there is no longer any virtue in virginity, so there is no longer any meaning in menopause. It requires fanatical determination now to become a Crone.

Women have thus, by imitating the life-condition of men, surrendered a very strong position of their own. Men are afraid of virgins, but they have a cure for their own fear and the virgin's virginity: fucking. Men are afraid of crones, so afraid of them that their cure for virginity fails them; they know it won't work. Faced with the fulfilled Crone, all but the bravest men wilt and retreat, crestfallen and cockadroop.

Menopause Manor is not merely a defensive stronghold, however. It is a house or household, fully furnished with the necessities of life. In abandoning it, women have narrowed their domain and impoverished their souls. There are things the Old Woman can do, say, and think which the Woman cannot do, say, or think. The Woman has to give up more than her menstrual periods before she can do, say, or think them. She has got to change her life.

The nature of that change is now clearer than it used to be. Old age is not virginity, but a third and new condition; the virgin must be celibate, but the crone need not. There was a confusion there, which the separation of female sexuality from reproductive capacity, via modern contraceptives, has cleared up. Loss of fertility does not mean loss of desire and fulfillment. But it does entail a change, a change involving matters even more important—if I may venture a heresy—than sex.

The woman who is willing to make that change must become pregnant with herself, at last. She must bear herself, her third self, her old age, with travail and alone. Not many will help her with that birth. Certainly no male obstetrician will time her contractions, inject her with sedatives, stand ready with forceps, and neatly stitch up the torn membranes. It's hard even to find an old-fashioned midwife, these days. That pregnancy is long, that labor is hard. Only one is harder, and that's the final one, the one which men also must suffer and perform.

It may well be easier to die if you have already given birth to others or yourself, at least once before. This would be an argument for going through all the discomfort and embarrassment of becoming a Crone. Anyhow it seems a pity to have a built-in rite of passage and to dodge it, evade it, and pretend nothing has changed. That is to dodge and evade one's womanhood, to pretend one's like a man. Men, once initiated, never get the second chance. They never change again. That's their loss, not ours. Why borrow poverty?

Certainly the effort to remain unchanged, young, when the body gives so impressive a signal of change as the menopause, is gallant; but it is a stupid, self-sacrificial gallantry, better befitting a boy of twenty than a woman of forty-five or fifty. Let the athletes die young and laurel-crowned. Let the soldiers earn the Purple Hearts. Let women die old, white-crowned, with human hearts.

If a space ship came by from the friendly natives of the fourth planet of Altair, and the polite captain of the space ship said, "We have room for one passenger; will you spare us a single human being, so that we may converse at leisure during the long trip back to Altair, and learn from an exemplary person the nature of the race?"—I suppose what most people would want to do is provide them with a fine, bright, brave young man, highly educated and in peak physical condition. A Russian cosmonaut would be ideal (American astronauts are mostly too old). There would surely be hundreds, thousands of volunteers, just such young men, all worthy. But I would not pick any of them. Nor would I pick any of the young women who would volunteer, some out of magnanimity and intellectual courage, others out of a profound conviction that Altair couldn't possibly be any worse for a woman than Earth is.

What I would do is go down to the local Woolworth's, or the local village marketplace, and pick an old woman, over sixty, from behind the costume jewelry counter or the betel-nut booth. Her hair would not be red or blonde or lustrous dark, her skin would not be dewy fresh, she would not have the secret of eternal youth. She might, however, show you a small snapshot of her grandson, who is working in Nairobi. She is a bit vague about where Nairobi is, but extremely proud of the grandson. She has worked hard at small, unimportant jobs all her life, jobs like cooking, cleaning, bringing up kids, selling little objects of adornment or pleasure to other people. She was a virgin once a long time ago, and then a sexually potent fertile female, and then went through menopause. She has given birth several times and faced death several times—the same times. She is facing the final birth/death a little more nearly and clearly every day now. Sometimes her feet hurt something terrible. She never was educated to anything like her capacity, and that is a shameful waste and a crime against humanity, but so common a crime should not and cannot be hidden from Altair. And anyhow she's not dumb. She has a stock of sense, wit, patience, and experiential shrewdness, which the Altaireans might, or might not, perceive as wisdom. If they are wiser than we, then of course we don't know how they'd perceive it. But if they are wiser than we they may know how to perceive that inmost mind and heart which we, working on mere guess and hope, proclaim to be humane. In any case, since they are curious and kindly, let's give them the best we have to give.

The trouble is, she will be very reluctant to volunteer. "What would an old woman like me do on Altair?" she'll say. "You ought to send one of those scientist men, they can talk to those funny-looking green people. Maybe Dr. Kissinger should go. What about sending the Shaman?" It will be very hard to explain to her that we want her to go because only a person who has experienced, accepted, and acted the entire human condition—the essential quality of which is Change—can fairly represent humanity. "Me?" she'll say, just a trifle slyly. "But I never did anything."

But it won't wash. She knows, though she won't admit it, that Dr. Kissinger has not gone and will never go where she has gone, that the scientists and the shamans have not done what she has done. Into the space ship, Granny.

A FUNNY THING HAPPENED ON MY WAY TO MIDDLE AGE

Evelyn M. Parke

Menopause happened to me when I was only 40 years old.

I didn't mean for it to happen to me that early, and neither did God.

It was an accident.

It came about this way: at 40, I was too old to have children and I couldn't take The Pill. I found other forms of birth control repulsive, and I was what we used to call (pre-AIDS) Sexually Active.

So I went to see my gynecologist and we made an appointment for surgery and I had a tubal ligation, otherwise known as having the tubes tied.

Immediately after the tubal ligation my periods became irregular and diminished in scope, if you know what I mean, and finally they disappeared entirely.

Meanwhile, I began to have spells of getting hot all over. I don't mean warming up a little: I mean HOT ALL OVER. And these hot spells went on and on and on, and when one ended it was only 15 minutes or so till the next one started.

Sweat dripped off the ends of my hair onto my clothes. I had to wipe sweat off my face as if I were running a long distance race in the sun. My glasses steamed up and then slid down my nose and stayed there, due to the hot salty stream pouring down my forehead and onto my nose.

Hot flashes, women call them, and the implication of the word "flash" is that they happen quickly and go away. Not so. (Some years later a different gynecologist took exception to my use of the term "hot flash," and corrected me, saying, "No, dear, they are called hot *flushes*." I looked him straight in the eye and said, "Well, *dear*, when you get one, you can call it anything you want. Mine are hot flashes, and so are the ones of every other woman I know." I also changed doctors—this was not our first difference of opinion.)

Meanwhile, back when I was 40 (and I am 54 as I sit here writing this), I took my symptoms to my family physician. I didn't do this right away, but after a while I began to feel I was getting psychotic from sleep deprivation: I would fall asleep and after about 15 minutes heat up with a hot flash, and wake up, throw the covers off, and go back to sleep. Then after 15 or 20 minutes of hot flash I would cool down and wake up, freezing, and pull the covers back up. This went on all night, every 15 or 20 minutes, night after night after night. Sleep deprivation can be used to torture prisoners. It makes them crazy. It was making *me* crazy.

My doctor didn't wish to consider menopause.

"You are too young," he said.

"Yes," I said, "But my periods have almost stopped, and I have these hot flashes *all the time* [as I lay sweating onto his examining table], and we have to *do something!*"

But he said it was most likely a symptom of stress, and would clear up in time, and don't worry; I dressed and went hotly and sweatily out the door.

A month or so later, miserably later, believe me, at the time of my annual PAP test, my doctor condescended to have a cell maturation test done. The analysis of my cells showed that I had indeed started menopause and if I was only 40, so what? (I have been told since then that this test is not totally reliable, and for that reason is not done a lot. However, the test results, combined with my hot flashes and completely stopped periods seemed conclusive.)

By this time I was spending a good part of my life crying and I was getting very bad tempered from the stress of being overheated and sweating all day, every day, so my doctor (against his better judgment), started me on ERT—estrogen replacement therapy.

First, he told me all the hazards of taking estrogen, which seemed to boil down to "increased risk of cancer and God knows what else." I hardly listened—I was too hot and sweaty to listen—and I said, "Give it to me. Give it to me NOW! I don't *care* if it kills me; there's no point living forever if I am locked away in a mental institution, and that's where I'm heading, believe me." By this time I had nearly lost my job because of my outbursts of temper—and who wouldn't have a temper under those circumstances?

My doctor believed in shots, not pills.

Relief came fast after the first shot.

After the third or fourth shot, however, relief faded away and the hot flashes came back. The shots, supposed to be given every three or four weeks, began to be needed oftener and oftener.

Finally, my doctor said I would have to wait three weeks for the next shot, regardless of my misery.

We discussed this. I showed him the lump I was getting at the site of the shot—a thing that always happens to me if I have too much medication by injection—which I felt indicated that my body was not letting the estrogen into my system.

My elderly and conservative doctor finally agreed to try giving me the estrogen in pills. Everybody else I knew was on the pills, but this man felt he could control the amount better if he gave shots. He yielded and gave me a prescription for pills. I promised never to take two in one day or anything silly like that.

The pills changed my life.

The hot flashes went away and stayed away, except for rare occasions. I slept all night, every night. My temper improved. My outlook improved. I felt like a new woman.

At last I was calm enough to appreciate the wonderful freedom from menstruation. No more tampons or pads. No more cramps. No more premenstrual stress. Freedom! I felt I had become myself for the first time in years.

No longer immobilized emotionally and intellectually by hot flashes, I got myself in gear and found another gynecologist. (The one who did the surgery had moved to another city.) This gynecologist was a woman, a new experience for me. She was so different from all the male doctors I had known, I could hardly believe she was really a doctor. It didn't seem possible that a doctor could be so uncondescending and unpatronizing.

She talked to me about my tubal ligation. I had not been conscious when it was done, and actually knew very little about it except that while people speak of having their "tubes tied," this isn't what actually happens. In my case, I had what was called "bandaid surgery," where a tiny incision was made inside my navel and another one at my pubic hair line, and instruments were inserted into each incision. When the instruments touched, they made an electric spark, which sort of cauterized the fallopian tubes, so that ovum couldn't travel down the tubes to the uterus. At least, that was my understanding of what happened.

My gynecologist said, and I do quote, "Ahah!"

"Yes?" I said.

"Oh," she said, "It's just that that explains your early menopause. We don't *do* that kind of tubal ligation any more, you know."

"No, I didn't know. Do tell me."

"Well, it's just that that particular procedure shuts off the blood supply to the ovaries completely, and they quit manufacturing hormones, and so you get a false, early menopause.

"What do you mean, false?" I asked. "This seems pretty real to me."

"Oh, yes," she said, laughing, "It's *real*, all right, it's just that it probably wouldn't have happened if you hadn't had that kind of tubal ligation. It's real but not real."

"Ahah!" I said. "How long will it last?"

"That's a good question," she said. "My best estimate is that it will last until whenever your normally-timed menopausal symptoms would have ended; say anywhere from 50 to 60—if they stop at all. Some women go on forever with the hot flashes, you know."

"Good God!" I was then about 42. And I hadn't known.

She was right. Some women go on having hot flashes forever. I am apparently one of them.

But no matter. Times have changed.

Today's gynecologist, ten years later, wants her 50-year-old patients to take estrogen. It may increase the risk of some kinds of cancer, but it is now believed that it also decreases the risk of osteoporosis, heart attack, and stroke.

In order to get the cancer risk back down to normal, the estrogen is taken in conjunction with another hormone, progesterone, after the patient turns 50.

Just about everybody knows that, these days.

What they *don't* know, and what their doctors don't tell them until they've already started on the estrogen-progesterone combo, is that once you get into progesterone you start having periods again. Once again, the uterus needs to discard its contents every four weeks. Once again, the uterus *has* contents.

Remember that gynecologist who told me it was hot *flushes*, not hot *flashes*? Well, he's the one who started my progesterone medication. I asked him about the periods.

"They aren't *periods*," he said, condescendingly. "You aren't ovulating. You're just having monthly bleeding."

Well, I now have this monthly bleeding, and I call it periods, and anybody who doesn't like it can lump it.

My new gynecologist wants me to stay on progesterone all my life, as far as she can tell now. When I am a 90-year-old bag lady (or whatever lies in my future), I'll still be stumbling into the grocery store once a month to buy my Sure and Naturals, or whatever.

I don't look forward to it.

I don't mind the monthly bleeding too much; it's less than I used to have when I was young.

But I hate the cramps.

My uterus got out of the habit of having periods, those ten years that I was taking only estrogen. I think my middle-aged muscles can't handle it any more. I take a lot of aspirin.

Can you learn anything from my experiences?

Yes, you can.

I learned that the practice of medicine changes fast these days. In 1976 my doctor thought it was radical to give me estrogen in tablets. Today I can't find anyone who takes it by injection. There was no progesterone then; there is now. Don't assume that what your doctor told you three years ago still holds true. If you have problems, see your doctor. There may be something to do about it now.

The big lesson I learned was, if your gynecologist gives you a hard time, get another one. Who needs to be patronized and condescended to, and told she is having a hot *flush*, not a hot *flash*? Misery is misery, and you need a doctor who understands that.

I also learned to stick with women gynecologists. I've had several of either sex, and the women tend to take my symptoms much more seriously. The men seem to prefer dealing with pregnancies, probably because that condition ends within a year, and patients don't return endlessly, complaining that it is too hot. (Also, pregnant women are usually young; menopausal women are usually not young. I wouldn't want to accuse male doctors of preferring younger, more attractive women as patients, but . . .)

My advice: Enjoy not having periods, and get ready to have them again. If your gynecologist or family physician is one of those who doesn't "believe" in ERT, seriously consider seeing someone else, particularly if the symptoms of your menopause are having a negative effect on your life. After all, reduced risk of heart attack, stroke, and osteoporosis can't be all bad.

Finally, don't suffer. No matter what your age, if you have the symptoms, find a doctor who will deal with them. There's no point hearing "You're too young," if you've already got the condition. By that time, *too young* doesn't mean anything.

SPLIT SECOND OF DENIAL

Marigold Fine

"You may be starting menopause," my acupuncturist announced after discussing my irregular periods. "I hadn't really thought of that possibility," I admitted— a little ashamed to be out of touch with reality. "I had thought fifty was the average age." "Yes, but the normal range is early 40s to early 50s. You're in that range."

Starting menopause. A distant and far-flung concept for so very long. That thing that happens to older women. Women who are greying, wrinkling, disappearing. To image myself as such a woman requires a leap. A leap from child, from daughter, reckless young woman, mother of a young girl, from one of a youth-crazed culture's circle of fertile beings.

A split second of denial. Like when you find out you're pregnant—even if you want to be. Of inevitability, finality.

Then came the surrender—taking refuge in the reality. I was to be joining an ancient sisterhood. A medicine hoop of age and wisdom. The knowers of the tribe. Admiring them from afar, I was soon to be one with them.

And this bloody bleeding. An end to that. The mess. The clocking and calculating. The worry and wondering. The cramping and irritability. The stained underwear and sheets. The mountains of paper products/forests sacrificed to absorb blood. Would I miss this? MAYBE.

I have newly come to savor these cycles. Almost enjoy them. The earthy, vivid blood from deep inside. Released by hormones talking to muscles, nerves and tissue. The *intelligence* of it. Knowing these cycles are short-lived suddenly makes them precious.

SOMETHING TO LOOK FORWARD TO

Marge Piercy

Menopause—word used as an insult:
a menopausal woman, mind or poem
as if not to leak regularly or on the caprice
of the moon, the collision of egg and sperm,
were the curse we first learned to call that blood.

I have twisted myself to praise that bright splash.
When my womb opens its lips on the full
or dark of the moon, that connection
aligns me as it does the sea. I quiver,
a compass needle thrilling with magnetism.

Yet for every celebration there's the time
it starts on a jet with the seatbelt sign on.
Consider the trail of red amoebae
crawling onto hostess' sheets to signal
my body's disregard of calendar, clock.

How often halfway up the side of a mountain,
during a demonstration with the tactical police
force drawn up in tanks between me and a toilet;
during an endless wind machine panel with four males
I the token woman and they with iron bladders,

I have felt that wetness and wanted to strangle
my womb like a mouse. Sometimes it feels cosmic
and sometimes it feels like mud. Yes, I have prayed
to my blood on my knees in toilet stalls
simply to show its rainbow of deliverance.

My friend Penny at twelve, being handed a napkin
the size of an ironing board cover, cried out
Do I have to do this from now till I die?
No, said her mother, it stops in middle age.
Good, said Penny, there's something to look forward to.

Today supine, groaning with demon crab claws
gouging my belly, I tell you I will secretly dance
and pour out a cup of wine on the earth
when time stops that leak permanently;
I will burn my last tampons as votive candles.

A JOURNEY HOMEWARD

Connie Batten

Over the past year or so the approach of menopause has been more and more a part of my consciousness. During that time I have come to realize that throughout my youth I had an overwhelming fear of this phase of life. I could not have worked with the fear ahead of time because I did not admit to myself that it was there. Only as my life has plunged me into the middle of my dread have I realized that it has been there all along. My story, I suspect, is not altogether uncommon.

The atmosphere surrounding menopause for women of my mother's generation was extremely repressive. I cannot remember even hearing the word menopause spoken out loud, though I was once, as a teenager, handed a pamphlet on the subject and told to read it. There was no discussion; only a lot of tension and confusing emotional messages. I reacted by distancing myself as much as possible, hoping menopause would go away if I ignored it.

In contrast to my unacknowledged fearful expectations about menopause and the years immediately preceding it, my actual experience has been a positive one in some very surprising ways. My accustomed sense of who I am has begun to slip, and while I feel a threat to my sense of security, I also feel a kind of excitement about my new awareness. This option of openness toward menopause is new to many women. For many of us it is easier now to be more conscious of what we are experiencing, and to share our insights with each other.

Since adolescence I have felt the ebbing and flowing of the ever-changing complex patterns of hormones in my body. I have known the mood shifting that takes place through the course of a month, so subtly at times that it is only in retrospect that I realize its cause. After a day when a brooding sadness had seemed ready to overtake me at the least excuse, my period would begin and I would suddenly realize the connection with the sadness. Or it might have been an irritability so close to the surface that I had almost no patience with my children. The onset of my period would provide sudden relief. The tide of hormones would have shifted and a sense of well-being would begin to build.

As women we are used to these tides. One way or another we've learned to live with them.

Now as I approach menopause the monthly pattern begins to lose its regularity. Another shift—this one of great magnitude—is taking place in my body, mind and spirit. I feel more closely in touch with the larger rhythm of the overall life cycle, and the awareness that this may be my last major life passage before death. Realizing this in my mid-forties, I suddenly feel wide awake. I am grateful for the years of experience from which intuitions and understandings are drawn.

For so many years, we as women are affected by the monthly changes which come to us and are beyond our control. This is probably what makes it possible for us to be more comfortable than many men are with the intuitive, the immeasurable, the inexplicable. Part of our being is ever responsive to natural flowings, which teach us in a profound, subliminal way that many very important things cannot be measured, controlled or explained fully. Our bodies speak to us in a primordial language which links us to the ebbs and flows of all nature. It is on this level that menopause speaks to me, although the message has been hard to decipher at times.

Menopause is not an easy time. We are faced with a number of challenges. Among other things we must adjust to a new sense of who we are. My identity is changing, and I don't know who I am becoming. Sometimes when I catch a glimpse of myself in a mirror by chance, I do not recognize the face of that middle-aged woman as my own. To whom is all this happening? A part of me is dying and someone else is being born.

I look down at my legs and hardly recognize them. They now have the dry, thin-looking skin I have always associated with my grandmother. The child I was when I took note of this characteristic of my grandmother's skin could not conceive of ever being that old. This new identity is not one I grow into easily. The muscles in these same legs with the strange skin have lost their clear definition and they are unwilling, this year, to hike as far in a single day as they always did before. These changes, so the books say, are due to the sudden drop of estrogen in my system. Whatever the reason, there is no escaping the fact that this aging process is happening to me—whoever I am. It is not some remote event someone told me about. It is my own direct experience, and there is no escaping it.

The irregularity of my menstrual cycles reminds me that I am moving out of the phase of my life in which my body could generate new human life. Seen from this perspective, the ability to bear children seems even more remarkable than it ever did before (and it always had seemed quite remarkable). Still, in some ways I had taken it for granted, as I rather thoughtlessly allowed myself to consider it part of my identity. Now it is leaving. There is a shock. Suddenly I am very alert. I am grieving a loss, and am also ready to explore what all of this may mean, what unimagined things may lie ahead. It is both frightening and enlivening to be going through this process.

Western culture does not support the kind of exploration I feel myself about to embark upon. In fact, every effort is made either not to notice this transition or else not to allow it to take place. Many of the books I have found on the subject of menopause give advice on how to go about remaining young. There are huge industries making lots of money selling replacement hormones, cosmetics, tranquilizers, surgery. The attack on menopause is formidable. Traditionally, in this culture there is little support for a woman who wants to remain fully conscious of all the implications of this passage so as to learn all it has to teach.

I do not want to counteract or cover up what is happening to me. I want to acknowledge it all and when I do, I will need to take time to grieve the very real losses I feel and to adjust to the new perspectives that will emerge. Western culture in general feels threatened by the process of aging, so it may be necessary for us to turn for understanding and support to other women who are going through the same transition. Those of us who were part of the baby boom of the 1940s are now about to discover menopause. Our generation has seen real movement on the frontiers of consciousness. In this same spirit we can, perhaps, offer each other a chance to change our culture's attitudes about menopause. We will need to give ourselves and each other the time and protected space in which we can absorb just how we feel.

Women who have careers feel the pressure not to disrupt the routines in their working lives. The temptation to take tranquilizers and replacement hormones is great. Women who are mothers feel the pressure not to stop doing all the things their families have come to expect. It is not easy to make room for ourselves to experience this transition fully. As I look back, I wonder if the so-called "crazy" behavior of the women in my mother's generation during menopause was not the inevitable result of the culturally-supported attempt to deny that anything was changing.

I think we need to do a lot of open talking with each other, so that the cultural taboo will be weakened. Already I see new kinds of menopause support groups forming. There seems a tremendous enthusiasm among women who begin to share their experiences, their fears, surprises, questions, and their realizations that they are not alone. There is such a feeling of relief at finally being able to speak openly about something which is so vital to them, yet so secret.

I remember the atmosphere I encountered twenty-five years ago as I prepared for the birth of my first child. A pregnant woman in those days was treated as an invalid. Following an inner guidance for which I found no external support, I insisted on being allowed to go through labor and delivery without drugs or other interferences. Then, I was considered a little eccentric. Over the past twenty-five years, however, a supportive birth community has developed. It honors the process of labor and delivery and allows a pregnant woman her dignity, by not intervening in ways that will remove her from the center of her own experience. There is no reason why this same supportive attitude cannot be brought to the process known as menopause. Perhaps twenty-five years from now there will be a widespread honoring of this phase, which itself seems to be a kind of labor and delivery.

Underlying all the identity crises and transitions we must face at this time is a deep message about the cyclical nature of all things in the universe, including human life. When we trick ourselves into thinking that human life is somehow separate from nature, that we ought to be excluded and protected from life cycles, we lose touch with the truth of our nature. Menopause is a strong force pulling us back to that truth.

In our late forties or early fifties, we women are stopped short in our illusory world by the inescapable fact of menopause. Until it actually began to happen to me I had felt somehow that it never would happen. Part of me felt special, as if I were to be excluded from the cycles of all life. I had managed to convince myself that this was something that happened only to older women, older than I would ever be. The thought of it seemed even more frightening than the thought of death, in some ways. Now, I am finding that the actual experience is nothing like what I had imagined, or more accurately, feared to imagine. I am feeling both frightened and enlivened, but not the least bit "crazy."

As my body prepares to leave the child-bearing years behind, my psyche feels the ancient messages that come in whisperings about mortality. For years, since puberty burst upon me, it has been relatively easy to feel caught up in the external activities of life. For the most part, the focus on things outside myself was appropriate and satisfying. But now, at menopause, those external things begin to blur a little, both literally and figuratively. They no longer command my attention as they used to. There is an inward call. A new note is struck. To the part of me that has become well-adapted to the work of the world, the note sounds somber, even threatening. To those around us, whether they are our colleagues at work or our family at home, this shift may also be unwelcome. Patterns of expectation are broken. There is pressure from within ourselves and from those around us not to change.

Even as I continue to go through the habitual motions of my various jobs, my perspective is different. I feel a certain new detachment. I watch with surprise and sometimes dismay as my old motivations begin to seem inadequate. I am becoming less patient with what does not seem deeply important to me. The focus is shifting. There is a new transparency to the things of my customary world: those familiar, necessary things which have helped solidify the illusion of my separateness, my importance.

18

When we reach this significant passage in our lives, we recognize the inexorable insistence of life's processes which pays no attention to our illusions, and does not wait for our permission. In this way menopause is like death. We all know on some level of consciousness that we are mortal, that we will die some day, but the knowledge feels unreal most of the time for most of us. Day-to-day, we function under the illusion that we, personally, will never die. We are not conscious of our deep connection with all the life forms the universe takes. When death seems unreal, our perception of reality seems dualistic, for life seems to be the opposite of death, not a changing manifestation of the same process.

When we are in the midst of the changes that signal the onset of menopause, death seems much less remote. This gives us a rare opportunity to see beyond our usual small ego-centered world. We can feel from a source deep within ourselves the wonderful rightness of the cyclical nature of the universe and can feel more directly than usual an awe and gratitude that we happen to be here to experience it. The fabric of our illusion rips and tears. We cannot help but see through it. We catch a glimpse of the Goddess without her veil. I feel myself pulled back, beginning to remember something I once knew but had forgotten. It is not entirely comforting, but it is deeply true. Experiencing that truth, I feel a substantial joy.

As I go through the changes leading up to menopause, I feel the pull back to a kind of pre-pubertal awareness, but it is also new. It has behind it the experience of half a lifetime. For how many generations has there been no place for women in our culture to express and use this very rich part of our experience? It is time for the context to change, and we are the ones who can change it by paying attention to our lives and by communicating with each other.

THE NEGLECTED CRISIS

Ann Mankowitz

Rites of Passage

Why is the menopause, ostensibly a momentous event in the life of the individual woman, so neglected by society, by history, by mythology and by religion? Why, for instance, are there no rites of passage recorded *anywhere* to mark out the menopause, as there are for other crucial events such as birth, puberty, marriage, childbirth and death?

The function of a rite of passage is to give significance to a crucial change in the life of the individual, to give one the support of society during this change and to attempt by means of the ritual to bring down the blessing of the gods at this time of danger both to the individual and to society. Rites of passage usually take place in three parts: first, the stage of isolation, withdrawal of the individual from society and into close contact with, and dependence upon, nature; second, the ordeal of severance, an event sometimes painful, involving physical or symbolic renunciation and confrontation with loss and death; and third, a ceremony of rebirth and renewal—the return of a changed being into society and the world.

It can be seen that the pattern of these religious rites (which is a universal one) reflects the inner pattern of individual experience in times of fundamental change. As Joseph Campbell writes:

> A great number of the ritual trials and images correspond to those that appear automatically in dreams the moment the psychoanalyzed patient begins to abandon his infantile fixations and to progress into the future. . . .
>
> It has always been the prime function of mythology and rite to supply the symbols that carry the human spirit forward, in counteraction to those other constant human fantasies that tend to tie it back.

It is the acting out of these rites that makes the changes bearable and valuable, and gives them a meaning shared by society and society's gods. The menopause, however, though specifically called *the change of life*, never seems to have had the benefit of this sanction. Why not? Let us consider some facts which may provide a partial answer.

In the Roman Empire, the life expectancy of a woman was twenty-five years; in the fifteenth century it was thirty years; by Victorian times it had only risen to forty-five years; and even at the beginning of this century it was only fifty years. Although these are of course average figures, brought down by the high rate of infant mortality, it does seem as if few women lived much beyond the menopause. There is some evidence that in earlier times the menopause occurred around the mid-forties rather than the fifties, but even so, fewer women would have experienced any length of postmenopausal life compared to those who do today.

There are other reasons for neglect in the past besides the generally shorter life span. One is suggested by Robert Richardson:

> We must ask why an event of such significance to the individual woman passed almost without notice sociologically, anthropologically and medically. And the answer thrown back from the silent past is that the menopause was a negative event of no importance in the life of the community. So when a woman's usefulness was seen to be ended, she ceased to be a woman.

This is a clear statement of a particularly patriarchal attitude: When a woman can no longer bear children, she is no longer of use. This attitude still persists overtly in many parts of the world, and probably unconsciously in many men and women everywhere, and it certainly accounts for much of the neglect of the menopause. But the belief that she loses her womanhood reflects less conscious attitudes of patriarchal society, which may have more bearing on the present day. These concern the sexual power the nubile woman has traditionally possessed, reflected in the taboos of menstruation.

. . . it was this taboo which reflected and increased the awesome power of the nubile women, and made them at their time of menstruation both sacred and deadly. It was the loss of this power at menopause which deprived women of their status in later life. Writes Paula Weideger:

> In our culture a woman is sexually desirable only as long as her sexuality can also inspire fear. Once she no longer menstruates, she is assumed to have lost her sexuality. . . . Our cultural inheritance has dictated that woman is valued and valuable only as long as she can reproduce.

This describes, not a conscious attitude, but a cultural inheritance which embodies the age-old universal image of the magical power of the fertile woman. As different as our modern rational notions of fertility are, we are still unconsciously influenced by archaic beliefs and taboos. Modern men may or may not be aware of fear, or modern women of magical power, but it is these elements, as well as the obvious social necessity for females to carry on the race, that give the nubile woman her special value in society.

History tells us that, with some exceptions, both the matriarchal, goddess-centered cultures, and the patriarchal, male-dominated ones have proved equally remiss in giving a position of dignity and worth to the post-fertile woman; the first because of the worship of female fertility power, and the second because of the repression of female power in general.

The Older Woman in Society

What is or has been the role, if any, of the postmenopausal woman in society?

Elaine Morgan's research into prehistoric times led her to the idea of the grandmothers as oral educators and storytellers of the tribe; indeed, she sees this as their evolutionary raison d'être:

> One of the most vital factors in human evolutionary success was the power to accumulate knowledge, to profit not only from personal experience but from the experience of others, even of others long dead. Before the invention of writing this was made possible only by the long life and memory of older members of the tribe. . . . The only way of accounting for the evolutionary emergence of the menopause in women is by the assumption that the tribe as a whole, and not merely the individual, derived some benefit from the presence of those females who, although sterile, lived to a ripe and healthy old age. In some way or other, and in a way that applied to other species that we know of, grannies were good for them.

In 1949, Margaret Mead described the situation in Bali:

> The post-menopausal woman and the virgin girl work together at ceremonies from which women of childbearing age are debarred. Where modesty of speech and action is enjoined on women, such behavior may no longer be asked of older women who may use obscene language as freely or more freely than any man.

According to Paula Weideger, in China before the revolution the post-menopausal woman had a secure and coveted position; for the first time in her life she could shake off male domination, and, with the approval of society, even assume domination over males.

American sociologist Pauline Bart, who studied anthropological accounts of the status of women in a great number of cultures, discovered that in spite of an enormous variation in concepts of femininity, the feminine role assumed in the fertile years of a woman's life was in all cultures reversed after menopause. The examples from Bali and China bear this out, and demonstrate particularly a reversal of sex-role.

The idea of the older woman losing her femininity with her fertility and joining the men, so to speak, may penetrate to inner feelings as well as to social practices. Vieda Skultans made a study of rural Welsh women in 1970 and found several at the menopause who felt they were changing structurally and anatomically into men. One said, "Women turn into men inside," and another reported that she felt "a turning and tightening of the thigh muscles."

Witchcraft was probably one way in which the old goddess religions survived after being driven underground. Historically witches have been of all ages and both sexes, but the concept of the witch that has come down to us in folklore and fairytale is that of a malicious and ugly old hag. There is a connection here with the image of the menopausal woman. "Many of the witches killed were old women since 'the devil walks in a dry place.'" So-called witch ointment, used by women in the menopause, was probably composed mainly of menstrual blood, and the only time when a woman could not be a witch was when she was bearing a child.

We often think of the wise women, healers and midwives of the past, as well as the priestesses, sibyls and oracles of classical times, as having been older women. History tells us that although there may be some truth in this (Esther Harding refers to the "ancient priestesses" of the moon goddess), in many cases these roles were filled by younger women, sometimes dedicated to these vocations in early youth.

In fact the evidence of the part played by the postfertile woman in the life of her society is sparse and often conjectural. General neglect and masculine bias can be partly blamed for this, but we know from the statistics that this is due also to the shortness of life in the past, which meant that few women lived for very long once they had passed the menopause.

Nowadays, however, an enormous number of women live for a long span after they have ceased to be reproductive . . .

Like every other adult in this society, the menopausal woman has to sort out for herself the most balanced advice from the conflicting information presented to her by pundits and experts. She can do this most effectively if she is supported by a positive attitude toward herself during the change of life, an underlying philosophy of life that can make of the menopause a progressive experience, in spite of conflicts and uncertainties. It is not in vain attempts to ignore the changes of age and to pursue the trappings of youth that strength and happiness for the older woman lie. On the contrary, that way leads to bitterness, exhaustion and instability. Even more destructive is a masochistic surrender to the inevitability of woman's "sad lot," a lifelong conviction that female biology has always been the scourge of women, and that the menopause is the final blow; that kind of feminine defeatism leads only to debilitation and decline into premature old age . . .

Each woman's experience of the menopause will be different, but if we can assimilate the shadows of the past and accept the realities of aging, it may be found that the menopause, though a difficult and demanding passage of adulthood, can also be a time of psychological integration and growth, increased strength and specifically *feminine* wisdom.

Vital ingredients of such wisdom are wit and humor, attributes not usually associated at the present time with the postmenopausal woman, but ones which traditionally represent a liberating factor in her life. In many societies the old woman was given a degree of license that was forbidden in her fertile years. She could join in with the men, tell bawdy stories and generally release her libidinal energy from many of the restrictions society imposed on the nubile woman.

This increase of freedom was accompanied by greater self-confidence and authority in the society outside the home, and in some cases a sanctioned domination over men. Such a situation does still exist in the American South.

Many of the women who tell vile tales are gloriously and affirmatively old. They transcend the boundaries—not by their station and employment—but by aging beyond the strictures that censure would lay on the young. The South, like many traditional cultures, offers an increase in license to those who advance in age, and ladies I have known take the full advantage offered them in their tale-telling. They seem to delight in particular in presenting themselves as wicked old ladies . . . . As the Southern Black comedienne Moms Mabley used to say: "Ain't nothin' no old man can do for me 'cept bring me a message from a young man."

NO MORE Xs ON MY CALENDAR, NO MORE PMS

Joanne Seltzer

Ruby-colored friend,
for forty years
you visited me

then fled like the flasher
who shames young women
by spreading his raincoat
blackly open

and I don't miss you
nor think of you

except once in a blue moon
when the sun defers
to the power of night

leaving me nothing
to howl about.

THE IMPETUS OF MENOPAUSE

Janine O'Leary Cobb

Menopause can be a disconcerting experience. Just when you think you have your act together . . . just when you have finally reached a comfortable level of poise and self-confidence, menopause causes you to sit up and take nothing for granted.

This is not the experience of *all* women, but it was certainly *my* experience. In my late forties, I was teaching college full-time and coping with a full house—husband and five children. The two oldest (aged 19 and 20) had just returned home after "drop-off" time to resume their schooling. I should have been delighted. Instead I was feeling rotten. My bones ached, my head ached, my digestion went to pot, and I was tired, really tired, all the time.

Hounded by my husband, I went to the doctor. She poked and prodded and found nothing wrong. My periods were more or less regular so I hadn't thought of menopause at all. However, when I finally realized that it was not arthritis, or ulcers, or a brain tumor, I said "hello" to menopause. For someone who considered herself fairly well-educated, I was woefully ignorant about the whole process. And, as I soon discovered, so was my doctor (who was five years my junior). My mother had had a hysterectomy at 39 and knew nothing about other women in the family. She also thought the topic rather vulgar. I checked libraries and bookstores and found that there was very little information available. Most of what I read told me that *I* was to blame—that active, well-adjusted women just weren't bothered by menopause.

But it wasn't only me. Many of my friends had complaints. We were all feeling *very* stressed and that stress was showing up in strained relationships with husbands, children, employers and employees, not to mention fatigue and burn-out. In fact, fatigue got in the way of organizing a self-help group. Who had the energy? Who had the time?

I figured I had two things going for me. I loved sitting in libraries and there was a good medical library in my city (such a nice change from my customary noisy surroundings at work and at home), and I had no reticence about talking about my troubles. I remembered that I was the first young mother to admit to having hemorrhoids. *I* had to bring it up but I soon found I had lots of company! Now it was time to bring up the topic of menopause. I spoke of it incessantly; I explained what it was (or what I thought it was) to my husband, to my children, to my friends, to other faculty members, and finally to my doctor. The more I talked, the more I was talked to—and the more I learned.

One day I bumped into an old friend who had just started having hot flashes. "They're so *funny!*"she chortled, "I can't help but laugh every time I have one." I liked her attitude and determined that I wouldn't try to hide mine, when and if they appeared. She also told me that she'd been told she had to have a hysterectomy for a prolapsed uterus but, drawing on her expertise in yoga, had devised an exercise program which used a combination of headstands and Kegel exercises. Six months later, the prolapse had disappeared.

When my own hot flashes started a few months later, I was prepared. I carried a fan with me at all times. When I was with my children, however, I didn't need it because they would grab a magazine, or menu or anything handy to fan cool air on my face until it subsided. I learned that talking about menopause or hot flashes in social situations caused heads to turn and I found myself—for the first time in my life—being outrageous and enjoying it. So much so that I only smiled when the president of my husband's company met me at a reception and smilingly greeted me as "the menopause lady." "Right!" I thought, "That's me."

After about six months of immersion in matters menopausal, I read about an International Congress on the Menopause, which was to be held thousands of miles away. This was when People's Express offered very low fares. I decided to go. There I heard eminent specialists talking about menopause and about menopausal women in ways that both shocked and offended. For instance, at the opening session, this declaration from an eminent Australian physician: "Menopause is a sex-linked, female-dominant estrogen deficiency disease, and I think these little old ladies should be given a better deal." *This* little old lady caught the eye of a few other "little old ladies" in the audience and we found each other after that session. From then on, there was a very small but stubborn group of dissenters at many presentations; we listened to doctors talking about their patients behind the patients' backs. We didn't like what we heard, and we had a hard time reconciling these images of neurotic, sickly complainers with the real-life women we knew—menopausal women in their late forties and early fifties who were vibrant, active and well.

The mystery was solved when we realized that medical science was basically not very interested in menopause *unless* it was a menopause induced by surgery. When they spoke about menopausal women, these doctors might be speaking about natural menopause or about surgical menopause: they appeared not to differentiate them. Hysterectomy (removal of the uterus) and, even more so, oophorectomy or ovariectomy (removal of the ovaries) offered solutions but also often created new problems. My reading (and my experience) had told me that some women sail through such operations, but that many others are forced to make repeat visits to their physicians after surgery. Such women are viewed by their doctors as dissatisfied nuisances, particularly when the complaints have to do with sex (desire or response) or with depression, both of which may—not *will*—be affected by the operation. Unfortunately, very few surgeons are prepared to deal with these kinds of consequences.

This was underlined for me when I was sent for a colposcopy a few months later. The young woman doctor who was examining me asked if I was nervous. "Not particularly," I said, "I was told that the worst that could happen would be a hysterectomy." "I wouldn't think of that as 'worse,'" said the doctor, "after all, you've had your family and you don't need your baby bag anymore." It was interesting to see how medical school had distanced this woman from natural possessiveness about body parts, not to mention the fact that she knew nothing about research demonstrating the role of the uterus in sexual response. Or perhaps she felt I was too old to be interested in sex? Wrong. Too bad for her and too bad for every woman who lay, as I did now, with her knees up and legs apart, at the mercy of one narrow medical opinion.

There is a double whammy associated with this cavalier attitude toward the removal of female body parts. Not only does the hysterectomized woman suffer more from menopause (as compared to a naturally menopausal woman), but she continues to be viewed very negatively by most doctors. So much so that the negative stereotype is carried over to reflect on *all* women in middle-age. Which begs the question: why do North American surgeons continue to perform so many hysterectomies? (At least twice and perhaps three times as many as are performed, for instance, in Britain.)

I learned that there were controversies over most of the treatments available for menopause and that ERT (Estrogen Replacement Therapy) and HRT (Hormone Replacement Therapy, which is estrogen plus progestogens) are prescribed freely by some doctors, particularly gynecologists, and very reluctantly or not at all by others. It was interesting to know that family physicians, those who were more concerned about the total situation of their patients, were among the most reluctant to use hormone supplementation—endorsing it only for younger women who have undergone surgical menopause. I later discovered that there was an underground network in each city and that, once you asked around, it was fairly easy to find a doctor who would support whatever decision a woman might make.

In this respect, ERT for the menopausal woman was like artificial birth control to the devout Roman Catholic. Some priests would consider family planning a mortal sin and wouldn't grant absolution. Others considered it a matter of conscience. The trick was to know which confessional in which church!

Through the women I met at the conference, I was put in touch with women activists concerned about various aspects of women's health. These were women who had agitated for the introduction of birthing rooms and rooming-in, who asked difficult questions about the inflated numbers of caesarian births and hysterectomies, who foresaw problems with aspects of the new reproductive technologies, who warned about the side- and after-effects of drugs prescribed to women—D.E.S., thalidomide, tranquilizers. Some of these women were now thinking about menopause and viewing with distaste the tendency to medicalize a very normal transition period in a woman's life. My contact with these women strengthened my feeling that menopause *was* important, that it should not be regarded merely as a "blip" in the course of a woman's life.

As the months went by, I recognized that I was emerging from a clinical depression, probably triggered by a combination of stress, quitting smoking (that was very stressful) and the "kick" of menopause. I found the fatigue and pessimism which had dogged me for months now lifting and realized that I didn't have to have an objective reason to feel depressed, that I was entitled to feel what I felt. I probably *should* have been treated with anti-depressants but because depression is usually self-limiting, I was now on the mend. I also realized that the weight gain which had contributed to the depression was a positive aspect of menopause. The additional pounds contributed to the manufacture of estrone and probably eased the severity of the hot flashes. I decided to relax, to accept the additional 15 pounds and to worry about it later, if at all.

Now that the hot flashes have eased and almost disappeared, the weight is starting to come off. Because I felt unwell some of the time, I have learned to ease up on my commitments, to make time for myself, and to think less of others' opinions. I have also learned to respect the needs of my body, rather than taking it for granted. I eat better foods, get more exercise and drink less than I did in my forties. I spend more time with my women friends—lunches, dinner and a movie, weekend visits. I left teaching to work at something else, which I find just as rewarding but not quite so stressful. I can't say that I look forward to old age, but I certainly regard it with more equanimity than I did five years ago.

It seems to me that menopause is feared not so much for itself but because it's a marker of aging. And aged women in our society are accorded neither the dignity nor the respect which they deserve. Menopause offers us an opportunity to appreciate and nurture our*selves*, to devote time to seeking the right physical and emotional balance for *us*. It's a time to reawaken old friendships and to foster new friendships, friendships which will enrich our lives for years to come. Menopause provides the impetus to get to know ourselves more intimately, a self-knowledge that is invaluable as we face the challenge of aging.

AS WOMAN GROWS OLDER

Carla Kandinsky

The body begins a backward gallop
towards adolescence, even baby fat
begins to appear again, soft over
bones like spongy mushrooms. Desire
either sleeps for weeks or reaches
out to grab you with merciless claws,
rattling your teeth. All the things
you've missed you crave, a Japanese
lover, learning to say fuck in Greek,
a week in Spain. You wonder why you
never lived in San Francisco, always
in the East Bay. You look at your
jade ring and cry for an emerald.
You wake alone in your vegetarian
bed ravenous for the taste
of bacon, a pork chop, a steak.
At times you reach out and grab,
you try to have it this time around,
just in case there's no reincarnation.
Just in case when the blood stops
flowing it really is the end.

GIVING UP THE RAG

Elayne Clift

When I was nine years old, my mother, a victim of the "We'll just take out the carriage and leave the playpen" fraternity, had a hysterectomy. Conventional wisdom in those days dictated that at the first pre-menopausal irregularity the female reproductive organs were dispensed with. I distinctly remember sitting on the stairs, my head in my hands, regretting bitterly that I had been born a girl, and terrified by what inevitably lay ahead. As I approached my own entry to womanhood, a stream of other terrors made their way into my subconscious, fueled by the whispered sharing of older girls and a variety of ominous magazine articles, usually conspicuously available in the doctor's waiting room.

Luckily, by the time I was staring down the M word, things had changed, and my own recent bout with pre-menopausal irregularity was less frightening than it might have been. Nevertheless, a four-month episode of heavy bleeding and clotting gave me pause. So did my (female) gynecologist's reaction. "We'll want to watch this," she said. "Fibroids. Of course, it's much too premature to even think about hysterectomy, but . . ." I couldn't resist prodding her. "You mean just the uterus, I'm sure?" "At your age, I'd take the ovaries. After all, who wants ovarian cancer?" (Not me. But I don't fancy a brain tumor either and I'm not about to cut off my head, just in case.) "Well, it's academic, as far as I'm concerned," I replied. "I plan to slide quietly into menopause and let the little buggers just shrink themselves into oblivion. And another thing, I'm not very big on ERTs!"

Like many other women, I would have found this sort of informed assertiveness impossible without the women's health movement of the 1970s, which I am fortunate to have worked in for more than ten years. Largely thanks to the women's health advocates who were my friends and colleagues, most of the mythology-driven attitudes and practices aimed at "normalizing" the reproductive cycle have been put to rest. But a few hard core neanderthals persist and I like to remind them that, unlike my mother, I am not, literally or figuratively, going to take it lying down.

I've gotten too smart. I know now, through sharing my own reality with other women, that middle age and over can be a time of invigorating energy and freedom. Many of my friends, to the chagrin of their fading male counterparts, take up artistic, business or service endeavors with talented fervor. My own career as a writer, producer and consultant began after age 40. The financial rewards are modest, it's true, but oh, what satisfaction! And contrary to the beliefs of those who still cling to Victorian notions of femininity, I have not fallen into a fretful malaise as I approach the end of my "biological significance" (as my daughter's high school biology teacher puts it). I celebrate it!

For not having had to face the very real issue of the biological clock, I now welcome the normal end of what was for me a very annoying monthly event. I mean, let's face it. It's been a nuisance crawling onto "Mickey Mouse mattresses" every 28 days or so, ever watchful for that awkward accident at exactly the wrong time. My husband tires of competing with a tampon and it's been no fun apologizing for being premenstrual, menstrual, or perimenstrual. It will be wonderful to pack a suitcase without consulting the calendar and to give up the midnight search for an all-night pharmacy. And I, for one, plan to work out exactly what I've invested in "feminine hygiene products" over the course of 36-plus years, making an equal and immediate contribution towards pampering myself.

Anyone who thinks this is an odd form of "involutional melancholia," as the menopausal years were labeled in my mother's day, needs to be reminded that times have changed. My own daughter, like many other young girls, does not fear her womanhood; she welcomes it. Like me, she is beginning to understand the gift of maturity, and to embrace its possibility. After all, she knows, like I do, that it's simply, and wonderfully, part of the life cycle.

CHANGING WOMAN

Jane L. Mickelson

If we lived on a planet with no cycle of seasons, we would miss the beauty and wonder of spring's renewal, of summer's bounty and fall's glowing moments. Winter's healing time of sleep and preparation for regeneration is also necessary to the human heart, if in more subtle ways.

As we glory in the changes of earth's seasons, so should we delight in the cycles of our own bodies, not only from month to month, but year to year and decade to decade, yet somewhere in our society something has gone wrong. We, as women, have been given the message that one of the most important times of change in our lives—the menopause—is bad. The drug companies, the physicians, and most of all the advertising media, have given us the message that this change, the climacteric, is a time to be dreaded, avoided and postponed.

We are encouraged to dress younger, wear more makeup to disguise our aging faces, dye our hair to hide the grey, undergo facial and/or body lifts, "cosmetic surgery," to fight off the inevitable pull of gravity and time. Worst of all, we are given drugs, synthetic copies of the estrogens and progesterones our bodies are no longer producing in as generous quantities, to postpone the inevitable, to keep us "forever young." For many women these drugs have brought about the ultimate form of non-aging—death.

Let's draw a parallel to illustrate how unnatural this denial of our normal changes really is. Our pre-pubescent daughter, on the verge of young womanhood, comes to us in tears. She's afraid of the changes happening in her body. Her developing breasts hurt; she has heard that menstrual cramps are painful, that getting her period will be messy and embarrassing and she simply isn't ready for adulthood. Her relationships with the other kids will change; the boys won't want to play sports with her anymore. She's alarmed by the dawning sexual urges she feels. She wants us to take her to the doctor and get some medicine which will stop all these frightening changes and let her stay as she is, comfortably enclosed in the garden of childhood.

Would any of us do this? Of course not. We would, instead, try to comfort her, to reassure her that as her body changes, her mind, her emotions and dreams will change as well. We would explain to her that the discomforts which she is experiencing are temporary, and that once she is established in her womanhood a whole new world will be open to her.

How can we be so gently understanding of our young daughters, yet so very hard on ourselves? Isn't the menopause as natural a part of the cycle of our lives as the onset of puberty? It is our conditioning which has made this time of our lives appear negative, and for women who wish all of life to be balanced and healthy, it is time to examine and challenge these negative stereotypes.

It is primarily in relatively recent, Western history that menopause and the menopausal woman have been viewed in a bad light. The world in which we are now living sees youth and beauty as being synonymous. Because of the fast-paced developments in technology, and the lack of interest in human development, the wisdom which comes with age is not so highly valued as it once was.

This was not always the case. In most pre-technological societies, the elder women were thought to be the most knowledgeable, in part because they did not shed their "wise blood" each month. They became the counsellors, the arbitrators, the leaders of important rituals forbidden to women still in the childbearing years. No longer so concerned with childcare, they had the time to become artisans, healers, musicians and teachers. A whole new phase of life began for them.

It is not possible for most of us to return to a less-industrialized culture. We are a part of our time. But it is possible for us to refuse to accept the conditioning forced on us by agencies which stand to gain financially if we back away in fear from the changes which nature intended us to undergo.

What, really, is so frightening about menopause? Our bodies were specifically designed to pass through it, just as they were designed to go through puberty, child-bearing and nursing. Many times fear can be disarmed by knowledge. Just as many of us read everything we could get our hands on about pregnancy and nursing, and just as we studied the printed inserts in the tampon box as adolescents, fascinated by this new insight (for many of us the first real education of our own anatomy), so should we prepare ourselves for this next grand step of our maturity.

Few major changes in our bodies occur overnight. Puberty was a gradual process; so is the menopause. For a few women, especially those whose uterus and/or ovaries are surgically removed, the menstrual period ceases abruptly, but for most it is a slower occurrence, with many variations, yet always leading to a time when the menstrual periods stop. The hormones which control and govern the monthly cycle are no longer needed in such powerful doses, so the body lessens its production gradually.

It is this process of hormonal change which can stimulate the classic symptoms of menopause: hot flashes, cold chills, fatigue, night sweats, sleep disruption, sensations of breathlessness, heart palpitations, dryness of the vagina, tingling in the extremities, and (in some women) temporarily high blood pressure.

What I have found the lessening of these hormones does *not* produce is: mental illness, loss of sexual urges, migraine headaches, need for a hysterectomy, promiscuity, depression, or anxiety. In a few extreme cases, such as for women who suffer very severe pre-menstrual tension, a similar menopausal pattern can occur, but rest assured that 85%–90% of all women progress through menopause without seeking medical help for symptoms.

The medical term *menopause* actually refers to the time when, for at least a year, the woman has had no menstrual periods, although popular usage of the word covers the entire process from being a menstruating woman to the time when the periods cease altogether.

What happens at menopause is that the ovaries cut back on production of estrogen, stimulating an increase of follicular stimulating hormone (FSH) to try and get the ovaries to produce eggs again. A side-effect (in some women a quite dramatic one) of these high levels of FSH is disturbance of the hypothalamus gland. Now, since control of normal body temperature, sleep patterns, amount of stamina and control of the autonomic nervous system (which regulates breathing, heartbeat, digestive processes, blood pressure and such) all depend on the hypothalamus to run smoothly, it is understandable why women often experience commotion in their bodies when the accustomed pattern goes through a time of adjustment. Few women manage to pass through menopause without experiencing some of these symptoms.

Here's the good news: to a fairly large extent, the severity of these side-effects of menopause is controllable—by us! In the same way that good nutrition, exercise, avoidance of undue stress and addictive substances (caffeine, nicotine, alcohol, "recreational drugs") can make such a dramatic difference in pregnancy or discomfort during menstruation, so can they alter the course of the menopause. If we were to treat our menopausal bodies with the same cherishing care and wonder with which we treat our pregnant or nursing bodies, this amazing time in life would be seen for what it truly is—another season in the cycle of our existence.

This is not to say that the uncomfortable symptoms of menopause are just in our heads. No one in the grip of a hot flash or trying to catch her breath after a series of heart palpitations can brush them off as psychosomatic, but it has been conclusively shown that the healthier the body the less distressing the symptoms tend to be for most women.

What is also becoming clearer, to women if not yet to the medical community at large, is that the healthier the *attitude* about menopause, the better off the woman will be. This is easier said than done in a culture which treats whole segments of its population (generally those people who are not in the midst of producing for large financial gain) as disposable or, at best, ignorable. It is hard to maintain self-worth when the society in which we live tells us we are past our prime. Is the fully-opened rose not just as beautiful as the bud? As hard as it may be to fight against cultural conditioning, we must claim our right to honor, respect and enjoy *all* of the seasons of our lives, not only a fraction of them, for we will not be given the chance to go back and do it all over again.

Fortunately (in this case at least), we are living in a time when the older sector of the population is growing dramatically in proportion to the rest. Sheer numbers, if nothing else, are forcing a re-examination of negative stereotypes of the older woman. We are also witnessing a renaissance of self-help groups, with a wonderful potential for helping others as well as ourselves.

Menopause support groups are now found all around the country. Taking part in such a group can lend not only reassurance that what is happening physically is normal, but also provide emotional encouragement, as well as insights into new directions for our lives.

JoAn Steinmetz, a therapist in Northern California specializing in menopause, is an excellent example of the new attitudes that are becoming more prevalent:

> I see it very much as a phase of a person's life when they have the chance to revaluate, because a woman up to that point is usually busy with family or a career. Menopause is a time for a woman to get the opportunity to go into herself deeper and realize what her values are, what she wants out of the rest of her life, moving up to what I would call a more spiritual level.
>
> Rather than a degeneration, a running down, which is the old model, what we're talking about is that it's all been building up, adding to what a person is. In that phase of the life it becomes rather service oriented. It's a giving out then, of being able to share the experiences, what a woman has learned. We see so many success stories of women who are still really active and doing good work in the world in their 70s and 80s.
>
> For me, it seemed to be a time when I had to go through a lot of evaluation of who I was, what was important to me in life, what I wanted to do with my life. In so doing, I became involved with a spiritual path.
>
> My theory on menopause is that whatever we are dealing with in our lives, whatever stresses or emotional problems, accelerate at that period. If we don't have any avenues to handle those things, they'll get out of hand. Perhaps, in the past, that's where the old [stereotype of the hysterical menopausal woman] came from. Now we have a lot of people working with their problems as they come along so they are not as acute.
>
> It's like adolescence where you're shifting into a whole new phase of being, and it brings up fears and anxieties. You don't know what to expect from your body. Acceptance helps a great deal. The more we fight the symptoms the worse they can become. Our minds are so powerful. If we can center, accept and be calm, through meditation of any sort, it is such a help.
>
> Take time to list the things that are important to your life. Take the time to go back in your life and tune in to the parts that touch you the most, that touch and open the heart—the times that have the most energy. Those are what we can learn from in

our lives. Those are the times our essence is able to flow. That's all spiritual, of course. It's getting in touch with our essential energy and when we are most alive. Then look at what we want and can do with that [energy] in the future, realizing that as much as we can incorporate that into our lives, our life is going to be that much more meaningful. *See that life is an expansive process as we grow older, rather than that life closes down.*

The concept of later life becoming more service-oriented should be examined closely. One need not view it from a purely altruistic perspective. Of course, volunteer work (either within one's own family or in the larger outside community) is rewarding, and mature women are the very backbone of America's volunteer force, but service can be seen in many lights. For some post-menopausal women, the new independence from their role as home manager and parent provides the chance to return to school and earn a degree, enabling them to take another kind of job. There is the fascinating world of local politics which appeals to many older women. Careers which were suspended during the child-rearing years can often be resumed. There is more time to share with a spouse, as well as the chance to renew the one-to-one relationship which existed before the children were born.

For women who choose to remain in the home, it is an opportunity to pursue an art or craft—weaving, pottery, painting, sewing—for which there was never enough time before. A number of cottage industries and home-owned businesses grow from such enterprises, although many women find ample satisfaction in the personal development of their own artistic nature.

A whole new way of life opens up to women after menopause. For the first time in our lives we not only have the time to develop ourselves, but the experience and wisdom to know in which directions we want to travel. If we do not know how to use these inner resources there are many others to help us. Not least of these is our peer group, which is why menopause support groups can be such a benefit. Working as a unit, women have the chance to explore every aspect of their changing, developing lives. For the fact remains that it is not enough to merely reject the negative concepts of the menopausal and post-menopausal woman. We need positive, strong role models to take their place, and it is here that we can turn to the rich heritage of cultures in which women have been traditionally viewed as powerful assets to their world. The Native American myths and tales often feature positive female figures, such as Changing Woman, one of the most holy of all the Navaho and Pueblo characters.

Changing Woman is symbolic of earth. Ageing with the year, she dies each winter and comes back every spring as a young maiden. It is she who teaches women of childbirth, of the cycles of their bodies and the seasons of the year. From her we can learn to respect and accept these changes rather than fight against them.

If we look back at the thousands of years of human history, we will find that many cultures had a female deity akin to Changing Woman. As long as there have been people on this earth, there has been wonder and awe concerning the body of woman and its seemingly mysterious cycles. We now understand some of the scientific reasons for these cyclic changes, but, ironically enough, our culture seems to have lost the sense of wonder. It is up to us to regain it, each in her own way, to return the richness to our lives and set aside the fear and misunderstanding which has been forced on us by those who stand to gain from our reluctance to age.

Let's examine one of those agencies. Just as we would not give a young girl a hormone to hold back her puberty, we must seriously question the use of estrogen replacement therapy in the normal, healthy menopausal woman. Drug companies reap literally hundreds of millions of dollars selling us chemicals which drastically increase our risk of uterine, breast and ovarian cancer, strokes and heart attacks, as well as less harmful but unpleasant side effects from the drug itself, such as edema (water retention), nausea, dizziness, weight gain, breakthrough bleeding, vomiting, cramps, nervous tension and excess cervical secretions. What's more, there is no predicting the effect this medication is going to have on our other glands, which, being somewhat interdependent, will undoubtedly react to the influx of artificial hormones. Suppression of the body's ability to produce its own estrogen (which the ovaries, adrenal glands and other extra-glandular sources continue to do well into our 80s!) is bound to occur, at the very least.

We must also remember that once the estrogen replacement therapy is stopped, the symptoms reappear and must be lived through. We cannot stay on medication for the rest of our lives when there is nothing wrong with us to begin with! Also, there are many natural ways of dealing with the discomfort of hot flashes, dry vaginal walls and any other individual symptoms. *Menopause Naturally* by Sadja Greenwood has excellent suggestions, as does the Santa Fe Health Education Project booklet. There are traditional herbal teas and infusions which can be found listed in herbals at the local health food store. If a menopause support group is started, one project could be compiling a lending library of books, pamphlets and articles.

Good all-around health is one's best defense for bodily changes at any age. There are hundreds of books available on nutrition and exercise, as well as meditation and relaxation. For some of us, menopause comes at a difficult time: our children are in deepest adolescence, perhaps our spouses are going through their own "mid-life crisis," and any help we can get from outside, be it a friend, a support group, a therapist or a well-written book, is a big help.

Be wary of any article, book or person (no matter how many degrees they hold) who tries to convince you that menopause is an illness or an estrogen deficiency disease. Your body, and the body of every woman since the dawn of history, was designed to go through menopause, just as it was designed to do all the other wonderful things it's done. When nature repeats a pattern for countless generations, it is usually because it works and is correct. Anyone who tries to tell us differently is wrong, and we should try to understand that they have something to gain (usually money) by convincing us that we need chemical and/or physical intervention.

It is time to follow our instincts with menopause as we have with childbearing and parenting. Women's bodies are strong and beautifully designed to do what they were meant to do. How exciting to think that a whole new life can open itself to us; that we can now use all that experience and hard-won knowledge to make our own world a multi-faceted, multi-colored place. It is a responsibility for the older woman to take on with pride—that of showing younger women how healthy and powerful the later years are. Let us follow our instincts and learn, and, in turn, teach. We all have so very much to gain.

OUR LEGACY:
MEDICAL VIEWS OF THE
MENOPAUSAL WOMAN

Mary Lou Logothetis

The menopausal woman seems to elicit a particularly virulent brand of negativity on the part of physicians. She has been depicted as being no longer attractive or sexually desirable, as being no longer needed, and as a degraded outcast no longer capable of achievement. In short, she has been portrayed as experiencing her menopause as a process of decay rather than development.

I reviewed medical literature from the 60s, 70s, and 80s to analyze its underlying imagery of the woman who is experiencing menopause. Sources included both medical textbooks and journal articles intended for consumption by other physicians and books and pamphlets intended for consumption by middle-aged women. I use direct quotations to elaborate three images of the menopausal woman found in the medical literature: as physically deteriorated, psychologically disabled, and socially worthless.

Physical Deterioration

The medical definition of menopause lies within a context of disease and pathology as opposed to a context of normal processes of aging. The menopausal woman is "a pitiful creature" whose body undergoes "dismal and catastrophic" physical changes (Rhoades, 1967, p. 349) which she watches with a "horrible fascination" (Davis, 1980, p. 44).

Defined as "not normal," the menopausal woman suffers from a deficiency disease (Wilson, Brevetti, & Wilson, 1963, p. 115). Her "dying or dead gonads" (Wilson & Wilson, 1972, p. 522) have made her in desperate need of medical treatment to replace the deficient estrogen and restore her "diseased areas" (Wilson et al., 1963, p. 115). Treating her deficiency with estrogen replacement is "just as natural" as giving "insulin to diabetic patients" (Rauramo, 1986, p. 185). Her treatment may also involve major surgery since hysterectomy "facilitates" hormone therapy "considerably" (Govan, Hodge, & Callander, 1985, p. 128), and "without doubt it is an advantage to a menopausal woman to be minus her uterus" (Easley, 1983, p. 372). Only with such advances in medical research and the constantly watchful eye of her physician can she be saved from these "unwelcome processes" (Davis, 1980, p. 3).

The description of the menopausal woman's body is often repulsive. Her spinal column is "hump-backed," her vagina is "a dry, rigid tube," and hair grows on her face (Kistner, 1978, p. 553). Her breasts are particularly of concern. They become "flabby and wrinkled" (Rhoades, 1967, p. 349), and "often the skin of the breasts coarsens and is covered with scales" (Wilson, 1966, p. 68). Further "unwholesome effects" of this deficiency disease include "ugly body contours and atrophy of the genitalia" (Wilson & Wilson, 1972, p. 522).

The medical terms commonly used to describe these changes in the menopausal woman's body create further negativity in themselves. For example, the word "atrophy," used above to describe genital changes, means to wither, to waste away. Other examples include "senile vaginitis," "estrogen starvation," and references to women as "castrates" or "hypogonadal." Implicit in such medical labeling is an extremely negative view of women as shrunken neuters with wasted bodies and of the natural process of menopause as a biologic withering.

The menopausal woman's image often includes a tendency towards obesity and an unkempt appearance. She is referred to as the "bedraggled, flushed, and flashed ash of her former self" (Berman, 1976, p. 5). She has "wrinkles where once there were dimples, and an egg-shaped torso is replacing her once trim figure" (Huffman, 1979, p. 213). Her most appropriate goal is to preserve her physical attractiveness, which is the "key to her fate" and "her starting capital in the venture of life—the 'ante' which lets her into the game" (Wilson, 1966, p. 57). To maintain her "appearance and charm" beyond menopause, however, she "may find that she has to frequent a beauty shop more often" (Davis, 1980, p. 22) and that makeup "used cleverly and subtly" can "take years off a face" (p. 21).

Because the menopausal woman can become obese "in a very short time," it is necessary to maintain "continuous vigilance" (Davis, 1980, p. 26). She is told to "weigh yourself *daily* on a bathroom scale" and to be alert for "any day the needle jumps up *only one pound*" (emphasis added), to assure she does not become like other women who "really let themselves go" (p. 26).

Her weight gain and untidiness, however, have consequences reaching far beyond just her physical appearance. Menopausal women who are "obese, sloppily dressed, and disillusioned," with "disheveled hair, random application of cosmetics, and depressed posture" are portrayed as having a more stormy adjustment to menopause than women who are "slimmer and trimmer" with a "new style of dress, confident upright posture, and a smile, not a frown" (Utian, 1980, p. 83).

Psychological Disability

The medical literature characterizes the menopausal woman as suffering from "neurotic and psychosomatic disability" (Kistner, 1978, p. 552). Her "encyclopedia of complaints" (Anonymous, 1972, p. 257) includes "depression and irritability . . . downright meanness" (Easley, 1983, p. 371), forgetfulness, anxiety, lassitude and a wide variety of psychosomatic aches and pains. She is an anxious woman, overwhelmed by her symptomatology, the etiology of which is her "hostility and rejection of the feminine role and envy of the masculine prerogatives" (High, 1962, p. 626).

The menopausal woman's fear for the loss of her femininity is depicted to be at the core of her psychological disability, since "to the feminine woman menopause is a narcissistic mortification" (Klaus, 1974, p. 1187). When her menstrual periods become irregular and scanty, she considers it "an insult to her femininity" (Kistner, 1978, p. 552) and she may be depressed, "reflecting the turning inward of anger and disappointment with one's self (Klaus, 1974, p. 1187). Thus, the "loss of feminine functions" is thought to precipitate serious anxieties about her feminine role (High, 1962, p. 626) and reveal a "first glimpse of panic" (Forman, 1968, p. 18). Her "decline in ovarian function and aging, coupled with the growing independence of other family members, creates a general loss of self-esteem" (American College of Obstetricians and Gynecologists, 1981, p. 141). The view of the menopausal woman mourning the loss of her menstrual periods is, of course, in sharp contrast to that expressed by the many women who admit they are rather relieved to be done with what they regard as nuisance and inconvenience.

The medical literature portrays the menopausal woman as emotionally handicapped by her menopause. She "dissolves into tears at the slightest provocation and sometimes for no reason at all . . . powers of concentration and decision are lost . . . which type of bread to buy becomes a major problem; attempting to plan the dinner menu, a chore" (Goldberg, 1959, p. 16). Her emotional instability causes her to acquire a "vapid cow-like feeling" (Wilson, 1963, p. 352) and become "a caricature of her younger self at her emotional worst" (Forman, 1968, p. 20). And the anxiety she feels will likely contribute to her obesity, since some women "are always nibbling to soothe themselves" (Forman, 1968, p. 19).

The degree of the menopausal woman's psychological disability is depicted as acute, "frequently amenable only to a carload of hormones or a lobotomy" (Berman, 1976, p. 5). Therapy to replace those hormones is most often proposed as what she needs. Medical journal advertisements promoting various estrogen products to physicians (*Journal of the American Medical Association*, 1976) are also revealing for their images of the menopausal woman's emotionality. In one, a miserable, disheveled woman of menopausal age is in the foreground, holding her head in her hands and seeming to struggle for control. Her family is watching her from the background, with father holding his yet unread newspaper. The copy reads: "Almost any tranquilizer might calm her down . . . but at her age, estrogen may be what she really needs." Another includes a woman holding airline tickets and her husband standing behind her impatiently looking at his watch. The copy reads: "Suddenly she'd rather not go. She's waited thirty years for this trip. Now she just doesn't have the 'bounce.' She has headaches, hot flashes, and she feels tired and nervous all the time. And for no reason at all, she cries."

The medical literature also portrays the menopausal woman as childlike, dependent, and in need of dominance by paternal physicians who know best how to steer her through crucial biological life events. Women approaching menopause are compared to young girls approaching menarche, whose anxieties will be relieved if physicians will only "sit down with them and explain what the menopause is" (Huffman, 1979, p. 211). In contrast, physicians are portrayed as omnipotent beings, "made in the image of the Almighty" and able to provide women with "a glimpse of God's image" through their kindness and concern to their patients (Russell, 1968, p. 25).

Social Worthlessness

The menopausal woman is defined in the medical literature by her sexuality and reproductive role. Unfortunately, without the estrogen that "produces the beauty, the allure which attracts the male" (Wilson & Wilson, 1972, p. 521), the "sexual fire burns less brightly" (Huffman, 1979, p. 212). She becomes "a shriveled shell of a woman, used up, sucked dry, de-sexed and, by comparison with her treasured remembrances of bygone days of glory and romance, fit only for the bone heap" (Sillman, 1966, p. 166). Her "intrinsic social value, femaleness, plummets at the menopause," when her "value as a sex partner is impaired" (Easley, 1983, p. 373). "The husband who not long ago came home with sex-oriented thoughts now falls into his easy chair and looks for his pipe" (Huffman, 1979, p. 214). Or, that husband may not even come home at all, for "it has become almost commonplace for men to desert menopausal wives for younger women" (Easley, 1983, p. 374).

The major portion of the burden for maintaining continued marital bliss is directed at the menopausal woman. After all, "if her menopause affects her sexual performance in any way, it certainly affects her husband . . . he may feel that he is not wanted" (Davis, 1980, p. 73). When her vagina becomes dry, making intercourse uncomfortable, she is advised how to "fend off sexual suicide" (Nachtigall, 1986, p. 90) and instructed to "run, don't walk, to your physician. The life of your marriage may be at stake" (Davis, 1980, p. 42). The remedy, emphasized in bold print, is estrogen therapy, credited with saving "untold marriages" (Nachtigall, 1986, p. 92), since "virtually every woman will eventually have to give up sexual intercourse unless she starts taking estrogen" (p. 85). Although estrogen won't make "fantasies come true," she is warned that without it, she "may soon have no sex life at all" (Nachtigall, 1986, p. 83).

The menopausal woman is portrayed as grieving for her lost youth and fertility as she "*reluctantly* (emphasis added) relinquishes her capacity to bear children" (American College of Obstetricians and Gynecologists, 1981, p. 193). No longer does she enjoy "the security of the potential mother, to be able to create at will" (Forman, 1968, p. 18). As menopause signals the end of her childbearing ability, she faces "a significant milestone" which signals that she is "getting old, approaching death," and losing her "position of value in the world" (Willson & Carrington, 1983, p. 59). She feels no one needs her, even "at times, in the way" (Wilson & Wilson, 1963, p. 356), as she loses the parental role of responsibility for her existing children who are leaving the nest. "The child who once sought her lap for comfort now merely wants spending money and the car keys" (Huffman, 1979, p. 214). But the physician can alleviate her grief by providing reassurances of her "motherliness" and discussing "styles of grandmotherhood" (Klaus, 1974, p. 1187).

As the menopausal woman becomes useless for her intended purpose in society, her image becomes that of a potential threat to some of society's institutions. For example, as an "unstable, estrogen-starved" woman, she is responsible for "untold misery of alcoholism, drug addiction, divorce and broken homes" (Wilson & Wilson, 1963, p. 355). Without family tasks to fill her "idle years" (Davis, 1980, p. 37), she "may interfere in her grown children's lives" (*Ibid.*, p. 2).

Her image improves considerably when she is given the estrogen therapy and can better provide for male comforts and pleasures. When healthy, "she can manage her own work easily and have a lot left over to give to others," whereas a sick woman may "snap at her children and irritate and upset her husband" (Russell, 1968, p. 25). With estrogen, she will be "much more pleasant to live with and not become dull and unattractive" (Wilson & Wilson, 1972, p. 523). And, best of all, with estrogen, her "genitalia can be preserved in a functional state" (Meier & Landau, 1980, p. 1658) to assure "super sex forever" (Nachtigall, 1986, p. 83).

By depicting the menopausal woman's physical, psychological, and social potential as limited by the declining function of her reproductive organs, the medical profession functions as a subtle form of social control to keep women in their place, thereby resisting change and maintaining institutions and customs that depend on the old view of women. Pronouncements about women expressed through the ideology of medical science carry prestige and authority. Thus, physicians hold enormous power to define and manipulate female reality. When women are perceived as physically, psychologically, and socially impaired by their menopause, sexism and biological determinism are perpetuated.

A fundamental point that influences how a woman will experience her menopause is her perception of menopause as a developmental phase or as a disease. A developmental perspective is essential, for it allows a woman the outcome of personal growth, whereas a view of menopause as a deficiency disease serves to change it from an expected stage in her life to a threat to her health. Women must work together to reject medical images of disease and reclaim menopause as a normal phase of their life cycle. Only then can each one experience her menopause as a process of development rather than decay.

References

American College of Obstetricians and Gynecologists. *Precis II: An update in obstetrics and gynecology.* Washington, D.C.: Author, 1981.

Anonymous, M.D. *Confessions of a gynecologist.* New York: Doubleday & Company, 1972.

Berman, E. *The solid gold stethoscope.* New York: Macmillan Publishing, 1976.

Davis, M.E. *A doctor discusses menopause and estrogens.* Chicago: Budlong Press Company, 1980.

Easley, E.B. "Important facts about the menopause." *North Carolina Medical Journal, 44* (6) (1983), 369-375.

Forman, J.B. "Hormonal vs. psychosomatic disturbances of the menopause." *Psychosomatics, 9* (4) (1968), 12-16.

Goldberg, M.B. *Medical management of the menopause.* New York: Grune & Stratton, 1959.

Govan, A., Hodge, C., & Callander, R. *Gynecology Illustrated.* New York: Churchill Livingston, 1985.

High, R.L. "Discussion: Menopausal flush syndrome." *Psychosomatic Obstetrics and Endocrinology.* Edited by W.S. Kroger. Springfield: Charles C. Thomas Publishers, 1962.

Huffman, J.W. "Counseling the menopausal patient." *Postgraduate Medicine, 65* (12) (1979), 211-215.

Journal of the American Medical Association, 232 (10) (1976), 992.

Kistner, R.B. "The menopause." *Advances in Obstetrics and Gynecology.* Edited by R.M. Caplan & W.J. Sweeney. Baltimore: Williams & Wilkins Company, 1978.

Klaus, H. "The menopause in gynecology: A focus for teaching the comprehensive care of women." *Journal of Medical Education, 49* (1974), 1186-1188.

Meier, P., and Landau, R. "Estrogen replacement therapy." *Journal of the American Medical Association, 243* (16) (1980), 1658.

Nachtigall, L. *Estrogen: The facts can change your life.* New York: Harper & Row, 1986.

Rauramo, L. "A review of study findings of the risks and benefits of estrogen therapy in the female climacteric." *Maturitas, 8* (1986), 177-186.

Rhoades, F.P. "Minimizing the menopause." *Journal of the American Geriatrics So-*

ciety, 15 (4) (1967), 346-353.

Russell, C.S. *The world of a gynecologist.* London: Oliver and Boyd, 1968.

Sillman, L.R. "Femininity and paranoidism." *The Journal of Nervous and Mental Disease, 143* (2) (1966), 163-170.

Utian, W.H. *Your middle years: A doctor's guide for today's woman.* New York: Appleton-Century-Crofts, 1980.

Willson, J.R., and Carrington, E.R. *Obstetrics and gynecology.* 7th ed. St. Louis: Mosby, 1983.

Wilson, R. *Feminine forever.* New York: M. Evans & Co., 1966.

Wilson, R., Brevetti, R., and Wilson, T. "Specific procedures for the Elimination of the Menopause." *Western Journal of Surgery, Obstetrics & Gynecology* (May-June 1963), 110-121.

Wilson, R., and Wilson, T. "The fate of the nontreated postmenopausal woman: A plea for the maintenance of adequate estrogen from puberty to the grave." *Journal of the American Geriatrics Society, 11* (1963), 347-361.

Wilson, R. and Wilson, T. "The basic philosophy of estrogen maintenance." *Journal of the American Geriatric Society, 20* (1972), 521.

THE RAGE OF WOMEN IN THEIR FORTIES

Penelope Scambly Schott

1

The rage of women in their forties
is predictable as weather; one way
or another, it's coming through.

All night long in the starlit
pantry, mason jars curtsy;
at sunrise, they leap from the shelves.

Syrup coagulates, puddles
under the door; the soft flesh
of peaches is gashed with shards.

The rage of women in their forties
unfolds from rose-scented drawers
where kidskin gloves hold hands.

We have practiced enough kindness
to last you the rest of our lives.
Our rage smells like thunder.

We no longer expect the lilacs
to open for us. The life
where you know us is old

furniture under dustcovers.
Our mothers, who have passed through
ahead of us, lack all patience.

The rage of women in their forties
baffles the angels. We tilt
on black lace wings.

More fearsome than gravity,
we rock the sea in its bed.
Islands disappear.

2
Topsoil lifting;
shell-less creatures
burrowing down
out of the brilliance . . .

The slippings at fault
lines: a collection of small
gestures gathered to . . .

I want to draw
from the center that
single end of twine that
unravels the whole ball that . . .

This earth is new and unconnected.
Out from the frozen dirt
a woman is digging onions.

Her rage travels through stones.
It rattles the stalks in the fields.

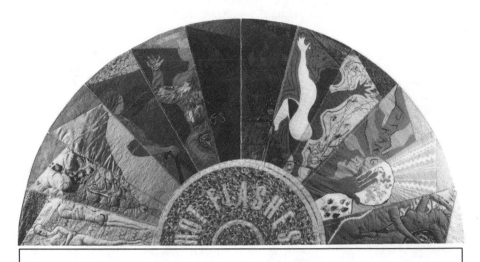

THESE FEVERED DAYS

The thermostat is off and I overheat like a stalled car.

—Judith Bishop

More and more frequently nowadays, my hot flashes have begun to feel like urgent communiques from the interior of a vast, dark continent—fast breaking news items from my heart of darkness. Sometimes hot flashes trigger sudden insights into previously obscure experiences. Other times, in reverse fashion, a rush of revelations will release the heat like thunder after a flash of lightning. Either way, I have come to trust the wired insights that hot flashes produce. Because I believe in epiphanies, I record most of these illuminations in a notebook I carry in my purse. Since hot flashes are often cryptic, I try to decipher their meanings as soon as possible.

—Barbara Raskin

MOTHER PREMARIN

Candida Lawrence

For the last six weeks I've been crazy, committable, and have used all energies in hiding this condition from my clever teenagers who would have noticed if they hadn't been so busy with their own hormones. We've now safely arrived at summer vacation and with my lovely dark green shiny Premarin pills in hand we'll bind again into a family of loving mother watching over her dear hostages, planning car trips up north, or to Mexico, long days on the beach.

I LOVE Premarin. It's my candidate for greatest discovery in all history. Just imagine the distance I've travelled in six weeks: There I was, earnest devoted teacher of thirty-two kindergartners, half of them bussed into my class because they were Spanish-speaking or black. I'm the morning teacher, twenty minutes for lunch, rush around preparing materials for the next day, then put in two hours in the afternoon class. Rose is the afternoon teacher and all of last year she was "in menopause." She'd be in charge of a group and suddenly I'd hear "Oh . . . oh . . ." and I'd look across the room and she'd be fanning herself with a workbook, her face swollen and red, her eyes staring. She would rise like a mourner from a bier and limp from the room. (She also had arthritis.) She didn't discuss her condition, never mentioned the word, but I knew. Who doesn't? There was my mother with her rages, her headaches, her exits from rooms. There was the tall teller in the bank where I worked in college who passed out on the marble floor on her way to the bathroom.

So anyway, that was last year and I thought I was safe. Common belief had it that if you started early you stopped late. Since I started at ten and a half I figured I had a few years—perhaps even many—before symptoms claimed me. But in mid-April I'm on my way to school and I begin to heat up. Neck first, then buttocks, private parts, thighs, underarms, back drenched with sweat, water streaming from my scalp into my eyes. I can see red bumps on my arms which are trying to steer during this assault. I pull over to the side of the road. I don't have time to go back home and put on dry clothes. I already stink of the ooze coming through my skin. I feel sick in my stomach and repellant, not at all the fresh, brightly colored teacher I like to present to my students.

That was my first hot flash. I prefer to call it my first sizzle. It's not a flash, which suggests speed. It takes forever and ever and while it lasts brain wires are disconnected. It is impossible to think or smile or move gracefully. It's my opinion that people faint because there's naught else to do. The governor has blown a fuse. You think you're dying because you connect dying with loss of control.

The day of my first sizzle I had six more during working hours (I could still count back then) which averaged out to about one each hour. The children's faces blurred and I couldn't remember their names, or my plans for the hour, the moment. That night I itched and couldn't sleep. I got out of bed and took a lukewarm bath which aggravated the rash and the itching.

In the weeks I was crazy, I was in a sizzle, or just out of one and about to go in again, constantly. My clothes and body were never dry and since I scratched, especially my neck and arms, ugly sores opened up and scabbed. They smelled putrid. I covered myself with Calamine lotion and told everyone I had poison oak, and oh how I wished I had a condition caused by an external poison. My condition was being a woman and this was the next event in a line of events— menarche, birth control, pregnancy and childbirth—which it had become fashionable to celebrate rather than deplore. Was I being punished because I thought and said, if asked, that if Nature was Mother Nature she was a misogynist? The design was clearly faulty. She was a lunatic and malevolent creator. Estrus would have been a fine plan—every six months an orgy—with a strong musk signalling our readiness, perfuming the rooms, the bed, our clothes.

During the crazy time, before my beloved Premarin, my green health pellets, I don't recall a single positive whiff of thought about what was happening to me. I didn't want to atrophy, have a dry vagina, get osteoporosis, be a Crone. I certainly didn't want to be free of the pregnancy risk. I'd been happily risking for years, playing my own Russian Roulette with sperm. Truth is, I wanted to get pregnant one last time, to be the oldest unwed mother in the school district, to nurse a baby again and risk getting fired for moral turpitude. As for the argument that since I would now be free of fear sex would be more fun, there was at least a possibility that the call to enjoy myself would prove tedious.

Why did it take six weeks to acquire my estrogen fix? I have "a cancer history." It's difficult to hide a missing breast, and every doctor I consulted said no, no estrogen, as soon as he saw my records, or my body. I said I'm going crazy, I'll lose my job, they'll put my children in foster homes. They said I'd adjust in a year or so. Ho! What did they know! I cried. In one office, I fainted. In the end, I arrived at our family physician's office at four every afternoon for one week. I would sit there and scratch and sizzle. The last day he asked me to design a quitclaim which would release him from responsibility. I created a masterpiece. I released him from all knowledge of me, all responsibility for me, all past or present connection with me, in exchange for a prescription for low-dose Premarin, those lovely shiny dark green pills. He sighed and signed. Twenty-four hours later I was free of sizzles.

Now I can again be nine years old, or eighteen, or early-married, or a young acrobat, or even a cranky crone. I don't have to be menopausal, a woman "in menopause," a woman entering a new time of life, a woman now free to enjoy sex without fear. I'm all ages, all pasts, all futures, as long as I take my beautiful pill each morning.

THIS IS LIVING

Pat Rhoda

My name is Pat Rhoda and I am a 50-year-old menopausal woman. Sounds like a participant at an AA meeting, but then most of us women over 40 have been reared in an environment where "women problems" were not openly discussed without first apologizing for bringing the subject up. Luckily, things are changing for our younger women—although some of the advertisements on television for everything from douches to diapers for adult women make one wonder if they may be going too far. Have you ever noticed how these ads come on at dinner time? But, it is in the best interest of each of us to read and learn what we can, either to avoid making mistakes or to gain comfort in knowing others have the same experiences, so here is my account of how I am handling menopause—or vice versa.

When recently at Kaiser for a pap test, instead of the usual male gynecologist, I saw a nurse practitioner and was amazed. She was like a doctor everyone dreams about—kind, interested, a good listener, full of information, competent— I couldn't believe it! Before we moved to Stockton, a previous doctor had persisted in prescribing .625 mg estrogen (Premarin) every day with 10 mg medroxyprogesterone (Provera) 14 days each month, even after I pointed out to him that the literature that comes with the meds suggests a much shorter regimen. But let's start at the beginning. . . .

On reflection, the big "M" was sneaking up on me a year or so before I made any connection. It started in 1983 when I was 44. The sneaky part was that my hair was getting dull and falling out more than it should, my breasts itched a lot and swelled before each period for a few days, and I was starting to have incontinence. I didn't know what that meant but a doctor wrote "incontinence" on my bill in November 1984 when I complained of losing bladder control when jumping, running, sneezing (I'm a big sneezer), etc. And, get this, occasionally a few fingers would go numb and turn yellow! Who knows if numb fingers have anything to do with menopause, but I thought it worth mentioning just in case. Remember, this was before I had any idea that any of these problems were linked to the beginning of menopause. A doctor suggested cutting out all caffeine and taking B$_6$ for the breasts, told me to do Kegel exercises for the bladder, and made no comment about my hair. Two out of three answers to questions is pretty good, don't you think? I mean for a doctor?

I had already cut out all caffeine, so wasn't helped by this advice. Vitamin B$_6$ and cutting down even more than humanly possible on salt intake must have helped, because for a few months my breasts didn't itch or hurt much at all. When I started doing the pelvic exercises, it was immediately obvious that they had to help since I didn't have any muscle control at all; but being a notorious procrastinator, I didn't do the exercises often so still had the bladder problem. My hair continued to fall out.

About this time, around March 1985, my periods were definitely irregular (41 days, 23 days, etc.), but I was still having them so didn't think I was menopausal yet—probably a common misconception. Actually, I was sort of looking forward to menopause which would mean no more menstrual periods. They had always been very heavy with lots of cramps. For some women, it would also mean no more messy bouts with birth control: diaphragms, pills, condoms. However, in my case, this was not a consideration since my husband had a vasectomy early in our marriage when I was having problems caused by birth control pills. What did make me unhappy was that now my breasts, in addition to itching, hurt increasingly often, to the point of my not being able to sleep at night. They were swollen (being small-breasted normally, this was not such a disadvantage), sore to the touch (my husband thought I wasn't any fun at all), and throbbed almost continually with little stabbing pains. But I still had a fairly good attitude, thinking that if I could just hit on the right combination, my body would get back to "normal" (whatever that means).

In March of 1987 I went to Kaiser for the first time. My husband and I had joined recently; it was the only health insurance that would accept him (another story) and I don't remember what my first appointment was for, but I ended up in gynecology talking about my extremely swollen, painful breasts to a male doctor, and he suggested a mammogram. I had no idea of what the procedure was, or I wouldn't have agreed to having it done at that time. The mammography technician said several times how firm and thick my tissue was as she squeezed the plates together, trying to flatten my breasts into pancakes but having to settle for less. I said that they were sore and swollen, but she didn't respond. She pushed the clamp as tight as she was physically able, ran to the controls and back, released my bruised boob, and went on to the right one. I didn't have guts enough to say stop (I've always been cowed by medical professionals), and I figured it was half over and couldn't get any worse. It was hard to believe that the next one would hurt even more—so bad that I couldn't stop the scream coming out of my mouth. My breasts ached constantly for several days afterward.

By February 1988 I had missed periods for five months, so went to Kaiser again to discuss whether to take hormones or go simply and quietly out of my mind—by this time I had developed hot flashes every 45 minutes, day and night, and was starting to hallucinate from lack of sleep. It seems that hot flashes/night sweats have an added effect of dosing the body with something like caffeine. It really is hard to separate which comes first, but usually a worrisome thought, being wide awake, and sweating occur all at once. Most doctors would like you to believe that the worrying comes first but I don't think so. A lot of the time I'm sure I haven't been thinking about anything at all—too tired or asleep! Some reading prior to this led me to use vitamin E to alleviate hot flashes, which helped at first but not when they got worse. In addition to the symptoms I mentioned already, my memory went (short *and* long term), my hair started feeling like shredded wheat and falling out by the handfuls, except on my chin and upper lip where it was growing with a vengeance. My body ached *everywhere.*

On my first visit to Kaiser Gynecology I picked up a pamphlet on menopause and read about possible side effects from taking estrogen replacement therapy (ERT), so like most women, I would imagine, my first reaction was to think "not me—I'll be strong willed enough and that will see me through the next couple of years of symptoms and then I will feel energetic and okay again." Superwoman syndrome. It wasn't long before all my resolve to not take ERT disappeared and I was ready for some relief at any cost; even the slight risk of cancer. I decided to take my chances because this was definitely not living! Instead of following the regimen in the pamphlet Kaiser puts out (days 1–25 on .625 mg estrogen with days 16–25 on 10 mg progesterone, leaving the last few days of the month off estrogen so as to avoid estrogen overload), the doctor said that the latest thing was to take estrogen constantly with 14 days of progesterone instead of just 10 days. When this caused increased breast swelling and pain, I decided to stop taking the hormones for a short time and then to try the regimen in the Kaiser pamphlet. They make a .3 mg estrogen tablet, but "Doctor" swore that everyone in the gynecology business agrees it isn't enough to stop bone loss in us susceptible types (fair complected anglo, tall, small boned), which is after all the main reason they prescribe ERT. He offered another regimen that I didn't try: taking .625 mg estrogen and 5 mg progesterone constantly to avoid any periods at all, but that seemed unnatural.

Getting back to the competent nurse practitioner, she said that she had never heard of using estrogen every day unless a woman had had a hysterectomy, and then rewrote my prescriptions to be taken according to the Kaiser pamphlet.

Another thing worth mentioning is that for several years I had been plagued with gradually worsening incontinence; recently, however, without doing exercises this problem is almost entirely gone, unless I drink alcoholic beverages fairly consistently or have a fit of uncontrollable laughter. God, the worst thing about all this menopause stuff is it requires one to be good to the body—since aging dictates eating fewer calories or we risk gaining weight with each and every chocolate bon bon (or whatever your fantasy food is), and now having to give up alcohol, what decadence is left?

All in all, the Kaiser pamphlet and another booklet from their waiting room were very helpful, so I'll pass along some of the information. Apparently, when the ovaries fail at the start of menopause, not all estrogen production stops. The conversion of adrenal gland hormones into estrogen, which before menopause had little importance, now is somewhat increased. This estrogen conversion occurs primarily in fat tissues, which may explain why overweight women often have fewer menopausal symptoms than thin women. Because of this conversion process, estrogen production appears to continue for at least 10 to 20 years after the start of menopause, but is quite variable from woman to woman.

One of the things I figured out for myself was that, at least in my case, there seemed to be quite a fluctuation in how much estrogen my body produced from month to month so if I took my estrogen as prescribed, it would be not enough or too much, causing all the side effects mentioned earlier. So what I did was vary the dosage as necessary, settling down to the standard routine after a couple of years.

Another thing that comes to mind, when I first entered college in 1957, one of the questionnaires required of new students asked if there were any physical/medical reasons why one might miss any classes, to which I answered yes, menstrual cramps and excessively heavy bleeding might on rare occasions keep me from class. The college doctor called me into his office to review my answers on his questionnaire. He asked if there was a family history of excessive problems with menstruation and I answered yes, thinking he was being understanding. But then he became very stern and started lecturing me on how cramps were all in a woman's head—that there was no scientific medical basis in fact for them and that my mother and sister had psychologically influenced me to feel pain when having a period! I was embarrassed to say the least, but knew intuitively that he was wrong. Of course, we know today that there are chemical changes in the body that can cause all sorts of problems, the least of which may be cramps, but it points out the typical male doctor's biased attitude toward female patients that persists even now. It seems to me that if a man has a problem that the medical profession does not yet thoroughly understand, the man is not told that it is all in his head. This attitude was obvious to me even in the Kaiser pamphlet and booklet on menopause. I have also read articles in magazines that seem to say the same thing. First they admit that scientific evidence shows that a rapid decrease in a woman's estrogen level can cause memory loss, nervousness, anxiety, depression, and insomnia, as well as hot flashes and night sweats, heart palpitations, aches, weakness and stiffness, weight gain, breast tenderness and fluid retention, wrinkles, gas and constipation, vaginal atrophy and sagging of other organs, osteoporosis, and decreased hair growth (except on upper lip and chin). But invariably as each symptom is stated as being caused by decreased estrogen, they find it necessary to add a "however" cause that sounds a little bit like "it's probably all in your head." For example: memory loss because you're easily distracted due to increased concerns at this time of life; and nervousness, anxiety, or depression because of lack of support from family and friends, increased outside pressures, and children leaving the nest. Of course these can add to the problem, but if anything can make one's brain sluggish and cause depression, lack of sleep from night sweats is on the top of my list.

It's time to bring my husband into this story. Since he has put up with all of my problems over several years, you probably would like to know how our marriage is holding up. Dick has always been a very caring person who gives me a lot of support and sympathy. It probably helped that he has had health problems too, which tends to make one more tolerant and understanding of others.

I've also been lucky to be able to work at home instead of having to drive for an hour in congested traffic to a hectic and demanding job (which I did until eight years ago), where having hot flashes, not being able to remember anything, etc., could cause problems. When I was working as a word processor years earlier, almost all the older women were hooked on tranquilizers, took long coffee breaks, and "kicked back" as much as they could get away with. It caused me considerable frustration when the work seemed to always end up on my shoulders. Had I understood that they were undoubtedly going through menopause and that the boss was just being sympathetic, I'm sure I would have been more tolerant.

People have called me a workaholic; it seems that I *need* to have worthwhile (translate income-earning) work in order to feel useful. My husband has had his own electronics business for years and eventually it needed quite a lot of my time as well. It has worked out well for me to be able to devote about half a day to the business doing circuit board wiring, bookkeeping, billing, etc., while the rest of my time is spent doing physical exercise types of things such as planting trees, gardening, landscaping, reworking our 30-year-old decaying house, and tending three kittens. Notice I didn't say housework. Our entire home looks like a playpen for the kittens, who shred kleenex, carry off small objects in their mouths and hide them from us for a joke, pounce on their milk dish, etc. But, being 50 now and living in a bad neighborhood in Stockton, I've noticed that we haven't made any new friends in a long time. This is an advantage in that there is no possibility that I can impress any of our friends of many years with my housekeeping, culinary expertise, etc.—they all know better. Besides, they're so glad to make it all the way to our house without being mugged or falling asleep at the wheel, no one notices the mess! You see, there are advantages to growing middle aged; one tends to adapt to a less demanding lifestyle, either by using tranquilizers or by getting away from the hustle.

All in all, what has caused most of the problems for me in the last seven years of menopause are feelings of guilt. Talking about myself in a physical way has always embarrassed me a little, but discussing menopause really threw me in a quandary. Women on TV and in the movies, and models in the magazines, never go to the bathroom, have periods or cramps, let alone hot flashes and night sweats. The message is that a strong woman should be able to overcome the body she inherited. This is pure bull, but more than that, it means everything has to be learned the hard way. If I had approached menopause as an enlightened, strong-willed woman, I would have researched each symptom, discussed it with other women before problems got out of hand, and not felt guilty for devoting time and effort to planning a strategy (keeping medical records of everything and visiting the doctor often with lots of questions). I guess I've always felt that my time belonged to someone other than myself, either my husband, or a boss, or even a cat! I hate to admit that at 47 years of age, I didn't even know what a mammogram was. This procedure is especially important for women who opt for ERT as I did, and appears from all the latest evidence to be quite safe. And, contrary to my first experience with mammography, it doesn't hurt at all when timed during the least breast swelling during the monthly cycle.

I even felt guilty for choosing ERT because it seemed I was cheating on other women. ERT slows a few of the aging processes that are accelerated by estrogen loss, so it seems as if you are cheating, kind of like dying your hair or having a face lift—things I would never do without feeling like a cheater. But, then again, the symptoms that caused me to take ERT were not frivolous. Constant hot flashes interrupting sleep every 45 minutes can really be incapacitating, as well as the depression that evolves from the lack of sleep. Looking at this in a broad sense, we didn't use to live much past fifty until recently; why should some women suffer during the second half of their lives if they don't have to.

There are risks with taking ERT, as there are with practically everything: the food we eat, the water we drink, the air we breathe. For me there is no question that the benefits are worth the possible risks. I feel better in every way now. My hair has stopped falling out, has regained some of its luster. And I don't have to pluck long protruding hairs from my chin anymore!

BODY BRIEFING: ESTROGEN REPLACEMENT

Marcia Seligson

The question here is clearly one of benefits versus risks.

There is no more crucial issue for women in mid-life than that of estrogen replacement therapy. And the essential question—Should I take it or not?—is so weighted with complexity, confusion, and fear that we have tended to make ourselves less informed, less fully responsible than we need be. If we are nearing or in the process of menopause, the subject is so important to the quality of the remaining years of our lives that we cannot postpone or neglect thinking about it; nor should we rely on our doctors to make the central decisions for us. Let it be said that there is no across-the-board solution. But there is more information than we probably imagined.

Although every woman is idiosyncratic and unique, the beginning of menopause often comes upon us in our late forties and is generally signaled by irregular periods and periodic hot flashes. Eventually, around the age of 51, menstruation will cease. What is occurring during this process is that our ovaries' production of estrogen, which began at puberty, is lessening. The reproductive organs are shrinking. The vagina is becoming dry and atrophying. Our skin and muscles are losing their elasticity and resilience. Our bones are thinning and losing calcium. All of these effects are due, in part, to the depletion of estrogen in our system.

In addition, 75 percent of us will experience an array of typical menopausal symptoms: depression or mood swings, insomnia, loss of sexual drive, and—above all else—the notorious hot flash. Again, these symptoms specifically relate to the body's diminishing supply of estrogen, and although for some women they may last for only a year or so, they can be remarkably uncomfortable and upsetting.

Like every aspect of menopause, hot flashes are so individual that some women have them five years before menopause, not identifying what they are, and others continue to have them for as long as 10 to 20 years afterward. Some women experience only a few occurrences each day, while others are overwhelmed three times an hour with the sudden heat and perspiration that herald the flash. Hot flashes are usually what propel women to their gynecologist's office to embark on a course of estrogen replacement therapy, or ERT.

Menopause hit me suddenly, dramatically, this year, at 51. One month my period was there, then it was forever gone. Concurrently I suffered frequent unexplainable sadness and emotional volatility. The hot flashes were so severe that while my husband was sleeping in a T-shirt under an electric blanket in our unheated bedroom (I could no longer tolerate any heating) I was nude on top of the sheets, sweating and thrashing about, unable to sleep. After two months I fled to my gynecologist, swearing to will him a substantial legacy if he could end my mid-life nightmare. He promised. After a few days on estrogen, the symptoms miraculously vanished. But I had no real idea of what I was doing, of the potential risks, the down side, the unknowns. I was not aware that there were alternatives to estrogen or that there are different types and various dosages. I was ignorant of how truly ignorant the medical profession is in this arena. Once again I had unthinkingly abnegated dominion over my body to The Doctor— ironically, in an area where there is more mystery than knowledge, more conflicting opinion than certainty. And then I became unwilling to be irresponsible. So I began this investigation.

According to James Waisman, M.D., an oncologist at the Breast Center in Van Nuys, California, "We *do* know what the advantages of estrogen therapy are, and they are vast. We *don't* yet know all the disadvantages. Menopause is one of the least understood conditions in medicine. Because the field is male-dominated, there has been a lack of commitment to research in this area. Symptoms have been discounted as emotional, with the profession demonstrating a reluctance to attribute them to physiologic changes." What studies have been done on ERT are relatively new, contradictory, and inconclusive.

Estrogen has been in common use for some 30 years, in birth control pills and for replacement therapy at menopause. In the 1960s and early '70s very large doses of estrogen were routinely given to menopausal women, until it was found that when the uterine lining was bathed in estrogen, an excessive buildup of cells occurred, causing hyperplasia, a condition that can be a precursor to cancer. (Indeed, among the women on ERT in those days, there was a tenfold increase in uterine cancer.) It was then that progesterone, the other major female hormone, was added to the therapy to return cell buildup to normal and thus prevent uterine cancer. Since the mid '70s progestin (the synthetic form of progesterone) has almost always been prescribed along with estrogen.

In America this is the most common regimen: One pill of conjugated estrogen (a mixture of natural estrogens) is taken in a dosage ranging from 0.3 milligrams to 1.25 milligrams for the first 25 days of the month and resumed again at the beginning of the next month. (Premarin and Ogen are the most widely prescribed brands.) Progestin (Provera the most popular brand) is added to the estrogen for days 16 to 25 in doses of 2.5 to 10 milligrams. Many women have opted for smaller doses taken every day of the month, or for the transdermal skin patch, applied once a week to the stomach or back (it is made of an estrogen called estradiol, which is absorbed directly into the bloodstream). Finding one's correct dosage is a highly individual and experimental process, and, in truth, nobody yet knows what dose will diminish the possible risks, like breast cancer, or produce the maximum benefits.

The benefits of ERT are irrefutably enormous: For the majority of women the disturbing symptoms of menopause are completely relieved very quickly as the level of estrogen rises and stays steady. Hot flashes disappear. The skin becomes more moist and retains elasticity, the vagina becomes lubricated, normal sleep returns, our moods even out. We feel as we did before. Yet the relief of symptoms is but a minor benefit (and can also be achieved by alternative therapies like acupuncture or a variety of vitamins or herbs) compared with ERT's proven ability to protect against heart disease and osteoporosis.

Characterized by a decrease in bone mass that predisposes its sufferers to breaks and fractures, osteoporosis is one of the true tragedies to befall women. Forty percent of all women develop the condition as a direct result of estrogen depletion. Ninety thousand osteoporotic women a year die from the systemic deterioration that often follows fractured hips. And osteoporosis, which begins *not* in our 70s and 80s but before the onset of menopause, cannot be reversed. Some women are at greater risk than others: those who are Caucasian, fair-skinned, small-boned, and thin; those with a family history of the disease; smokers; those who don't exercise, drank little milk, or reached menopause before age 40.

Estrogen, which is vital to the absorption of calcium into the bones, is a potent preventative, indeed the best preventative, against osteoporosis. And it must be taken forever, experts now believe, or the bone loss will begin and then accelerate.

ERT is also thought to be helpful in the prevention of heart disease, the leading cause of death among postmenopausal women. (After menopause the rate of heart disease among women jumps precipitously to nearly equal that among men.) What the estrogen does, it's believed, is raise the level of HDL, the "good" cholesterol, and prevent the formation of fatty deposits on arterial walls—a process that can result in a stroke or heart attack. According to Walter Willett, M.D., professor of epidemiology and nutrition at the Harvard School of Public Health, "Many studies now show profound protective effects of ERT for women. The magnitude is on the order of a 50 to 70 percent lowering of the risk of coronary heart disease."

There are, however, disadvantages to ERT too, and they fall into the category of unknowns, or possible down sides. According to many gynecologists, some women feel worse on the hormone rather than better. Unpredictable bleeding can go on for weeks, triggering the need for a biopsy or D & C.

Gaining weight is not uncommon. Depression, rather than being alleviated, can be exacerbated. The monthly menstrual cycle is mimicked as the uterine lining builds up with estrogen and then is sloughed off due to the addition of progesterone.

Then, too, we may have an intuitive, discomforting sense that we are not meant to play such games with nature as drinking in estrogen when the order of things has been set up otherwise. We may feel like female laboratory mice as we remember DES and Thalidomide and the role that estrogen itself played in the early days of uterine cancer. *But the biggest disadvantage is that we simply do not know the long-range consequences.*

The question of breast cancer looms most large these days. Since the early 1960s, there have been 20-odd studies examining the relationship between estrogen and breast cancer. Most experts agree that there has never been a significant study showing a conclusive connection but that the issue is muddled in controversy.

Last August, when the results of a Swedish study were published in the *New England Journal of Medicine*, the question of ERT and its role in breast cancer rang out with great alarm. In the study more than 23,000 Swedish women above the age of 35 who were taking various kinds of estrogen replacement—not birth control pills—were followed for an average of six years. The largest group of women (56 percent) were taking estradiol *pills*, which are not used in the United States. For those women, the rate of breast cancer was double that of the women not taking estrogen. The rest of the women were taking either conjugated estrogens like Premarin or other types of estrogen, mainly estriols, and in those samples there was no increased incidence.

The most disturbing part of the findings centered on the ten women using estradiol along with progestin. After taking this combination for more than six years, they showed a rate of breast cancer that was 4.4 times that of women using no hormones. The red flag had gone up regarding progestin.

The Swedish study contradicts prior research, in which this same regimen was found to *reduce* the risk of breast cancer. An important study published in 1979 observed 168 American women, for ten years, who were randomly given either estrogen replacement or a placebo. According to an editorial in the *Harvard Medical School Health Letter*, "None of the women receiving hormone had developed breast cancer, whereas four of the untreated controls had. In other words, the result was precisely the opposite of the Swedish finding."

One of the confounding aspects of this subject—confounding to doctors as well as patients—is the amount of contradictory evidence. Then, too, most studies did not follow women for an extended period of time, and many cancers are quite slow-growing. "Long exposure or latency may be necessary to show any association between hormone use and breast cancer," wrote Elizabeth Barrett-Connor, M.D., chairman of the department of community and family medicine at the University of California, San Diego, in a postscript to the

Swedish study. "A single study rarely proves anything," she says, "but I have been concerned about progesterone for a long time, simply because we don't know very much about its long-term effects."

The Swedish findings, then, are definitely worrisome but will not be considered definitive until further studies corroborate the research. But doctors and researchers now are reversing their previous endorsement of progestin, and that is the loudest alarm issuing from the Swedish study. In addition, the newest research that extols the value of estrogen in preventing heart disease suggests that progestin may cancel out that particular benefit. But if we stop the use of progestin, we are once again facing the proven risk of uterine cancer.

As my own personal bias in medical matters follows more the natural, alternative path, I set out to see if there were options and possibilities beyond the medical model. I spoke to acupuncturists, homeopaths, practitioners of Chinese herbal medicine, nutritionists, and medical doctors who practice alternative therapies. I discovered that nonmedical methods do help relieve menopausal symptoms; far less comforting, though, is the fact that there is no hard evidence that any of these will prevent osteoporosis or reverse the tendency toward heart disease, at least not with the certainty that estrogen does. And of course, all the data are anecdotal, as nobody has ever conducted a major study of these approaches. Nonetheless, a menu here might help us make more informed choices about our own course of action.

For hot flashes the medical options include belergal (addictive) or clonidine (lowers blood pressure and causes drowsiness). Many experts, physicians as well as "alternative" practitioners, have seen that vitamin E and pantothenic acid are quite helpful. My own gynecologist recommended dong quai, a Chinese herb that contains natural plant estrogen in a very low dose. Says Janet Zand, a holistic practitioner in Los Angeles: "No one in the West has done substantial research on dong quai. I know only what I see from a large percentage of thousands of patients who swear that it works to lessen the discomfort of hot flashes. In Chinese medicine, menopause is viewed as a blood deficiency, and dong quai nourishes the blood. Of course all my information is anecdotal and historical, handed down via Oriental history. Menopause is at a very low roar in the Orient, compared with our culture, as is osteoporosis. We don't know if that's because of different genetic body types, nutrition, or because aging is considered very differently in the Orient—as a natural and not unwelcome part of life."

For vaginal lubrication, water-soluble lubricants like Astroglide, Lubrin, Replens, and Crème de la Femme are good substitutes for estrogen. These are better than petroleum jelly, which is greasy, but will have to be used forever, as they do not provide natural continuous lubrication.

As for osteoporosis—let us be clear that neither a calcium-rich diet nor a calcium supplement will guarantee prevention of this terrible condition. This is why most experts agree that if a woman fits the profile for severe bone loss, she should be on ERT. Those of us who are chubby, do regular weight-bearing exercise, and do not smoke are at lesser—but not, by any means, zero—risk.

Which brings us to cardiovascular disease. I come from a family with a history of strokes (both my parents died of them), so I am particularly focused on that genetic pattern. I do all the things a responsible woman should do for my well-being—exercise regularly and rigorously, have annual stress tests, watch my diet and cholesterol intake. But I am aware that, as my natural estrogen diminishes, my rigor may not be sufficient. I have made my decision about ERT based on an array of benefits and risks, but the proven advantage is, for me, the clarion call.

Each woman is idiosyncratic in her experience with menopause. I will tell you the regimen I have arrived at, after six months of mixed experiences—total relief from hot flashes and angst but a gain of 10 pounds and bleeding on a dosage of 1.25 milligrams of Premarin and 10 milligrams of Provera that signaled the need for a uterine biopsy. I cut the dosage in half; then I cut it in half again. Then I went off it completely. The bleeding stopped but the hot flashes returned along with headaches. Now I have finally created for myself a satisfactory modification (and I had to enlist my doctor's support in *my* choice). I am taking, I believe, the smallest amount of ERT that will probably make a difference, combined with natural substances as an adjunct to the program. I take 0.3 milligrams Premarin and 2.5 milligrams Provera, dong quai, and a larger-than-usual amount of vitamin E and pantothenic acid. I feel physically wonderful and comfortable with my well-thought-out recipe. And I might change it at any time that new information becomes available.

I offer this in no way as a prescription, simply because there are no two women whose systems, history, and concerns are the same. I offer it only to illuminate the choices we do have—more than we probably have been told. My formula has worked for me, for the moment. I do recommend that you investigate all the possibilities. And before going on an ERT regimen, if that is what you and your doctor decide, I strongly advise that you submit to a reading of your hormone (FSH) level, a cholesterol workup, a family history, and a new mammogram.

The best we can do, at this moment in time, is make the smartest personal choices available to us.

LOSS

Joan Joffe Hall

Hot flash. I wake,
my body steams.
Tossing my covers off
I lose my dreams.

THESE FEVERED DAYS

Frances Ruhlen McConnel

I wake up, heat rising in my body like the evening desert dissipating the heat of the sun. I throw off the covers to let the night air at me. May, and by noon the thermometer will be hitting the high 90s. Across my husband's shoulder the digital alarm says 1:55.

When a hot flash is starting, I always have to pee. The bathroom is just to the right of the bedroom. Light from the streetlamp comes faintly in the distorted glass of the window. Cars go by as they do all night on the busy street behind the house. Back in bed, I turn on the small electric fan on the night stand. There's also a box fan near the door, my husband Glenn's fan. He lived for years as a graduate student in a mouse-ridden, stereo-throbbing apartment building in Boston. The fan is his sleep machine. I sit up in bed so the sheets can cool. What was my dream?

School days. Home sick from Elm Grove Elementary. Feverish, a slight echo and buzz in the air. A radio is playing a woman's program my mom is half listening to. "The first call to breakfast" and the invisible company marching around a table.

My mom's in the kitchen, humming slightly, rattling kitchen things—pans, paper. The refrigerator door opens and shuts. She has made me what she calls a milk shake, though it isn't really. No ice cream, just milk and crushed ice and sugar shaken up. But it's cold and sweet.

The passing lights of cars sweep through our bedroom, catching on the ceiling fan. Cool again, the spell past. The clock reads 1:57. It was about a year ago when I had my first bout of missed periods, hot flashes, moods where I snarled at everyone; moods that plummeted me into a tunnel of misery at the end of which seemed only the white light of death.

I think of the hot flashes as my spells. My Nana had spells which kept her in bed all day, the room darkened, her head propped on her hand, her radio tuned to a Baptist station. To me she was just old, and the old were a more delicate species. I had never heard the word "menopause," but I knew that some years earlier Nana's younger sister, my Great Aunt Lily, had taken to her bed with "female troubles"—a mysterious and dangerous phrase that suggested being female was enough to doom you.

My "spells" last only a couple of minutes, but on bad days they come every hour. So I am up and down all night, remembering how as a kid, I would hear the bathroom door close or see the light go on in the hall, and know my Nana was on the prowl.

"The old don't sleep so good," Nana would apologize. "The good Lord should have made us wakeful when we were young with kiddies underfoot and a pile of ironing to do." But my mother said there were plenty of kiddies for both of them and let her catnap if it kept up her strength. It was a natural, animal way to sleep. And sure enough, you'd think Nana was down for the day, in the dark of her room with the fan going, but, next thing you knew, you'd look out the window and see her bent over, weeding strawberries, the summer sun baking down on her white head.

I drift off pretty quickly. And wake again, feeling sick to my stomach. I've pulled up too many covers with the chill that sometimes comes over me. The clock says 3:09. Now the fever comes and I turn on my little fan and sit up. On the bedtable is a glass of water, chapstick, lotion for the soles of my feet, reading glasses for doing the crossword puzzle—which Glenn and I do each night to put ourselves to sleep—about a dozen burned-out matches, and a row of candles, for romantic interludes.

(I'll still have them, won't I? These are the Eighties and sex is supposed to follow you right to the edge of the grave, that fine and private place. Though this is one of the symptoms of age I can't yet bear to think on: the drying up of the body's juices.)

My husband is snoring softly. Thank the Lord. In pollen season his snores rage and anguish, so I have to exile myself to the couch.

Turning up the cool side of the pillow, I wake him. "Still bouncing?" he asks and I give his shoulder a poke. He reaches for my hand, but I can't bear it long; it's as if I were a space heater plugging myself in.

Earlier in the year I was having trouble with bursitis in my right elbow, then that went away when the asthma started in, and then the asthma was replaced by the hot flashes. I have a theory that disorders like these are all one disorder, only they take different forms. But it's all the same thing I think. Stress, my daughter would say. Though it's just life, isn't it? Stress, I mean. And when was life something else, we wonder. When I was a kid and the world seemed a mellow enough place, without jet planes and express lanes and not on the point of self-destruction, my dad still developed ulcers. And his dad, who lived on a farm all his life, had to have "nerve treatments." And his mother, my great-grandmother, took cocaine, like many a Midwest farmwife in the 1850s.

And they had asthma worse, from haying.

Whatever "it" is, the archetypal disorder, it explains why you don't usually catch a cold and the stomach flu *at the same time.*

The bursitis in my right elbow got worse last summer from gardening—but originally it started up when I had the first attack of hot flashes and started using a fan. I had a small Oriental folding fan in my purse—beautiful, with black and gold butterflies. I would snap it open and start fanning myself in mid-sentence, eating lunch out with friends. That was when I discovered how taboo a subject menopause is, even jokes about it. Forget male friends, you don't want them to know anything. Younger women friends suddenly look at you differently. You're an "older woman." You've seen the look before. You've given it yourself. A couple of years ago when my friend Barb, who's ten year older, had migraines and hemorrhages and mood roller-coasters and insisted on discussing them, I couldn't look her in the face. But now I search out frankness. My artist friend Catherine says for her it's like being doused with gasoline and set afire. For me it's as if I'd just run five miles. You can cringe at such images if you want to, but, hey, this is a public service announcement.

How long does it go on? I asked them, my older women friends. Barb said five years, so far. So it's not acute; it's a chronic disorder. Is that supposed to make it worse or better?

My mother went through menopause early, when I was still little. I didn't know about menstruation until I was eleven and going off to camp and she warned me it sometimes started in strange settings, packing into my suitcase a box of Kotex and a belt. That was gratifying too, like something from a secret society: the paraphernalia and the words *blood* and *cramps.* I looked forward to it. Though I had it easy when it came to periods and was in awe of friends who moaned and took to their beds.

Of course I also secretly scorned them, as if they willed their own infirmity, like my little brother, the serious asthmatic, asking for special pampering.

And when weakness is really power in disguise, like a usurping baby brother, oh, the rage that can come over you. But, when it's your parents' weakness, oh, the shuddering.

My own daughters are sympathetic about my symptoms of upcoming menopause—but they don't want me to dwell on it. Can't the doctors *do* something, they say, and they mean *stop you from aging.*

Of course, I've wondered that too. When I first was forty and having my little ups and downs with drawn-out periods and depressions and what not, I had gynecologists who couldn't wait to slap the hormones to me. But when I went back last year, begging for hormones, suffering severely from hot flashes, sleeplessness, and the impression I was turning into a witch, they said I hadn't skipped enough periods. Instead, they gave me a prescription for pills that were supposed to keep my blood vessels from expanding and running my temperature up. "But what are they?" I asked, "and what are the side effects?" Oh, not to worry, dear.

So when I got home and called up my daughter, who is a medical assistant, to look up the medicine in the PDR, she said it was basically a barbiturate. "And they gave you three refills?" she asked, "and here I am, a diabetic, and I'll always be a diabetic and my own doctor only gives me two refills on syringes. I guess he doesn't want to hook me."

But this reminds me of troubles friends of mine have been having with their elderly parents. For one reason or other, during a visit, their mothers or fathers—usually their mothers—will complain of constipation, or lack of energy or fuzzy vision or that the prescription for their "nerve pills" has run out, and the son or daughter will discover the prescription is for valium and the parent has been on it for five or six years. A doctor will have prescribed it for some kind of upset—a death or a trip—years ago, and then just kept renewing it.

That's what it means, ultimately—having hot flashes. They're going to start treating you like somebody's pet creature that needs to be kept subdued.

Though they were right about the hormones, as my period started back up after a couple of months. Meanwhile, I threw out the barbs and took up fans. Good old female doctoring, I thought, remembering summer evenings back in the South, with all the older women out on their porches fanning themselves with newspapers. Or in church, when the sultry August air just closed in and, up and down the pews, the programs were being folded into fans. It was always the women doing it, not the men, even though they were dressed hotter, in their dark suits. I thought then men's dignity was more important to them; it awed me about men, like my father, who was in pants and undershirt and shirt and shoes and socks no matter how hot it was, while my mother ran around barefoot like us, in shorts and a halter. Of course, once you've gone through pregnancy, you can see what little use there is for dignity, what with hordes of people—doctors, nurses, medical students—looking up into your sacred parts, and prodding and commenting on them in Latin, as if you weren't there. To say nothing of delivery—the farting, the shitting, the moaning, the screams—right out there in public. But, nowadays, I think it's not something lacking in women—like dignity—but some extra gumption they've got, some bold imagination, to turn a church program into a fan. Surely women invented fans—the comfort and the beauty of them—a beauty I discovered at Pier One. Why have we no beautiful fans in our culture? I was thinking of buying some paints and decorating the plainer ones in my collection when I got the bursitis from all that vigorous fanning.

How did they get around that—those older women? Or did they just suffer, softly, with the sound I associate most with elderly women, a kind of gentle, day's-end moan, my Nana's sound, even when she was feeling well enough to let me sleep with her. In the middle of the night, I would stir awake to her soft groan, the click of the radio going on, and the rhythmic rant of a preacher.

She was far past hot flashes herself, unless they follow you to the grave, waking you from dreams of the past, and so far, no one has promised me that they won't.

Maybe a century ago, there was a spell some ancient crone could give you, a folk remedy passed down generations of women who lived past menopause. Or maybe, haunted by dreams, they just walked their camps and villages at night, leaving their families alone in their beds, letting the cold air blow down the wicks of their fevers.

The clock reads 4:15. My husband mutters in his sleep and turns on his side. It is a different universe he inhabits, both by day and by night. Things are more solid, more separate from him, as if the male body had less connective tissue than the female's—between itself and the world, itself and the past.

Dreams swirl around me: mummies and caves and the heat of beloved bodies long since gone out, or gone over to the Other World, a world promised me by grown-ups, but a world with absurdities more childish than flying reindeer and Easter Bunnies—harps and wings and stairs of clouds and eternal bodiless bliss.

A rush of anxiety announces another hot flash—death closing in against my heart. Heat fans out to my ribs, my wrists, my under-arms. Sweat pops out on my skin. 5:45. I throw away the covers, and spring up, naked. It is light enough in the bathroom to see in the mirror and I stare at myself, feeling my skin flush hot, the moisture on my upper lip, but there is no other outward sign. Our black and white cat comes in, stretching and mewing and nipping at my ankles to be fed. Morning traffic has revved up and soon the alarm will ring.

Up the street a few blocks, the six o'clock train is blowing and clanging at the crossing. The train always makes joy rise in me, a child's joy. Can it be so long ago, the vacation cabin next to the railroad tracks in the Smokies, thirty-five years? My father in his short-sleeve summer shirt, showing his upper arms, pale and vulnerable, unlike ours which are brown and tough. He's teasing us that if the train jumps its tracks, it will land right in our laps. My mother shushes him up. She is standing at the rickety pine table, spreading mayonnaise on sandwich bread. Wisps of grey hair come floating from the French roll on the top of her head, and the caps of her shoulders are freckled and peeling. I've also had too much sun and the smell of Spam makes my stomach turn. Lying on my sleeping bag on one of the camp cots, my face tightened with sunburn, my temperature shoots up and down, as it does now, making me sick and dizzy.

I burrow back down beside Glenn, dreaming my brothers there to wake me: Teddy, bounding up and down on the bed and starting the dog barking; Lamont, giving me a mocking look as if I'm faking it and if I try to smack him with my pillow, he'll swear he didn't *say* anything. "Come on, Frankie," they'll nudge me. "Don't be a slug-a-bed. Let's go fishing." And Glenn will slip out of bed first, as he always does, to fetch the morning paper from the driveway, feed the cat, make coffee, then roust me out. "Get up, lazy-bones. Day's a-breakin'."

My dad's voice. My mom's kiss. And I'll throw off the hot covers and pretend it's nothing, it's natural—my spells, my female troubles, my aging.

WORLD CLASS MENOPAUSE

Pat Miller

I welcomed the first hot flushes as a rite of passage and expected this manifestation of menopause's purely physical process to be anything from as bothersome as menstruation to as tedious, but endurable, as the last months of pregnancy. I was pleased to have a real experience of what I'd been reading and hearing about, and hoped I'd be among those who pass through the hot flush stage quickly. After a year, I figured I must be among those who go on with hot flushing for two years. After three years I began to suspect that the information that menopause lasts about five years meant hot flushes for five years. After five years of hot flushes that did not seem to show any sign of diminishing, and after hearing about other women's real experiences, such as still having hot flushes at age seventy-five, I began to despair. In the sixth year of my "menopausal symptoms" I said the hell with it and got onto estrogen replacement therapy, ERT, which I had been avoiding because of its uncertain effects, such as uterine cancer for those of us who have not had hysterectomies. By this time information about osteoporosis was being widely circulated and ERT was a possible preventive. Given that I had long-lived women relatives who suffered from their bones aching in the last ten years of their lives, I decided to trade the then-diminishing cancer risks for an increasing assurance of freedom from osteoporosis. The ERT immediately got rid of the hot flushes.

If there's pride to be had in having the most flamboyant of hot flushes I claim that pride. I suspect that descriptions of hot flushes are toned down in articles which try to reassure women that menopause is not a miserable thing. Probably it's felt that describing worst case hot flushes will have the power of suggestion to make a reader have them in a more potent way than if she just expects to have a nice little pleasant warm feeling once in a while for a few months or so. This was one time in my life when the reasonable and realistic books and articles failed to prepare me for what happened. Maybe I'll be subject to hot flushes until I'm past a hundred. I'm sixty-two now, and any time I try leaving off the ERT, back comes the heat.

Here's a day in the life of a worst case hot flush victim. The flushes go on day and night, as often as three per hour, and lasting for as long as five minutes. They dominate my attention and debilitate my energy. At night a person sharing the bed with a hot flush victim suffers cold flushes as the blankets are thrown off. A hot flush is often preceded by a surge of extreme anxiety that makes one almost gasp in day-time, and wakes one up in the night. The sweating is so profuse that clothes or sheets are soaked. During the day the hot flush sufferer learns to dress in quickly removable layers, the bottom one, for decency's sake, being a light sleeveless blouse. T-shirts cannot be worn because their knit fabric is too warm when the heat goes on. Room and automobile temperatures become subjects of cross, grumpy arguments as the hot flush victim wants coolness when she tosses off the clothing because her internal, infernal, heat mechanism has kicked in. Hand-held fans become a necessary piece of equipment. The hot flush sufferer may do seemingly odd things such as hurriedly going outside in icy weather for a few minutes every half hour or so. Legend tells of the woman who would frequently stick her head into the freezer to cool off. Having read anthropological reports of elderly Eskimos voluntarily going off into the icy cold to commit suicide, thus leaving the scarce food for baby Eskimos, I wondered if some of those elders were perhaps desperate menopausal women trying once and for all to get cooled down.

I took an easier way out and went on ERT. I had tried dietary sanctions of caffeine and alcohol, and ingestion of ginseng, and deep relaxation and other suggestions without success. I did not try any esoteric or peculiar diets, nor did I try acupuncture, meditation, or complex herbal remedies. But I am prepared to believe any stories I hear of women who have added to their basic healthy diet a daily portion of some foodstuff which reduces the frequency and potency of hot flushes or eliminates them altogether. Also I will not discount acupuncture, meditation, hypnosis, daily head stands, or deep psychoanalysis to find out why one is obsessed with having hot flushes. The medication of ERT is so minuscule, a patch with a tiny bit of estrogen and worn for as little as eighteen days out of a thirty-two day cycle, and balanced with progesterone for ten days. Such tiny amounts make such a big difference that it leads me to believe that somewhere there is an herb or a dietary supplement which can be taken to cope with hot flushes.

Living in this present time when knowledge about our animal selves is still so new and limited I am happy to have ERT, even though it is still, in a way, experimental. I'd like to think that with the computer marvels of data-collecting possible, vast numbers of health records would be accumulating to indicate the effects of ERT. I'd like to contribute the record of my individual struggle with hot flushes and subsequent use of ERT, and whatever becomes the consequences of this therapy which I am happily using now, and may come to regret later, or may continue to value as something which made me secure from osteoporosis as well as giving relief from those hellish hot flushes.

This health issue might receive a lot more attention if hot flushes happened to men. The entrance of females into roles formerly held by males will perhaps engender (pun intended) more extensive research.

Now that I am on ERT life is not idealistic. ERT has its own effects, simulating the menstrual cycle. In addition, age does creep in. I do not have the energy I had when I was forty. I have finally had to reconcile myself to the fact that I am not going to have a career as a brain surgeon. There was a bit of propaganda, as I would call it, about menopause back when I was just getting into it. It was said that most women had something called "post-menopausal zest." Perhaps that is true, but perhaps, also, "zest" has to be carefully defined. The reality of life for me is that energy diminishes. Time becomes more precious because one can do so much less within it. I cherish something I learned long ago, and that is to realize that every life is limited, no one can possibly do all the things that a human mind can imagine doing in one lifetime. The compensation for that limitation is that each of us can appreciate the multitude of wonderful things that other people are able to do.

NATURE'S PLAN

Jean Mountaingrove

I was shocked when the doctor casually said I was pre-menopausal. I was only 43. I wasn't thinking of growing old until some far distant time, and in my mind, menopause was definitely the gateway to "old." I was there for a PAP smear, not any gratuitous predictions about wrinkling, withering and shrivelling up. "Well, you've been pre-menopausal since you were born," I joked to myself to cover my anger . . . and dismissed it.

In fact, he was correct. Four years later my hot flashes began. My periods were not as regular and menstrual pain was a little less than I had suffered previously. And I had changed. In those four years I had become a feminist and a lesbian and was considering the importance of menstruation for women's psychic development and wisdom.

So I watched menopause come upon me. From feminism I learned that all our life experiences are valuable. I knew I should keep a diary of my menopausal experiences, but I didn't do it. I did write a poem, "Aging Amazon."

How fortunate to "do" menopause with a mid-life woman partner, I congratulated myself. How odd and alone I would feel with a husband. No matter how "understanding" he was, how could he possibly understand as another menopausal woman could?

Our first hot flashes went unrecognized. We attributed them to the hot day, to the electric blanket, to the steep climb. Eventually we figured it out. You see, we were the first women in our social circle to reach menopause. It was at least three more years before an older woman arrived. She was still having hot flashes and sweats that woke her at night when she was 55.

Now it is 16 years later and I am still having hot flashes that wake me at night. When my lover visits, we laugh as we ask each other, "Is this your hot flash or mine?" And then we move a little apart until that heat passes.

With each hot flash I wonder if it will be my last one, or if they will go on forever. I'm sure I'll miss them if or when they ever end. Like breastfeeding, they are an intense and often pleasurable sensation. And when the experience is over, it will never return.

I have tried to describe my hot flashes to curious younger women. I considered using silver paint on canvas to convey the tingling sensation that often starts on my legs and flows upward, circling my thighs and then my arms, flushing my throat and face, moistening my upper lip. And each time a little different. Very wet hot flashes are recent for me. In the past when I began to feel hot, I would ask if others noticed it too (meaning: Is this room hot?). Then I realized I could just draw my finger above my upper lip. Damp? Hot flash.

Sometimes that gradual sensuous tingling doesn't occur. The first warning then is vague irritability. I don't like what's happening. I want to leave. But as soon as I'm aware of my impatience, the heat begins and I realize my discomfort is due to inner events, not outer ones, and the hot flash follows.

"And how frequent are they?" is a favorite question of my fortyish friends. From a few each day now to more than twenty a day in the beginning, I tell them. This is a guess because I didn't keep that diary. I hope others are. From sharing experiences with other old women, I believe we are as individual in menopause as we are in menstruation.

I am sweating now. I fan myself with my papers. I have pulled my shirt above my breasts. I wipe my face, throat and chest. When I have a hot flash and am alone, the urge to pull off my shirt is irresistible.

Now two minutes later, I am cool and dry.

When I was about 50 with very frequent and intense hot flashes, I sometimes had brief thoughts of suicide. And I mean brief. I would be writing and suddenly think, "It's no use. My life is meaningless. I can't go on." Just out of the blue I would feel utterly hopeless. I would put down my pen and tell my partner. By the time she could come across the room to comfort me I was all right, cheerful and ready to resume my writing. This happened perhaps once or twice a day for a few weeks. It convinced me that hormones affect my feelings powerfully.

Lowered levels of hormones also affect my energy. Mystified at first by sudden fatigue, I have gradually identified that "all gone" feeling unlike any other kind of tiredness as a hormone drop. I have to rest a while until my energy returns.

Hot flashes and tiredness sent me to the clinic. I was in fine health so the doctor offered estrogen replacement therapy. I accepted his prescription slip but couldn't bring myself to get the pills.

I am a skeptic about the latest medical miracle for our problems. I have witnessed the Salk vaccine: it gave polio to some of its users. I witnessed the birth control pills: they gave embolisms to some of their users. I witnessed the IUDs: they perforated many a uterus. I'll never know what life would be like for me if I had chosen to take the estrogen, offered to me with hints of eternal youth and never osteoporosis. I'll stick with nature's plan.

Medically, menopause is defined as having occurred when a woman has had no menstrual flow for one year. This is a tidy definition for statistics but difficult unless a woman keeps a careful calendar. Even when that year is over, our hormones keep changing. The phrase women use, "going through the change," better describes my experience of a long transition. The obvious change that I ceased to bleed monthly was all that I was told to expect, but there are other significant changes.

I had heard of "the middle age spread" with the inference that women just let themselves get sloppy. I learned that estrogen is stored in fatty tissue, so the increased fat around my hips stored estrogen to ease the effects of my irregular and lowering estrogen production.

In response to my body's changes and the new sensations I experienced, I had to notice that some things were ending for me. I had to realize that even as my periods ended, someday my life would end. Far in the future, I hope, but closer than I thought during the years of my familiar monthly cycling. I looked for a new way to gauge my time and pace my aspirations.

This society dismisses these profound shifts in my body and consciousness as "post-menopausal." As if menses are what is truly significant in my life and after they end—the next 30–40 years—are just a "post" script. But I asked myself, what are the potential benefits inherent in this natural unaltered process?

Menopause is not just a single event or ceremony, it is really a long transition, a change on all levels of a woman's inner life. Beyond the obvious changes in our bodies there are other profound changes—in our interests, focus, direction, and aspirations.

AN ACT OF FREEDOM
For Grace Butcher

Ann Menebroker

My friend stapled
a used estrogen patch
onto a letter she wrote
to me;
a thin, clear plastic circle
releasing chemicals
into her system, creating
extended cycles,
protecting her heart,
the bones and worth
of this woman.
She wore it
against her skin
between belly button
and crotch
like a second pulse.
She runs competitively.
Her legs hurt.
The Achilles' heel aches.
Her tendons are sore,
but she keeps running.
She is fifty-five years old
and won't give up.
I go down by the river
where I live
and toss the patch
off the H Street bridge,

watching it move along,
like my friend, a
silver glimmer
in the sun.

COMING OF AGE

Henrietta Bensussen

At age 47, this is what I thought menopause would be like: periods would gradually come later and later, finally stopping after a year, maybe two. The hot flashes I was already subject to would also gradually disappear, certainly they would be easy to live with. I read about estrogen replacement therapy and thought it was a good idea. I looked forward to freedom from menstruation.

This is what really happened: four more years of sporadic bleeding, lasting anywhere from three weeks to three days, requiring a large investment in mini-pads. Acne. Burning-up hot flashes, sometimes in waves every 20 minutes. Foot cramps in the dead of night.

The constant slight bleeding made me anxious, but when I consulted doctors either they advised estrogen therapy or told me it was nothing to worry about. For acne I was given a topical prescription; wearing socks to bed helped the foot cramps a little. Eventually, I just accepted all this as a natural part of menopause.

But there was freedom. I was at last done not only with child-bearing but also with family responsibilities. I had fulfilled the obligations required of a woman growing up in the 1940s and 50s: married young, successfully raised two children, had not divorced even though tempted, worked and used the extra income to help finance my daughter's education at a women's college (my own dream when I was young).

Now my son was preparing to leave home for college, and I realized I had another 25 years of life to live, at the least, and that I was finally free to focus on my own needs. One of the first things I realized was that I did not need or want a husband, or any man, and that what was really important to me was the community of women. I came out to myself as a lesbian.

Menopause is like going through adolescence a second time: changing hormones upsetting the body's measured responses; questioning one's future and place in life. But now, one has the knowledge and experience to face these questions in a positive way. The long view back helps light up possibilities for the future.

It is quite a step to go from a heterosexual 27-year marriage to being a single lesbian. How did it happen? I am still trying to coherently answer that question. Remembering my youth, I can see the signs of lesbianism that were never acknowledged as such because I had no words for the behavior I expressed, other than the critical words of my family and my culture.

As a child I distrusted boys, except for those that were gentle; maybe they were the boys that would grow up to be gay, now that I think of it. I knew by age three that boys had power and girls didn't. I desperately wanted to be a boy, dressed in boy's clothes as often as my mother would let me get away with it, acted like a tomboy, and felt bereft when my best friend shunned me in favor of boys, when we began junior high school. When my body started filling out, and the usual boy's clothes no longer fit me well, I came to the realization that I would never be a boy and would just have to make the best of it as a girl.

When a proposal of marriage came on my high-school graduation night from a boy I had been introduced to by a friend, and had only been with, at parties, twice before, I accepted, because I thought no one else would ever ask me. My mother was ecstatic at this turn of events: the unpopular daughter who was never asked out was suddenly engaged, no matter that she hardly knew this boy. As for me, I had made a promise and almost immediately regretted it, but kept telling myself this is how one shows maturity: grow up, get married, have babies. Besides, this was the first time in my life I had done something that had made my mother uncritically happy.

When I told a special friend the news, she abruptly turned her back on me and wouldn't speak to me for weeks, and then only to give me a speech that I didn't understand. From my vantage point now, I realize she already knew she was a lesbian, and had committed herself to that, but the whole issue of homosexuality was so dangerous in those days of the early 1950s that one did not come out and speak clearly about it. I was so unsophisticated on this issue, that when a girlfriend told a joke about "queers" I didn't understand it, and she refused to explain what a "queer" was.

Yet, one of the first books I read after marriage at age 18 was Radclyffe Hall's *Well of Loneliness*. I'd heard of this book somewhere and knew I had to read it. I identified with Stephen in the novel; she was an outsider, the one who didn't fit in, and she led a tragic and self-sacrificing life.

My marriage was not especially happy, and I often felt depressed. I gave birth to two children and loved them fiercely. I knew I didn't have the emotional strength to care for them alone, and so did not consider divorce an option. I was not a person who could easily express anger to my husband, because he was stronger than I was. I was afraid of the consequences. Eventually, after a stint of therapy, I accepted that a "comfortable" marriage had its value.

My husband encouraged me to go on to college (I finally got a degree after 20 years of sporadic classes), and was supportive of my need to go out to work, where I could meet and interact with a wide variety of people. I managed for many years to live a double life, an inner, personal place of my imagination, where I was independent and free, and an outer place acting the role of wife and mother.

As my son came closer to graduation from high school, I began to have very dramatic, lurid, and disturbing dreams that symbolized to me my unhappiness and the deterioration of the marriage. My husband and I began couples counseling, where I was told it was okay to be angry and to show it. I learned things about the way my husband thought that I hadn't been conscious of before. I was active in N.O.W. (National Organization for Women), and there I met women who had divorced and become lesbians. I changed jobs and began to earn a better and steadier wage. All this was leading to a feeling that if I chose, I could support myself. I could walk away from this marriage if I really wanted to. All that was lacking was a good reason.

That summer, my husband and I spent our vacation in the mountains. One day we became lost while hiking snow-covered trails; I had an intuitive insight about our interactions that illuminated how I had been living my life: blindly following someone whose sense of direction was very different from mine. I remembered my original feelings as a young woman of 16 and 17, when I was capable and self-sufficient. I felt deep anger at how I had perversely accepted and followed the agenda that patriarchal society had set for me.

Soon after we returned, I attended a N.O.W. convention and saw women dancing together for the first time, and saw how much they enjoyed each other. The woman I drove to the convention with told me she was married (like me for a long time), but that she also had a woman lover. The movie "Lianna" had just come out, and I went to see it, and was deeply affected. That night, I bought and read *Rubyfruit Jungle*. Another book by Radclyffe Hall, *The Unlit Lamp*, described how a woman ended up old and embittered by always subverting her dreams in favor of following society's roles for women. I rummaged through all the feminist books I'd been collecting over the years and read everything having to do with lesbianism. At the university where I worked, I went to the library and checked out armfuls of books from the homosexuality section. In these books I found myself, and found out how other women had found themselves, and how they lived their lives. With all these books, and the movie "Lianna" giving me a script for living a new way, I gave up a split and shattered life for a whole one.

After telling my husband of this revelation, he suggested we divorce and I heartily agreed. For the first time I moved out to an apartment and lived alone, an exhilarating feeling, as well as a scary one. Very soon I began a buddy/love relationship with a woman who initiated me into all facets of lesbian life. This led me to question every belief that any group put out as being "politically correct." I told my children of my change; my daughter said she suspected as much, and seemed to consider it quite exotic and fun to have a lesbian mother. My son had no comment, but over the years has treated my lovers and friends in an accepting and friendly way.

In the years since this great change in my life, the big question around menopause has been, for me, the threat of osteoporosis. I've been suspicious of estrogen replacement: take these pills for the rest of one's life, deal with the usual periodic discomfort, and the prize is strong bones and eternal youth. Breast cancer may be a side-effect, but doctors tell you results are inconclusive and not to be worried about (doctors are always telling you not to worry, and seldom focus on long-term side effects of medication; it is left for their patients to deal with those, and of course to again have to seek treatment).

I've read that calcium pills do not have an effect on bone strength, and that the only consistent preventative of osteoporosis, besides estrogen, is weight-bearing exercise. (My sources are *Science News*, a weekly digest of the latest in scientific research, and the news releases of medical research institutions.)

I make it a point to do a lot of walking during my workday, and to go hiking on weekends, and try to get in some cross-country skiing in the winter. I enjoy gardening. Though not interested in eternal youth, I do want to remain as flexible as possible for as long as possible. I'm learning through my own efforts what's best for me, gaining my own wisdom in the process.

At 52 I've survived this long journey bridging my mother-self to my apprentice crone-self. The bleeding has stopped and the hot flashes have almost died away. I've been initiated into a new life. I am an active woman in my community, helping to put out a monthly newsletter, keeping in touch with and trying to get other women in touch with the many groups that make up the lesbian/women's community. It took time for me to become this new person, but maybe, if I had come out as a lesbian in 1955, I would not be as open and optimistic as I am now.

THINGS THE WIND DOES

Pat Schneider

Lifts a spatter of last night's raindrops
and flings them in my path.

Lifts a dozen leaves
and spins them for no good reason.

Lifts the sound of my neighbor's voice.
(She is seventy five. I am fifty four.)

> She: Let me see your new clothes.

> Me: These aren't new clothes,
>   I've just not worn them much.
>   They're too hot.

> She: Too hot?

> Me: Yeah, I'm having hot flashes.

> She: (Primly tightening robe around her)
>   Are you wearing underpants?

> Me: (Surprised) Yes.

> She: Take them off. Let the air
>   blow up under your skirt.

Lifts the sound of my youngest daughter's voice
singing, "Blessed are the last days of summer."

IT'S TURNING OUT OKAY

Clara Felix

I had my first menstrual hemorrhage at age 32. I had just started working as a secretary in a large architectural firm, so the shock of finding that I was flooding underpants and clothing with blood was nothing compared with the agony of having to exit through a roomful of draftsmen to get to my car! The doctors said it signalled the beginning of an "early menopause." I think they used the term as an umbrella catch-all for poorly understood female symptoms. (In fact, I had my last period at age 58—a rather late menopause. Started early at 11, ended late—not unusual.) After the first, the hemorrhages happened intermittently and unpredictably, leaving me apprehensive at work and in other public situations. The gynecologist suggested that whenever I didn't ovulate during a cycle, my body tended to make too little progesterone hormone to control the bleeding. Why didn't I ovulate? Well, maybe it had something to do with being divorced and alone with three small kids. Maybe it was related to my nutrient intake which wasn't all that great. Maybe the hemorrhages were caused by fibroid tumors in my uterus. (But then, why did I have normal, light periods much of the time? The fibroids were still there.) Or, could it be hereditary? My mother had had fibroids, hemorrhages, and finally a hysterectomy in her early forties.

In what I thought would be a happy ending to my life as a divorcee, I married an architect at the firm. Tom was a widower with a son close in age to my 5-year-old daughter, my youngest. We were both 33, crazy about each other, passionate as all hell—but monumentally unsuited for family life together! He was of the old strong, silent, macho school, and I thought I needed a leader, but quickly found myself dealing with a tyrant. We had agonizing fights in which issues were never resolved. Instead, we'd reconcile by making love. We never were able to discuss our problems. We never were able to be *friends*.

Early in the marriage, I read my first Adelle Davis book on nutrition, which prompted a grand reworking of the whole family's diet and, to my surprise, a rapid upgrading in everybody's health—even the dog's! My periods became more normal. Hemorrhages were infrequent and tended to occur only during exceptionally stressful times. The years went by; the children grew up;

the marriage lasted twenty-two bittersweet years, alternating between brief interludes of passion and long ones of alienation.

My adoption of good nutritional habits probably saved me from a lot of extra grief. I say that because, when Tom and I lived for six months in Italy, after our supply of vitamin supplements ran out I hemorrhaged with every period, just like my mother. I was 50 at the time. Back in the U.S.A., I took my courage in hand and went back to college to earn a degree in nutritional science. The marriage had run out of steam; it no longer made sense for me to give up becoming a nutrition researcher in order to devote myself to a man who didn't want my devotion!

In my early 50s, I began needing to throw the covers off my feet at night FAST! My feet suddenly would get uncomfortably hot. It happened only once in a while. I never connected it to menopausal hot flashes. Tom thought I was nuts; *he* didn't feel any surges of heat under the bedclothes! I was still menstruating in my usual late, irregular pattern of 35 to 40 days between periods as before. Few hemorrhagic periods, thank goodness, but I began to notice staining for a week or more after the periods ended. A few years later, I began skipping periods. By then, the sudden sensation of heat was happening often enough to clue me in. So *that's* what they meant by hot flashes! I never became drenched with perspiration or felt faint; I just got intensely and rapidly warm, usually when a room *was* warm and my clothes too confining.

At age 55, I graduated from U.C. Berkeley with a B.S. in nutritional science. Tom and I were divorced a year later. I met Clay, who's more than twelve years younger than I, and he's been "my main man" ever since. He's a writer, cartoonist, and all-round lover of life. We talk each other's ears off. We bask in each other's company. We share our lives. *We are friends.*

Fullblown menopausal symptoms hit me after my last period at age 58, when I would feel waves of heat that reddened my face and neck if the room got too warm. Working with other women, I constantly faced "thermostat struggles." No one agreed on settings! I settled for a small but powerful fan at my desk and readily adjustable clothing, such as layers I could peel off quickly and blouses I could unfasten at the throat.

But I never suffered incapacitating symptoms. Sure, it's tiresome to realize the natural body thermostat that all one's life functions too smoothly to notice is now playing tricks. Particularly annoying is the uncomfortable heat that sweeps over the upper part of my body and face when I am experiencing some emotional stress. It passes quickly, though, and I shrug it off, just as I've learned to do with graying hair and aging spots on the back of my hands. It took me a while, but I can accept them now as part of an inevitable natural process. For the last five years (I'm 68), the overheating moments have considerably lessened, both in frequency and intensity. My "thermostat" seems to be working better again. (My hair is still gray, though!)

I've never had to take medication or hormones for the uncomfortable times. Medical checkups inform me I'm okay. The fibroid tumors dwindled down to nothing, as they often do after menopause. I don't suffer from vaginal thinness or drying. My bones are strong.

Most important, I've kept good emotional equilibrium and avoided any tendencies to dreariness of outlook. That's supposed to be the big pitfall of menopause. I had enough to last a lifetime when I was younger, so I know what it feels like. Some of the reasons I've been able to skirt any emotional or physical abyss have to do with the marvelous people in my life: Clay, my children, children-in-law, grandchild, friends and colleagues; and the fact that at the age of 60 I began the absorbing work of publishing the bimonthly *Felix Letter*, co-authoring a medical nutrition book, and working as a nutrition consultant.

But a big factor in the good health that sustains me is dietary. My studies have given me a key to the foods I should eat, those I shouldn't, and the kinds and amounts of vitamin, mineral, and herbal supplements that work for me (and, of course, for others). Healthy tissues at any age depend on the nutrients that bathe each cell. Older cells and tissues sometimes require a little extra, because our ability to absorb and process nutrients can dwindle with age. Our *thinking processes* depend on neurotransmitters. These have to be made in our bodies from components in our diet. By taking supplements of lecithin I make sure, for instance, that I get extra choline, which our system uses to make the neurotransmitter acetylcholine.

Fragile, demineralized bones can make a lot of trouble for women, especially after menopause when estrogen, which protects us from osteoporosis, diminishes. I not only get plenty of calcium from food and supplements, I make sure that I and my menopausal clients choose foods each day supplying the mineral *magnesium* in bountiful amounts. Without plenty of magnesium, calcium, instead of keeping bones strong, gets stuck in joints, where it hurts!

Foods such as broccoli, peas, garbanzo beans, corn tortillas, peanut better, sardines, salmon, tofu, brown rice, Cheerios, raisins, and almonds happen to be a few of the many foods that are superb sources of both calcium *and* magnesium. More than that, they supply the additional vitamins and minerals that the bones of everyone, but especially older women, need to maintain strength and resilience: nutrients like potassium, zinc, silicon, manganese, boron and vitamins A, B, C, E and folic acid.

Popular traps midlife women easily fall into are weight-loss diets. Did you know it pays to be *zoftig* after menopause? Forget the Nancy Reagan image! Our fatty tissues make *estrogen* for us, helping to fill in the void after our ovaries quit. Not only are those rounded contours a comfort to the grandchild on your lap (or the man in your arms), they actually make you more womanly! And help to keep your bones strong.

I began working as a co-author with Donald O. Rudin, M.D., in 1984 to adapt his biomedical nutrition manuscript into a popular-style book. He's one of the pioneer researchers on the Omega-3 essential fats, establishing in his pilot studies that most of us (even well-educated nutritionists!) are sorely lacking in these nutrients. Case studies in *The Omega-3 Phenomenon* (Rawson/Macmillan 1987) show that a number of bothersome menopausal ailments, which had resisted standard treatment, cleared up when his women patients added Omega-3 oils to their diets. Food-grade flaxseed oil and fish oil supplements brought about improvement in vaginal dryness, chronic bladder infections, arthritis, and so-called menopausal depression. These oils are related to good circulation, less sludging of blood, and better chances of avoiding heart attacks or strokes after menopause, when women become as susceptible as men to these disorders.

The Omega-3 fats happen to be needed in large amounts in the *brain*. Yes, fish *is* brain food! I eat a lot more fish now. I need all the active brain cells I can get.

Lately, the medical literature is full of references to antioxidants. It seems our tissues, including brain and nerves, are subject to oxidation—a fancy term for spoilage! The more oxidation our cells are subject to, whether from normal metabolic byproducts or environmental insults, the faster we age. Or get cancer. I'm happy to report that certain nutrients are our best defense: beta-carotene, vitamin E, vitamin C, the mineral selenium, and the sulfur-containing amino acids cysteine and methionine. With care, we can get nicely protective amounts from good foods, except for vitamins E and C. With these, I'd rather not take a chance, so I've been using supplements for at least thirty years.

My mother and father, whom I loved very much, had unhappy lives and a sad old age. I didn't look forward to menopause—the door we enter as still young women and emerge from as old ones. I feel differently now. Free of the burden of menstruation, I think of my body as being under my control, rather than subject to omnipotent hormonal forces. Thanks to good nutrition and, oh yes, I forgot! ample physical activity, my physical health is fine. My emotional health is far better than it was through all the tumultuous years of my youth, love's agonies, young motherhood, divorce, and dreary jobs. I no longer live for the promise of *tomorrow*. My todays are my life. I love it.

FANFARES:
AN ARTIST LOOKS AT MENOPAUSE

Ann Stewart Anderson

The woman relaxes in her black wicker chair. Her skin, glowing with heated energy, contrasts with her languid body which is wrapped in a blue print dress. One hand rests on a table strewn with cosmetic containers and a hand mirror. The other holds a bright orange fan with a green aura, exactly one inch from her face. The painted surface extends on either side toward crisp folds of a fan, constructed from taffeta. The painting is called *Chrysalis*.

It is one of a series created to depict and to celebrate women in menopause.

The project began in 1984 when, during the presidential campaign, I read an article about Geraldine Ferraro which said that she was unqualified for the

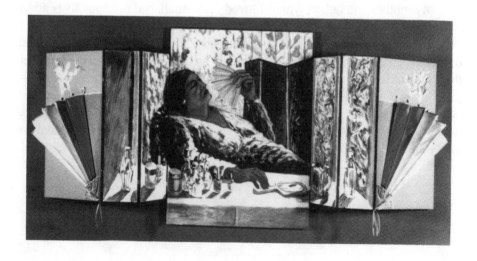

position of Vice President because she was fifty, and thus, in her menopausal years. I found this attitude deplorable.

I had been asked to participate in a project in which artists invited other artists to work with them on collaborative efforts. I invited Judy Chicago, and ultimately she, I, and about fifty other artists, in response to our concern about typical attitudes toward menopause, created a large fabric hanging, the *Hot Flash Fan* (see cover of book).

The extensive research I did in preparation for the Fan showed me that there was virtually no other art, past or present, which dealt with this subject. Working on the collaboration stimulated me to consider the imagery from a number of angles, and when the Fan was completed, I began to work on an individual series, which I call "Fanfares."

Each of these works consists of a number of panels, hinged together, so that the viewer may open and close them, making individual visual, emotional and aesthetic decisions. The inside panels are painted, oil on canvas, while the outside panels are covered with needlework—quilting, embroidery, trapunto, etc.—in each case, referring to the fan shape. In the painted areas, the fan again occurs, along with mirrors and cosmetic containers, symbols of the transience which women face with particular drama at this biological cusp.

Night Flash begins with a fabric quilt pieced in a fan pattern. Opening the first two panels, the viewer sees a painting of a bed covered with a quilt which

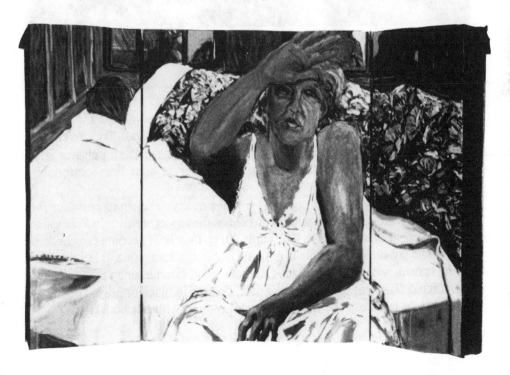

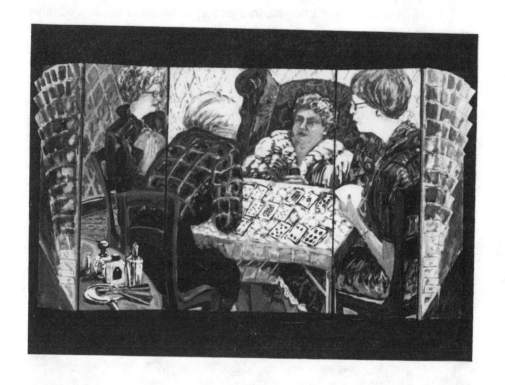

repeats the actual one. Finally, the innermost painted view shows a woman, dressed in a white nightgown, seated on the edge of a bed. The covers are thrown back, one hand is held to her hot brow, her red flesh pulsates with energy. Behind her, with his back to the viewer, a man lies comfortably snuggled under the fan quilt.

But, not all hot flashes occur in virtual privacy. I began to consider the common activities of women which can take on the aspect of ritual. In *Foursome*, four women sit at a card table. The cards which they hold become fans in their hands. The lay-out on the table is not, one realizes, a card game. It is a fortune-telling spread, with the cards placed so that a good fortune for an aging woman is predicted. Three of the women are pale, dressed in black or gray. The fourth wears bright pink and her face and arms flow red with her hot flash.

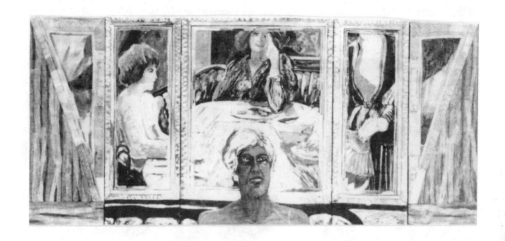

In *Hot Lunch* a friend fans the red woman who dines with her friends in a restaurant, while in *Ladies' Room* many women crowd toward a common mirror, leaning across pink washbasins to apply makeup, ignoring the menopausal woman who stands in the center, her hand held against her hot face.

As I worked on these paintings I was inspired by my own recurring hot flashes. I laid layers of transparent red color, one over the other; I worked to show the richness, the incredible depth of this experience. While I drew fans in the hands of my women, I considered their dual purpose. The fan can cool hot flesh, but it can also be used to fan a fire to make the embers glow more strongly. My women became both individuals and archetypes—modern women in fashionable clothing, energized and transformed by their universal biological destiny.

I pushed the concept of ritual further. *Crowning* shows a large glowing woman, dressed in white. A woman on her left places a crown on her head; to her right another woman ties a pendant, the magical Tet, Egyptian symbol of the genitalia of Isis, around her neck. Around the group appear white lilies, familiar symbols for resurrection. The background is a strong green, indicating life. The title refers to beauty pageants as well as the instant in which the baby's head emerges from the vagina at birth.

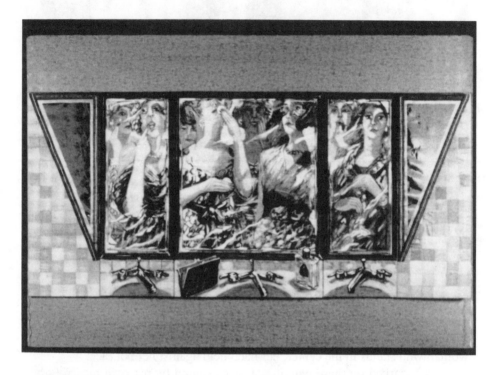

Fan Dance shows two women supporting another, who is apparently overcome with the power of her hot flash. The attending females clasp hands, and wield fans close to the glowing form of the central figure. Actual strips of light-weight fabric are sewn along the outer section of the work so that even the normal breathing of the viewer activates them, enhancing the rhythmic movement of the dance.

Since prehistory, art has been created which recognizes the power of woman the mother. Fertility goddesses with wide hips, rounded bellies and full breasts appear in virtually every culture. Rituals for puberty are legion. The process of giving birth has been depicted by primitive cultures and more recently in the work of Judy Chicago. The bearer and sustainer of life has rightfully received her honor.

The extraordinary next task for our times is to create images which extol the woman in midlife. She is the person who has lived within the biological confinements of the bearer of children, the giver of birth. She emerges, not as tradition often decrees, as a hysterical silly shriveled nonentity; on the contrary, she is strong, confident, experienced, filled with new energy and wisdom. She is the woman in menopause. She is the woman in "Fanfares."

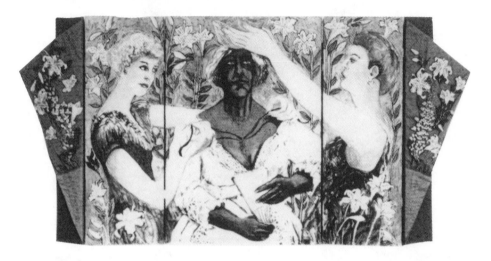

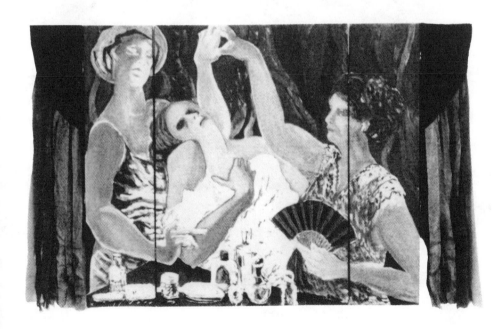

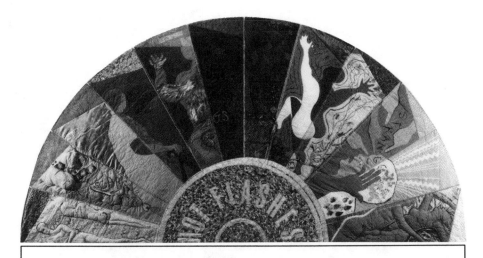

SWEET INSANITY

If a woman's going to blow a fuse, she'll do it during menopause.

—*Elaine Goldman Gill*

Some forms of madness are no more than failed transitions from one vision of life to the next.

—*Sheldon Kopp*

It is not in vain attempts to ignore the changes of age and to pursue the trappings of youth that strength and happiness for the older woman lie. On the contrary, that way leads to bitterness and exhaustion and instability.

—*Ann Mankowitz*

A WELCOME CHANGE

Constance Mortenson

Melanie Grey decided to see the doctor. She was not sick: just tired to death. Sleep evaded her. She courted it, wooed it, suck holed to it, and it stayed just on the periphery of her consciousness. She got up and ate. She pulled the covers back until she was half frozen and then cuddled down hoping that the warm coziness of her comforter would entrap old Morpheus and tuck him under her belt. Nothing worked. She suspected it was a final symptom of the menopause and she had decided years ago she would sail through the Change of Life as her mother and grandmother had always called it and ignore the whole thing like the natural phenomenon it was.

She hated the idea of taking pills but the lack of sleep was getting to her. She picked up her essay on "The Four Day Week." Perhaps she would get time to type it up at the office. She rinsed her cup under the faucet and strode to the car.

The day at the office went well enough. She sweat a bucketful only twice during office hours. If she completely ignored it, did not wipe her brow or fan herself with her shirt front, the men in the office didn't seem to notice. Not that it really mattered except she didn't like the idea of them looking at her and thinking she was a dried up old woman. She wasn't. If they meant sexually at least. She had never had more fun between the sheets than now. The nurse at the clinic had assured her she was past getting pregnant and had with those few words unlocked the frozen lump of her sexuality. So, she was mixing a metaphor. It was like being born again. No more fear of pregnancy. The pill had made her swell up and stagger and she needed one hundred percent reassurance which no contraceptive she knew of had given. After nearly forty years of praying for menstruation to come on time, *vive la menopause*.

She remembered to make a doctor's appointment for four-thirty. As the time approached she mentally listed exactly what she would say to him. She would stick to the subject of sleep. When she had been in for a mammogram she had asked about a new vaginal gel for use during intercourse and embarrassed the hell out of the young man. Probably thought that now I was creeping up on fifty I should *abstain,* Melanie muttered to herself. Damn young punk!

Herb complained, "Since you started The Change you've taken to contradicting me." Melanie considered his complaint. It had some merit. But she was delighted to discover she didn't give a clam's cuticle. He could complain until the tides ceased to ebb and flow for all of her.

Her "damned cheek" hadn't come only from the liberation of menopause. It had also come from the fact that her nest had emptied at about the same time. Pamela graduated in June and was away to Europe for an extended vacation before settling into a research lab somewhere and Duncan was firmly entrenched in a good job. It was a great relief to have both children settled and at the end of the month she had quite good sized gobs of money to put in a holiday account; also there was time to study. Which reminded her she had forgotten the cinnamon buns she had meant to bring to the office. She had been studying and they had raised into huge sticky masterpieces that made Herb ask what happened. He muttered about her damned nose in a book but she ignored him while she planned her next Sociology paper.

Melanie left the office early, a perk that came after twenty years of service and leaned back against the warm leather of the car seat. She thought again about how lucky she was to have a job, and University, and a comfortable old farm house. She loved her children and a twinge of guilt clawed at her for enjoying her empty house. Things were looking good though. She was in her second year of University and though three night courses were really too much, by getting up at five and starting her papers the very day they were assigned she was managing. Her marks were satisfactory, mostly B's with a few A's to warm the cockles of her heart.

Dumb phrase. She saw the cockle shells cuddled up under her breast bone and was driven to looking the word up. She flipped her always open dictionary to the C's and waited for the next stop light to find the exact page. "Cockle" also meant to pucker or wrinkle so maybe the phrase meant the puckers of her heart. Not near so pretty though. She saved the knowledge for an English paper; Ian Johnston liked to be confounded by odd and archaic usages. She jumped as the driver behind her gave a mean blast on the horn. She really must stop using the dictionary as she drove.

The doctor's office was full but she didn't mind. She settled down with Marx and tried to concentrate on the introduction of the assembly line while kids howled and mothers shushed them, cajoled them, and got all hot and sweaty over them. One woman was grey and looked more like a granny than a mother and Melanie offered a silent prayer of thanks that she had not had a Change Of Life Baby as her grandmother and her mother both had. She had thought it might be genetic and had peed in a bottle and rushed it off to the nurse at the clinic for a pregnancy test so often that the nurse had finally told her about the tests you could buy at the drugstore and perform yourself. She had bought them by the gross, but the closer she had come to the final periods of her life the more frightened she became of having one last baby. You really are an ass, Melanie Grey, she chastised herself. You only had two children and you act as though you had produced dozens. Another lucky break. She hadn't wanted more than two. But they had been born so close together in the earliest months of marriage that she had looked down the years expecting to have at least twelve.

"The doctor will see you now," the nurse said loudly and Melanie winced. She could tell by the tone that she had been called at least twice but she had got back into Marx and his labor theories.

She was moved into a cold, small cubicle and she knew it was one of three or four that held waiting patients. The doctor had taken Marx's assembly line theory to heart and the thought irritated her. She could remember when doctors had one examining room and were always accompanied by a nurse. But that serene service had vanished with white linen napkins. All the grace was going out of life, Melanie thought wryly. Women like herself who worked and kept house and gardened and had hobbies like going to University helped destroy gracious living. Warming up a fast plate in the microwave or grabbing a quick sandwich between classes contributed nothing to the heavy-white-linen-and-silver-teapot scene. But if she got a little help from his Lordship she could manage more of these things. Herb, however, belonged to the "if the little woman wants to amuse herself with a job" school of thought. He did allow her to pay for the groceries and the utility bills plus the mortgage payment, though. In fact she thought with some surprise she had gradually taken over all the household expenses except a few like taxes and insurance. She'd have to speak to him about it.

"And how are we today?" the doctor said as usual.

"I need to get some sleep. I am not sleeping. It is imperative I get more rest." Melanie was babbling. No wonder doctors seemed to disbelieve every word she said. She got nervous and repeated herself and acted flighty. She took a deep breath and he stared fixedly into her file as if giving her problem the deepest consideration.

"Well now. How old are you?"

At least he didn't say "we," she thought as she said, "forty-seven," though she couldn't see why he didn't know if the file contained any information at all. She suspected sometimes that they held the latest stock market quotations or the next chapter of a book he was reading.

"Well sometimes women of your age feel this way. We will just have to get you busy at something. Too much leisure time is bad for us."

Melanie's heart stopped. Rage threatened to rob her of words. Then her good manners took over as usual and she said as sweetly as she could manage, "I have a full time job as office manager. I take three courses at the University during weekday evenings, I have a house and garden, I cook and can, and bake my own bread and freeze vegetables for winter," her voice was rising perilously.

The doctor held up his hand and she subsided but he did not apologize; he did not even blush. He merely wrote her a prescription which she presumed was for some sort of sleeping dope and said, "Come see me next month if the condition doesn't improve."

Melanie was half way home before she relaxed. She had got the prescription filled and picked up a few groceries. She noticed she was very low on gas but didn't have time to stop. Tonight was one of the few nights that Herb was home for dinner and he liked to have it early. Thank god it was Friday.

Herb was fixing himself a drink when she came in and the phone was ringing. She dropped her groceries and grabbed the phone wondering why Herb couldn't have got it. He was closer. She listened to her boss tell her why it was imperative she come in tomorrow to check over the bid figures on the Hospital extension and agreed to meet him there at nine in the morning.

"There goes your day off, eh?" Herb said.

A wave of heat stormed through Melanie's body. Sweat broke out on her forehead and she grabbed a clean table napkin and mopped her face.

"Hot flushes? Or are they flashes? I never knew for sure," Herb said. "How long do the damned things last? You had one at the club the other night right in the middle of dinner."

Melanie said nothing. She was too tired for an argument. She put lamb chops in the pan and got down the rice. She should run pick some new peas. Maybe she'd just have a drink first, there would still be time.

She fixed her own. Herb would never think to do it for her unless he was feeling particularly amorous. She joined him in the den and sat back trying to plan her weekend. Damn John for wanting her to come in tomorrow. She had planned to pick and freeze the main crop of peas and start on her next English paper.

"While you are in town, pick up my new suit. It should be ready and I want to wear it to the Kiwanis dinner tomorrow night. I hope you haven't forgotten we are going." Damn the Kiwanis, Melanie thought tiredly. "Oh, and your car is due for an oil change. You'd better see to that too."

Melanie looked down the dirt road that cut a path through the distant trees arrowing straight north for as far as the eye could see. She thought about getting her oil changed. The garage Herb insisted they patronize didn't give you a courtesy car and it would mean waiting for a taxi. She'd have to leave early.

"If you're heading for the kitchen," Herb said as he always did when he wanted her to get busy on dinner, "get me another drink will you?"

Melanie got up and went quickly to the kitchen. She turned the heat off under the chops. Mixed Herb his drink. Delivered it. Went to the bedroom, changed into her one hundred percent blue denim outfit and her best jogging shoes. Stuffed a small pack sack full of clean underwear, fished her wallet out of her purse, put her bank card in her shoe under the insole and walked out the door.

She looked at the dirt road and said aloud, "North or south?" "North to Alaska," the song, came unbidden to her head and she turned north. She had never hitchhiked before but there couldn't be much to it.

She should have left Herb a note, phoned the University, and the office, arranged for her neighbors to salvage the peas. The list was endless. She'd let the children know when she was safely away so they wouldn't worry but fuck the rest of them. It was her turn for The Change Of Life.

AUNT LENA IS COMMITTED TO BELLEFONTE STATE HOSPITAL

Ginny MacKenzie

Because he'd heard menopause was hard he forgave her
the unmade beds, the cold meals—
what he couldn't accept was the way she looked:
the slip all yanked down below her dress,
the hair pasted with grease and sweat
to her neck like wet crepe paper.
The hospital would have to come and take her.
In those days, in those small towns, what else
could you do with a wife like this—a good wife
and mother falling into the things around her.
No matter what, it does matter what people say
and their breath was full of accusations . . .

That was all thirty years ago now. I don't
know any more of the story, they're all dead
or gone away, or why it matters to me,
why I lie awake nights sometimes thinking about it,
imagining Lena still alive somehow,
though delirious, senile by now. I see her there.
I visit her there: I sit across from her
and watch her scrawling a crayon over
some scratchpaper, which she asks me
to slip out the window as if there were
someone down there, waiting for a message.
Sometimes I try to read them. Here
and there I make out what seem to be words:
"blouse" or "searchlight" . . .

Sometimes in the mornings I wake up
from a dream of her and start to worry the things

in my house are like hers were back then,
when her bad time came—a sinkful of dishes,
the laundry-hamper spilled down the stairs . . .
Or I'll hear someone at the door:
only the deliveryboy probably, wanting his money,
saving up to go to college. There's just
no future, he says, in these small towns.
There's a place for everything but you
can't find it in its place. He's out the door
before I can say yes, yes, I agree.

THE CHANGES

Fionna Perkins

In July I was back home. The border of poplars, the locust in Mother's flower garden and the willow in front of the framing for the house we never had money to finish had leafed into shimmering greens. The bluebells were in bloom, and the scarlet and pink and purple petunias spilled over the rock terrace we'd built our first summer in Hillview Acres. Peas and new potatoes the size of marbles were ready to eat. But the cow had been sold, and the electricity was off.

At breakfast my first morning Dad asked if I wanted to pick the raspberries again this year. "Good crop," he said. "Any you sell, the money's yours."

"Sure," I said, beaming, remembering that last summer I made enough for dress goods and new shoes for Mother.

This way I wouldn't have to take another job doing housework to buy clothes for school. Our last had been a real bad winter, worse than the ones before, Dad with no work and Mother seeming off somewhere, and at school in Latin and geometry my brain had stalled. I quit and took a job, but after sweeping and mopping all spring, I wanted to go back and finish high school so I could go on to college.

As Dad went out to keep on with the irrigating, I stood up to clear the table. Mother bounced over and gave me a hug, then held me at arm's length.

"Let me look at you," she said, all smiles and her black eyes sparkling. "I've missed my girl. You've grown, and you're thinner."

"I worked a lot, Mama, about all the time." We sat back down for a visit, and I said, "How's everything?"

"A little better now. Dad has work starting next week at the Olney ranch, and Brodie was hired to clerk at the feed store. First thing he did, he and Nancy ran off and got married, and they're living in town."

"Where's Wallace?"

"Logging on Black Mountain. Juana's with him."

"Heard from Laurel?"

At mention of my sister a shadow clouded Mother's eyes. Laurel, the oldest, had been gone from home a long time and seldom wrote but occasionally sent a box of clothes she was tired of.

For answer Mother's clasped hands fell apart, and she said, "Your cat, Feisty, sure missed you."

I was on my way out the next morning with a bucket dangling from my waist and a crate to dump the berries in when I remembered what I'd meant to ask.

"Where did Hettie Temple go," I said to Mother, "after she was in the hospital?"

"Back to her mother, I guess."

"Hettie's mother died. That's why she came to live with her father and stepmother."

"I don't know, Freda, only that she wasn't to be with Mrs. Temple ever again."

"But isn't Mrs. Temple in the insane asylum at Sweetdale?"

"She was the last I heard."

Walking to the berry patch, I thought about Hettie, remembering the other kids at school making fun of her thick woolen socks and long skirts and the twang of her hill speech. If insanity was inherited, like everybody said, Hettie was lucky one way, that Mrs. Temple wasn't her mother.

I didn't like thinking of what had happened to her and put my mind on berry picking. Dad had been right. We'd never had a crop like this. Every bush was a mass of white blossoms, green berries, pink berries and ripe berries. It took me two days to pick halfway through the patch. By the time I was to the last bush, enough more berries had ripened that I had to start over.

Before I could sell any, I had to pick our share, so every so often I took a filled crate in for Mother to can and make into jam and jelly. Near the end of the week, as I reached the stoop, I heard Dad's voice from inside, loud as though he was angry, saying, ". . . old enough to be on her own. Face it, Edith. We might have a chance if we sell out and go somewhere else."

I was fifteen. If he was talking about me, that meant back to mopping floors and no school in the fall. It's what we'd done for years, move from place to place, and I didn't think Mother wanted to go back to that. Where we lived was just a shack, but the land was ours, and we had the start of a nice house that was Mother's dream.

Not hearing anything more, I went on in. Dad looked up with a scowl, and Mother seemed pretty upset.

Sunday evening Dad tossed his knapsack into the pickup and drove off for the Olney ranch somewhere to the east about 50 miles. With him gone and the stillness and dusk settling around us, Mother and I, who only talked when we had something to say, didn't speak at all.

She was already at work when I got up in the morning, boiling sheets and washing our clothes by hand. While I picked, she canned. The shack with its one thickness of boards was sweltering. At our evening meal Mother's place was bare of even a glass, and she looked tired and preoccupied.

"Don't you feel good, Mama?"

"I'm fasting."

"Raw eggs and beef scrapings?"

She just smiled. She'd tried that one on me the spring I whooped for weeks. It was from a book we had called *The Ralston Method*, which recommended fasting to rid the body of poisons. I suspected that Mother fasted as much to keep her weight down as to stay healthy because Dad didn't like her to be fat. Usually she didn't eat for a day or two and drank juice and lots of water.

In the morning she was out irrigating her flowers but again at the wood stove in the afternoon, making jam and ironing our clothes with the heated flatirons she used when we couldn't pay the light bill. Little rivers of sweat ran down her face.

Out in the berry patch I wore a halter and shorts from Laurel's last box of castoffs. If I got too hot, I went to the well back of the shack and filled up on cold water and stood a while in the shade. But mostly I just picked. Clouds of bees crawled and buzzed around my hands, and I was never stung. I liked bees, and I liked picking; it left my mind free to travel.

While moving from bush to bush, I zoomed off in my head in a movie-star wardrobe, driving my new *Cord*, which I'd only seen a picture of in a magazine, being a foreign correspondent in China and Paris or autographing the books I intended to write, which everyone wanted to buy.

Then coming back to earth on our two acres in Hillview, I'd take more raspberries to Mother's long workbench. I was used to her being quiet in a warm, comfortable way, humming to herself and smiling when I appeared. This afternoon she didn't smile or look up, and I hadn't heard her sing once since Dad left.

"Sure hot," I grumbled and rubbed sweat off my face. "You drinking juice?"

"No."

"Water?"

Mother shook her head, and I felt a prickle of fear. She'd been a nurse and was hipped on the body's need for water by the quart. In summer around Middleton the only things that didn't burn up and die without being watered were juniper, sagebrush and jackrabbits.

"You'll get sick, Mama."

"It's the way I'm to do it this time."

I went back to the berry patch thinking that she'd never done a fast like this before and that something seemed to be pressing on her mind. A little black ball of worry bounced into my daydreams.

At noontime on Thursday I dangled on the workbench eating a slice of bread and fresh jam and watched Mother living somewhere else. I spoke up so she'd hear me.

"Drinking water now, Mama?"

"I'm to abstain from all food and drink for three weeks." Suddenly she flung her arms wide. "I've had a wondrous vision, Freda."

I looked at her askance; our family was already overrun with visionaries. We imagined Christmases in a house that was only stud walls on a stone basement, trips we never went on and noble deeds of Scottish ancestors centuries dead. Dad envisioned better governments and political systems, and all of us, even Mother, were haunted in the midst of the Depression with a vision of better days.

"What kind of a vision?"

"God is calling his people home."

With a look of rapture Mother pointed to the tapestry sent to us after Grandmother died, which hung over the studs on the back wall above her sewing machine.

"The lost tribes of Israel," she said in a hushed voice. "God showed me a vision in the tapestry. I saw all the vanished tribes gathering and moving together. I was among them. We were on our way to the Promised Land. I have to be ready, cleansed and purified."

Was this like the stories I'd read of Joan of Arc's *voices*? As I stared at the shadowed tapestry, the jousting knights began to move, and I quickly shifted my gaze, not wanting to see any of Mother's lost tribes emerging from the gold and black threads on their way to heaven or Palestine. One of us, I thought, better make sense, as Dad was always admonishing.

The next night I watched Mother at her cleansing, and my back hair lifted. She stood in the round tin washtub pouring streams of cold water over her body without a quiver. Her skin just seemed to sop it up. Her wild, fiery eyes burned holes in my head. I stared back, speechless.

A week of her fast was nearly over. By tomorrow evening Dad would be home. I was sure he would put a stop to whatever madness had taken Mother.

Dad brought a piece of beef for Sunday dinner, which Mother roasted. She made a cream sauce for the little potatoes and new peas, a canned milk and vinegar dressing for the leaf lettuce and sponge cake to go under sweetened, crushed raspberries. I set a place for her, and she said grace but didn't eat. Dad told funny stories about the haying crew, and Mother and I laughed. In the afternoon he drove away in the old pickup.

Monday morning I awoke to heat pressing down; we were in for a scorcher. Mother was at the stove fixing poached eggs when I went to the tin basin to wash. At seeing only one plate, I lost my appetite.

"You've got to start eating, Mama," I pleaded.

She turned, not hearing me, and overnight her eyes had paled to a faded brown. She moved as if she had weights on her arms and legs, and her dress fit like a tent.

With an effort Mother straightened. "We have to get the place cleaned up, Freda. The Sunday school is coming for a picnic Friday."

"Here?"

"Yes, it's all planned."

"But, Mama, we can't have that whole bunch at a shack like this. Are we supposed to feed them?"

Her face had that unearthly look. "God will provide, Freda. There'll be a great feast and a miracle."

Now, I was scared. This was something more than a fast. Mother had taught Sunday school at Calvary Baptist in Middleton for years and at Easter made the kids a special breakfast in the church basement, but never were they invited to our place in Hillview. Cummings were too proud for that.

In a loud voice I said, "You've fasted long enough, Mother."

"No, it lasts till Friday."

She had said no water or food for three weeks. Had she been fasting before I noticed? I had counted on Dad to put an end to it, and now he wouldn't be home again for a whole week. She'd start a task and seem to forget what she was doing. At night I couldn't sleep for trying to decide what I should do. The Olneys might have a telephone, but this was Dad's first job since last fall. Wallace, the one I wanted, was as good as lost driving a Cat somewhere in the woods. My brother, Brodie, in town, was closest.

At first sight of Mother in the morning I was afraid to leave her for long enough to walk the five miles to Middleton to find Brodie.

"Why don't you stay in bed, Mama?" I urged.

"We've work to do for the picnic."

Her voice had a whistling sound, and her dimples and rounded cheeks had sunk to hollows; her bones stuck out. Her eyes shifted restlessly, bewildered, as if she were searching for something lost.

Picking would give me a chance to think. Three bushes down a row my only thought was that Mother would die before Friday without water. If the picnic was tied in with her fast, and I could stop it, she might start eating. I walked out of the berry patch, over under the willow in front of the stone basement and the wood framing sticking into the air and out to the road up to the Gerstles. They had the only telephone around, and I didn't care that Dad said a Cumming should never be beholden.

My fingers shook finding Mrs. Baker's number. I was violating another rule, butting into grown-ups' arrangements, but she was the one in charge of the Sunday school.

Her sticky-sweet voice turned sharp when she heard who I was. "Why on earth are you calling me?"

"About the picnic, the picnic at our place Friday. We can't have it."

"Freda Cumming, did your mother tell you to call?"

"Not exactly." I wished I could lie and say a sentence without stuttering. "Mother's not feeling good."

"But this is only Tuesday. I'm sure she'll be all right by Friday."

I pictured Mother as I'd just seen her and screamed at the deaf woman, "My mother's *sick*."

Mrs. Baker hung up.

Old Mr. and Mrs. Gerstle had been listening, and I explained that Mother had been fasting and with the heat and no food or water, she was in terrible shape. I hoped they would think of a way to help or come home with me and talk to her, but they only asked questions.

Scuffling down past the Cloud place, I clenched my jaws to keep from bawling and thought of Marie Cloud, Mrs. Gerstle's daughter, and the time her baby had convulsions. They had come in the night for Mother to go with Marie to the hospital. I began praying to God to make Mother's miracle happen early. But no one came all day.

She was swaying on her feet next morning.

"Please eat something, Mama," I begged. "Drink a little water."

Her only words, "Not till the Father comes."

By her eyes she didn't know me. As her aimless wanderings began, I followed. She dropped to her knees to pray, struggled up and outside, clinging to the chairs, the table, the walls for support, then back inside to flop a few moments on her bed. The old green smock she wore hung on her like an empty sack, and she had no clothes on underneath, which with Mother was unheard of. I was terrified that any minute she would drop dead at my feet. When I moved too near or reached for her, Mother's vacant mad eyes warned me away.

Hot as it was, she was bound to pass out. Yet by afternoon she was still on her feet, making her way to the well. She lay across the handle, pumping water to pour over herself, and I watched, numb. How could I make her go inside and lie down? I couldn't hit her, she was my mother.

At last Mother fell and lay gasping on the ground. I bent to help her up, but she pushed me away and got to her feet. Staggering back to the well, she drenched herself again and again. The sopping smock clung to her like wrinkled green skin, gaping open where she had torn at it in her agony. Stumbling, falling to her knees and pulling herself up, she reached the skeleton of the home she had dreamed of for so long. With an arm hooked around a two-by-four, she hung swaying there for the Gerstles on the hill and Marie Cloud across the fence to see. Not once had they been outside all afternoon.

Stepping closer, I peered into Mother's eyes. Whatever had been driving her drove her no more. Still, even helpless, she couldn't just collapse and let me carry or drag her inside. To see her brought to this and no one caring, I wished us both dead. Trembling, I held out my hand. She clutched it and let me help her across the dirt yard, up the steps and around the cluttered table past the tapestry to her bed. She lay staring at the rafters, taking air in through her mouth. Her stringy wet hair on the pillow looked black again. In moments she was asleep.

By now it was nearly dusk, already night in the shack. I couldn't think what to do next or where to go for help. It was no use praying. How could I believe in a God that had told my mother to kill herself? Striking a match, I lit the coal oil lamp and started a fire to heat water to wash the dishes, then carried the surplus raspberries to the cooler.

Mother was sleeping, and I was still cleaning up when I heard an old rattletrap pull into the yard. In it were Wallace and Juana. Out in the woods, how had he known we needed him?

"Where's Ma?" said Wallace.

"In bed. We have to do something or she'll die."

"I got the doc coming."

Before long a new coupe swung into the yard, the doctor's, and he and Wallace talked together in low tones. Juana stood in the shadows against the wall, silent.

I was still scared, but the worst was over. I went outside for air and was startled by the lights of a third car. Inside were two Baptists I saw only on Sunday, the summer preacher and Mrs. Baker. I wanted to tell her she was a day too late.

"How's your mother?" said the preacher.

"Everything's fine now. My brother's here and the doctor. It's been hot, and she wasn't eating much, that's all." To get rid of them quicker, I said, "I'll run see what the doctor says and come tell you."

Wallace had opened the cretonne curtains that hid our beds and moved the lamp to a chair by Mother's. She was awake and talking, and I hoped she wasn't telling them her vision. The doctor stood over her, his face flushed, and he looked angry. I hesitated a moment, then hurried out to persuade the Baptists to leave. Just as I reached their car the door of the shack slammed. It was the doctor.

I ran over to him to ask, "How is she?"

"The woman's crazy!" he shouted, and his voice could be heard around the world. "She belongs in Sweetdale."

"Don't say that. She's my mother. It's not true."

He shrugged and climbed into his coupe, backed out and roared away. The dust drifted back over my face and bare arms. I turned from the watching Baptists and looked up at the hogback that rose black in the night straight up behind Hillview like the clenched hand of God, as it had for a thousand years, a million.

From inside I heard the sound of boots. Wallace stalked from the shack carrying Mother wrapped in a blanket. She hung over his arms like a bundle of rags.

The windows still showed black outside when voices roused me. I was in an auto court cabin in Middleton and couldn't even remember leaving home. Juana and Wallace sat at a table with Brodie drinking coffee.

"I no sooner hit Middleton than I heard about Ma on the radio," said Wallace. He sounded old and cold and tired. "Out in the yard naked and starving to death. A neighbor'd called the sheriff."

"Dad couldn't figure it," said Brodie. "When I went out to tell him, he said she was all right Sunday."

Wallace snorted. "Well, she wouldn't eat for the doctor, said she'd had a vision, and it was God's will. She didn't weigh nothin', seventy pounds, if that. If I hadn't got her to the hospital, Ma'd be dead."

Through the thin walls of the cabin from outside came a sound I'd never heard before, my father sobbing as if all his insides were tearing loose. But when Laurel arrived in the afternoon, hair frizzled and teetering on spike heels and giving me a cold stare, he seemed to have recovered.

"Your mother's in the change," he told her. "She hasn't been herself all winter."

"Wallace said the doctor told him she's insane."

"Happens to a lot of women, Laurel. A year or so ago a woman out at Hillview went the same way and had to be committed."

Listening to them, I learned that Mother had been force-fed in the night and had started eating on her own once Dad had visited her in the morning. I wanted to say that Mother hadn't acted crazy till she'd gone I didn't know how long without water, but I was still too numb and scared, and they never paid any attention to me anyway.

More than once I heard Dad say, "She'll never live through it."

With all their talk of death and insanity, I didn't know what to expect by evening, when they let me go to the hospital to see her, whether she would be in worse shape than yesterday or if I'd be seeing her for the last time.

Mother was in bed but sitting up with her hands clasped around her knees. Her hair had been washed and fell loose in silvery waves over her shoulders. At sight of her whole family trooping in, her face was radiant.

"Why, here's Freda," she said. "How's my girl?"

I searched Mother's eyes. Wherever she'd been, she was back. The madness was gone. I wanted to sink down beside her and put my head on her shoulder. But the Cummings wouldn't let me close, and in a few minutes Laurel edged me out the door.

"You might upset Mother if you stay too long."

Later, when we were all back at the cabin, Laurel talked a mile a minute. "We can't afford anything private. We can't even pay the hospital. What else can we do? She'll need care for a long time."

They were still talking and drinking coffee when I fell asleep with my clothes on. In the morning I asked to visit Mother again.

"Better for her if you don't," said Laurel.

"She coming home soon?"

"Not for a while."

Juana fixed breakfast, and afterward Wallace and Laurel and Dad left for the hospital. I helped Juana with the dishes and made the beds. Then she put on another pot of coffee and told stories about her Indian grandmother. I watched the expressions change on her beautiful dark face, heard her hiccupy laugh and didn't know a word she was saying. I listened for footsteps and remembered that it was Mother's day of *feast and a miracle*. She was the only miracle I could think of, that she was alive.

In late afternoon just Dad and Laurel came back.

"How's Mama?"

"Better," said Laurel. Neither she nor Dad would look at me.

"When's she coming home?"

My sister glanced at Juana and Dad, then at me, her eyes cold and her face like a piece of blank paper.

"Mother's not coming home. She has to be taken care of."

"Where?"

"Now, Freda—" Laurel's voice sharpened— "don't get hysterical. We don't have money for her anywhere else. She's in the change. That's what happens to women—they go insane. We just did what's best."

"Mama's gone? Where?"

"To Sweetdale."

Turning my back on them, I went over and stood at a window and stared out at the dreary street in the ugly town. Didn't they understand that Mother's vision wasn't real, that it was just something she'd imagined, like my trips around the world being rich and famous? I couldn't believe the Cummings had heeded the unfeeling doctor and sent Mother away without even letting me say good-bye. After a while I sat off by myself pretending to read a magazine and wished I had my cat for company.

"Freda?" Dad said suddenly. "You remember Mrs. Temple?"

I looked up and nodded. I didn't think I could ever forget. Mrs. Temple going berserk and taking after Hettie with a horsewhip, beating her unmercifully from room to room and out into the yard till Hettie to escape ran back to the bathroom and swallowed all of a bottle of poison that burned her around the mouth and down her insides.

"She came to the train to see your mother off."

I supposed that Mrs. Temple, like Wallace and the Baptists, had heard about Mother on the radio.

"How'd she get out of the nuthouse?" I muttered.

"Over her change. You'd never think to look at her she'd ever been insane."

But what about Hettie? What had happened to her? She'd be seventeen now. Barely saved and left scarred, would she ever find anyone to marry her or even give her a job?

Dad was on his feet, pacing. "What say we pack up and get on out home?"

Laurel and Juana were coming with us to stay the night. My brother still wasn't back. I'd heard Laurel tell Juana he was the one who signed the papers to send Mother to Sweetdale.

Wallace was probably somewhere getting drunk.

AN INDISCREET THING

Miki Nilan

There was a woman I knew during my teen years who one fine morning abandoned her family and stayed at her mother's for a period of weeks. This was unheard of. I didn't know of another such case. She was loving, kind, an excellent mother, active in the church, highly regarded by everyone. In fact, I think it's safe to say her family was our town's model family. One explanation was whispering hotly around. The woman was going through her change. I overheard my mother and aunts before they noticed me listening. Later, when we were alone, my mother attempted to appease my curiosity by explaining that some women, even the most respectable and charming, when going "through the change" went a bit mad. That's as much as she would say.

I filed this information away in my brain the way we do those bizarre bits that are almost too incredible to deal with. From time to time I'd think about it when any older woman showed fits of temper or did anything out of the ordinary. The term older was wildly flexible because I had no idea when this unmentionable change occurred in a woman's life. Change from what, was what I was curious to know. And why go mad? I badly wanted to know but there were too many signals that this was not a proper subject for conversation and since I never saw an article about it, my ignorance remained intact. Then, in my forties, I began noticing how hot I was when others complained of chills.

Steaming dish water was sending me to the door. I'd open it, someone else would close it. "It's freezing in here, what's the matter with you?" they'd say. The heater came on, like a flash I'd be at the thermostat. "Turn it on," my husband would yell. Or one of my daughters would come into the room and say, "Why is it so cold in here?" Throughout my thin teens I was one of those people who shiver while eating ice cream. Swimming turned me blue. In between these moments of heat that seemed to be triggered by particular, almost psychological, things I'd still be chilled and was forever putting on or taking off a thermal undershirt or flannel nightie.

The advent of heat was pretty insidious. Not like later, when in the full throes of menopause, my body was a burning oven much of the time, day or night. By my mid to late forties there was no longer any doubt what was happening. My menstrual periods, regular as clockwork most of my life, were irregular bouts of staining. I had nursed both my daughters, but in the third month of nursing my second daughter, my milk just trickled away until there wasn't any. My periods were like that, diminishing until they were scant tissuey stains not even requiring napkins. There never was a final spill that more often, so I'm told, signals the end of menses.

I remember visiting my terminally ill brother in the hospital. He took a year to die and when he died was one month short of his fiftieth birthday. He was three years my senior. This is my landmark for keeping track. I would park my car in the open sun of the parking lot, make the blocklong trip over endless grey sidewalk, take the elevator up, up, up, then walk the long long hallway to his room. By the time I reached his bed I had to sit and fan myself. My face would be violently red. My brother would laugh. We all knew the sun bothered me, and I was gaining weight. Add a fair measure of trauma, and it's very easy to see why everyone smiled a little disbelievingly when I whispered, catching my breath and dignity, "Hot flash!" Sure, they'd say, embarrassed, if you'd stop getting fat . . .

The surprised look of "Oh for god's sake, don't talk about THAT!" was almost more stunning, and annoying, to me than the hot flushes. I quickly learned, even with the openness of the seventies, this still was not a fit subject. I found men like my father would often chuckle and shift about as though an offcolor remark had been made, but women would freeze their faces and get the subject changed rapidly.

Once, during a hospital visit to an aunt, I noticed my cousin was also huffing and puffing and getting red in the face. I lived far from these relatives and it was only at funerals and visits like this that I got to catch up on gossip. My cousin and I very obviously were in that indiscreet thing, "the change of life." To our mothers' dismay, we laughed and joked about the turmoil our bodies were in. While we bubbled over about our stealth in opening the windows in our bedrooms after our husbands had closed them again, her mother and mine were pooh-poohing the whole notion. They both disclaimed any personal experience, they'd never suffered a whit, it was all mind over matter. The exchange with my cousin during that hour was one of the most meaningful I'd had since the onset of menopause. I wasn't the only one.

Off and on I'd had occasional flashes of another kind—I'd suddenly see my mother's face, or my aunt's, flaring red. I come from hardworking stock, but I began remembering it wasn't only after a day in the fields when their faces would be glowing. My aunt would whiz into the house with a pie or cake, and stepping from the comfort of her car, beneath her short blond curls her normally pale skin would be flaming. I would go downstairs in the morning to the smell of coffee, and would find my mother, brown hair in a soft bun, her stout ordinarily tight little body loosely spread in a chair, sitting in the open doorway, cold air blowing into the kitchen. I could hear my own voice, "Mom, it's cold in here!" and her voice, "I'm just getting some air." Lately I've come across a snapshot of her sitting on the porch and her white face is distorted by more than summer temperature. In that distortion I recognize my own face when a rivulet of heat spreads itself in a wave across my entire being, pushing my nerves and skin as it goes, unmercifully shattering all composure.

I was a nontraditional student, which means I began college life late. My teachers were the most considerate of anyone I've run across. My blushes were a fixed, traumatic, part of the school day. Younger women were curious. Many were surprised at my willingness, my need, to talk about it. They would tell me how their mothers were going through it, how some of their mothers were open about it while others maintained silence. Most, like girls of my generation, had never heard of it.

My daughters, feminists, developed mixed feelings. An article in *Ms.* magazine, like my mother and aunt, denied any distress in the menopausal woman, or, if there were any little problems, modern medicine made short shrift of symptoms. Any negative notions about menopause belonged to the realm of myth. That was the day from which I staunchly refused to read *Ms.* magazine. I needed their support and the support of my daughters. What I was suffering was a lonely thing, and to have it made light of by a publication opening up possibilities for women was devastating.

My family has a history of stroke. Several maternal aunts died in mid-life as the result of cerebral hemorrhage. My father's mother, a short-lived woman, passed along migraine to me and my daughters. Migraines have been my only major illness. They've had a life of their own, and little by little, over the years, I've learned techniques for stemming their fierceness. With them I have had auras, fainting, and vertigo. With such a history it would have been a bad idea for me to have received hormone therapy, what may still be the ideal treatment for hormone depletion.

The positive side of menopause for me was a diminishing both in number and intensity of migraines. That was good news and now there is more good news. While my own menopause was longer than average, ending only recently following my fifty-seventh birthday, there is the other side of the mountain. Perhaps if I had known the symptoms would have lasted so long or been so devastating, I might have made the decision to take hormone replacement. But here I am, I have made it through.

One young woman I met along the way, a fellow student, gave me hope. She told me about her aunt whose menopause had an end and that the aunt was kicking up her heels, claiming she felt better than ever. Somehow the idea that someone else made it, and had become revitalized, re-energized, "better than ever," was my carrot on the stick. Sometimes when I was thoroughly depressed, crying in my doctor's office about feeling so bad, having no energy, being unable to lose weight, but not having the kind of depression that needed therapy (I never lost the will to do things, only the means), I'd finally remember the woman's aunt. Such things can sustain us.

Now I am as good as new. The hot flushes are gone, the night sweats are gone, the depression is gone. I'm walking without huffing and puffing. The least exertion, like vacuuming, getting out of a chair, talking, or having a rush of thought, no longer saps my strength or leaves me demolished. My weight is stable, walking is a pleasurable exercise, and life is good again. Now when people smile at me it has more to do with my quaint habit of giving a phrase an archaic turn, or because I have taken a tumble playing badminton or volleyball. I am not a bit mad, as sane as ever. Yes, life is very good.

MAKING BELIEVE: A TRUE STORY

Marylou Hadditt

Once upon a time there was a mid-life woman. She was tired and she was discouraged, she thought it was the end of the world. She'd lost a job she loved; she'd had a nervous breakdown; and she was in the throes of a shattering divorce. She'd almost given up hope. She wanted to sit in the middle of the freeway and get squashed. By an eighteen wheel semi. Brrmmm! Splat!

On a sudden impulse, she decided to go to college. For the first time ever. (She was afraid she was having another nervous breakdown because, like many mid-life women, she trusted neither her impulses nor her intuitions.) But her daughters and son encouraged her and so did lots of other mid-life women she met at college. She was very brave. She enrolled.

"After all," she asked herself, "what do I have to lose?" "Only four years," she replied to herself, "and I'd lose four years anyway."

So she signed up for the easiest courses she could find: Mime, Drawing, Swimming—the kind of classes which did not require exams or term papers. She was terrified of being tested because she knew everyone would find out how dumb she was.

In the easy classes she got A's and began to feel just a teeny-tiny bit smart. She dared difficult courses like Algebra, English 301, and Philosophy. She wrote a short play about mid-life and menopause. "Well," she thought to herself, "maybe I'm not so dumb after all."

She sharpened her brain for four years in college. When the great day came, her grown daughters and son put on their Sunday best and came to Mamma's graduation. She was proud of graduating and proud of being certified smart. She showed off her piece of paper and danced down the aisle, singing

> I could while away the hours
> While conferring with the flowers
> Consulting with the rain.
> And my head I'd be scratching
> While my thoughts were busy hatching
> If I only had a brain.

She was excited about her life. So many things to try. So much to look forward to. She dreamed of doing something important. "Not big important, but little important. Or maybe even middle size important," she said secretly to herself. She dreamed of being a great writer and began work on her great novel, but women stopped her wherever she went and said they'd really like a copy of that play on mid-life and menopause she wrote back in college. She made copies for these women, charging them only for xeroxing the text, plus postage. Although she was convinced she was smart, like many women, she wasn't convinced she was worth money.

Then, one bright summer day between Solstice and full moon, when important things happen, she said to herself, "I am going to take the advice of my very first writing teacher, Alta. And with quiet determination, I will publish my play, myself."

And she did. She felt brave.

She smiled at herself in the morning mirror. "I have my piece of paper which certifies me smart and I have bitten my fingernails which proves I think.

"Ah. I believe in me."

She waved her magic wand which is the same pen with which this story was written because she knew she was doing something important.

She was making believe in herself.

SWEET INSANITY

Claire Braz-Valentine

1

My mother looks at me,
the way only my mother can look.
I have just purchased a bright red jacket
to wear with my bright pink dress.
How old are you now she asks?
She knows.
She is testing me.
45 I say . . .
She shakes her head. "That's right.
And when the women in our family go crazy,
and the women in our family do you know,
they do it at 46," she says.
"Be careful," she says as she stares at the jacket.

2

One year to the big ticket,
then I won't have to explain red jackets anymore.
One more year to pay the bills on time,
and take showers every morning,
to stand in line at Safeway
One more year to figure out the phone bill,
to have two checking accounts because one has to rest
while I use the other so they balance themselves.
One more year of going to bed at a sensible hour
so I can wake up at unreasonable ones
to get to a job that was crazy before I was.
Twelve more months to have good manners,
to keep secrets,

to comb hair that doesn't want to be combed,
to keep a spread on my bed,
and to feel guilty because I read junk novels,
and don't clip coupons from the newspaper.
52 short weeks
to believe one oven cleaner is better than most
to think I have to cook hot dogs before I eat them.

Oh madness, sweet insanity,
smoking cigars and eating chocolates,
pinching men's asses,
shop lifting,
setting fire to my desk,
peeing on it first,
learning at last how to spit.

Pink plaid jackets over red polka dot dresses,
lounging in bed
watching Godzilla movies on a VCR for five days in a row
because I'm too damn crazy to go anywhere,
telling people who want to help me for my own good
to just fuck off,
letting the cats sleep on the kitchen table
for the rest of their lives
the way they've always wanted,
not planning to wash my car next week
when I know I'll never wash it,
never being called reliable again.

Madness,
my sweet heritage,
you sure as hell owe me,
and if you don't arrive on time,
I'll just go crazy without you.

Lord God how I pity
those families of sound mind.

OFF THE EDGE

Amber Coverdale Sumrall

My mother keeps the doors and windows locked in her house. The curtains are drawn all day. She says it's to discourage prowlers but I say if it looks like no one's home they'll break in for sure. Besides the air is stale and warm; it's like a funeral parlor all closed up. She looks at me as if she can't believe I came from her very own flesh and blood.

"So, college is teaching you to criticize your mother is it? Maybe a funeral parlor suits my mood these days." She heads for the kitchen, the only room she's comfortable in, and opens the refrigerator.

"What can I fix you, Kathryn? A hamburger?"

"No, thanks, Mother. I just had lunch with Susan and besides I'm not eating meat anymore."

"How ridiculous! God wouldn't have put animals on this earth if they weren't to be eaten. It's not the Garden of Eden anymore, you know."

"Maybe they have a purpose aside from serving human beings."

"I can't believe your father and I waste money on your college tuition. So what *do* you eat Miss Contrary? I hope you're not turning out like Nora, your godmother's housekeeper. Imagine, a cleaning woman who can't kill a bug or a fly because of her backwater religion. Well, can I fix you a cottage cheese plate with mandarin oranges?"

"No, thanks. I just ate."

"But you can certainly have some sourdough toast with marmalade. Some fruit perhaps. I have ripe pears."

"Mother, I . . ."

"Can't I tempt you with anything? At least some orange juice."

"A glass of water please."

"With lemon, yes, and some English butter cookies?"

She dashes to the pantry, skidding on her black high heels.

At the glass dinette she bows her head and makes the sign of the cross over her tuna salad, watching me with half-closed eyes as I lift my water glass.

"What, you don't say Grace anymore, either? You can't take the time to thank God for His infinite bounty?"

"It's only water, Mother!"

"People are dehydrating and starving all over the world because they've turned away from Him."

"That's *not* why, Mother."

"And you're one of them, my own daughter who thinks she knows more than her mother. Or God." She suddenly lunges across the table, grabs my glass and cookie plate and slams them in the sink. Shards of glass and china fly across the floor. She slumps, holding on to the breadboard, staring out the window at the wall of bamboo she planted years ago for privacy.

"Mother, what's wrong? What can I do?"

"Go to your room."

"I don't live here anymore," I say softly.

"Well I'll go to mine then," she shrieks, storming out of the kitchen.

I hear her muffled sobs, knock on the locked bedroom door, begging her to come out. She yells at me to leave and finally I do.

It is my mother's first visit to the house of my failing marriage. I come out of the kitchen where I have been preparing lasagna, drenched with sweat. I am having another hot flash, angry flashes I call them because they leave me feeling rage, deep and all-encompassing.

"Why dear," my mother says, "what's the matter? Are you coming down with something?"

I sip my iced tea. "I think I'm coming down with menopause."

"Good Heavens! That's not possible. How old are you now?"

"Forty-two, almost forty-three."

"Yes, well, I guess it *is* possible. I went through it at forty-three. I didn't know what was happening to me. I wanted another baby but your father . . ." she sighs, stares out the window into the forest.

"Did you have a difficult time, Mother?"

"At first I thought I was losing my mind, but Dr. Harvey put me on estrogen and it got better. Your grandmother had a horrible time of it though. She almost went crazy. Poor Grandpa, he very nearly did too. And your great grandmother was institutionalized, by her own husband."

"Oh God, Mother, I . . ."

"Unfortunately dear, I'm afraid God won't help you either."

"Maybe women should leave their husbands," I say. "Instead of taking drugs."

"Hormones keep you off the edge," she says. "With our history estrogen is insurance."

"But you'll have a period for the rest of your life. I think I'd prefer to leave my husband."

She laughs, not realizing how serious I am. I think of my floundering ten year relationship. How I've kept hanging on like a tired fish at the end of a hook. My hot flashes begin with the heat of anger. I need to harness this energy, to free anger from my body where it lies like a stone over my heart. Heed the warning signs. Leave my marriage before menopause begins in earnest.

Over the next few months my marriage collapsed like a tent when the air is allowed to escape. I joined a gym and started working out three times a week and I got a massage twice a month. This allowed the energy to circulate in my body instead of accumulating and turning into tension. I stopped drinking coffee and drastically reduced my intake of alcohol, sugar, dairy products and meat. My anger as well as my hot flashes abated. The *I Ching* advised, Work on What Has Been Spoiled. I was afraid to begin the long process of menopause without changing myself. I wanted to be sane and aware and to allow my life to reflect the spontaneity and chaos of freedom.

I remembered my mother's rage and ensuing depression, the emotional unavailability of my father, her many prayers. Menopause was unmentionable, a taboo subject. There were no outlets. The feelings were all internalized. Estrogen was her saving grace. Now we have books, resources, women doctors, women's voices, friends and lovers to guide us through this transition. We have choices, alternatives to hormones and hysterectomies.

The prospect of an early menopause has been the catalyst for me to move in a new direction, which means losing the security of what is familiar. I trust in this process, knowing that I carry inside or will discover along the way everything I need to insure a sane and exciting passage.

I call my mother to tell her I have fallen in love with a man in New York, a younger man. That he is moving out here to live with me and that I have never felt happier.

"New York!" she says. "Everyone in New York has AIDS."

"Not everyone, Mother."

"Well, be careful. How well do you know him? Men can't be counted on during these times. They think menopause is catching. They trade in their wives for women their daughters' age. Or start a harem. They fall asleep on the couch. How old is he, your young man?"

"In his thirties."

"Oh my goodness. Does he know you're having hot flashes?"

"I think I'm in remission, Mother. I feel like a teenager."

I am amazed by my new-found sexuality. Lovemaking has never been so intensely pleasurable. I continue to open and expand. Much of my past anger had been connected to fear. The combination resulted in paralysis: an inability to act on my intuitive knowledge or to acknowledge the power of the erotic and its potential for healing.

My mother sighs deeply into the receiver. "I wish I had felt that way at your age. There seem to be so many choices now. The women in our family had such a difficult time during the change. So don't get too confident, young lady." She laughs. "At least we don't have to pretend to be saints anymore. Not that *you* ever did."

GOING TO BEAT FIFTY

Doris Bircham

Last month I turned fifty. Just a short time ago, I considered fifty to be absolutely ancient but now *old* is at least fifteen years from now. I reinforce this belief by reading the obituaries and carefully taking note of the eldest deceased.

A family get-together was planned for my birthday. The first card I opened looked promising. The cover, in bold print, stated, "Wine improves with age. Cheese improves with age." And inside, "It's not your fault you're not wine or cheese." My daughter's Hallmark greeting suggested I have a snooze as soon as the day's festivities were over. My daughter-in-law's choice was a card emblazoned with fireworks and a message that read, "Let's face it. At your age, sex isn't Fourth of July anymore," and inside the cover, "more like Thanksgiving."

A few weeks prior to the big day my mother discreetly handed me a book entitled *Coping with the Menopausal Years*. Her birthday gift was a wheelbarrow. After all a fifty-year-old back needs all the help it can get when it works in the garden. Another gift was Bill Cosby's book, *Time Flies*, and written when Bill reached the big 5-0. This book makes light of middle-age problems like forgetfulness. He suggests that when you go into a room to get something and promptly forget why you're there, you should sit down and meditate. The idea being that the thought that was in your mind has gone to your behind and by sitting on it and re-thinking your steps, the thought by some slight chance may go back to your mind. If that fails, jump up, slap your behind to loosen the thought, but don't ever let your kids catch you doing this.

Turning fifty has been costly. One rude surprise was the price of a partial plate. Plastic must have jumped on the inflation band wagon. Along with the partial plate came root canal number three and a week later, bifocals. "Nothing we didn't expect at your age," my optometrist told me. In addition my driver's license was a hefty $120 due to a too-close encounter our truck and I had with a corner fence post. My son, with his dubious driving record, had the audacity to phone and ask when I'd be available to teach defensive driving. On the plus side, I was told that since I've reached this "mature" age, I'm *now* eligible to receive 1/2% higher rate of interest on a term bank deposit. What a safe gimmick that is. With all my expenses, how could I possibly have anything to invest?

There's some grey showing around the edges now. Wrinkles are less noticeable in the mornings when my face is a bit puffy. Perhaps an after dinner siesta would improve my evening look.

People my age seem obsessed with oil of olay, sit-ups, cholesterol and oat bran. In spite of this I have acquired a few extra pounds, not spread around like you would butter a piece of bread, but all in one undesirable blob. So when my daughter asked me if I'd mind shopping for some maternity slacks for her, I was a bit hesitant. Finally I said, "Okay, but if you think I'm going to try those things on, forget it!"

There are a few good things about turning fifty, like becoming a first-time grandmother and the fact that my spouse and I, both in the same decade, are so far doing our aging at approximately the same rate. So I'll just take those hot flushes or flashes or whatever they are and face the challenges on each calendar page.

THE CHANGE

Linda Nemec Foster

At fifty, she's the quick-change
artist resembling anything but herself.
Even her shadow becomes nothing more
than a thin cape stitched in place by air.
Her body assumes the posture
of a stranger while the children
grow away, the husband simply
leaves and she's stranded holding
a picture of her once ripe cervix.
A tiny mouth with slick lips,
bubbles along its edge. Probably
cancer, but she keeps the picture,
frames it on her bedroom wall,
anoints it with moist breath.
Her body now stops flowing red,
rarely flows white unlike those two
lucky princesses named after the two
rosebushes growing in the backyard.

Her body now creates its own
fairy tale. She groups holy cards
in families of eight. She saves
the dust that settles on the blue
Virgin's head. She knows her soul
inhabits the eyes of mute dogs.
She wears red lipstick. Redder.
Reddest. Until her wild, loud
face becomes slowly dormant:
the perfect smooth and quiet of mask.

ONE MORE AWKWARD AGE

Gretchen Sentry

Some times I talk to myself, out loud and uppity. I don't know if that's a direct result of menopause, or if talking to myself just aggravated menopause. There is a connection, though, between the two. About ten years ago I started this process of talking to myself. It started quietly. Whispers, really. Like the signs of aging. Lines barely there. A thickening in the middle that had nothing to do with weight, a changing of the flow. Mostly, I asked rhetorical questions, like "What's happening here?" "What *do* you want?" "Are you nuts?" Remember, these were whispered questions and there was no one answering. It took a long time to get through menopause. I took the stiff upper lip, New England backbone route. I sweat in silence, switched to Light Days panty liners and looked forward to the benefits listed in supermarket magazines. "When, oh when," I asked, "will I feel the promised surge of passion, the blossoming of sexual abandon now that child bearing is not an issue or a threat? And when it gets here will I recognize it? Will I know what to do with it? Will there be someone to do it with?" Questions, questions and no responses. It took a few more years and a few more symptoms before a dialogue really got going. There were written explorations on reams of blue lined paper; tortured soliloquies crammed into the three ringed binders I called a journal. Seems the journal is the menopausal woman's repository of questions, stations of the cross, primal therapy and her myopic mirror, mirror on the wall. It wasn't until I started reading journal entries aloud that I started trusting my own voice. Out loud, I could hear the anger, the whine, the humor, the friend. Occasionally, I would hear small notes of sanity and truth.

That's pretty much how I started hollering and giving myself arguments and sass and backtalk. Now I discuss everything with myself, like the belief in the connection of modern words and their ancient definitions. Like menses and mensch. Some old meanings of menses, besides monthly flow, are humanity, propriety, grace, to do honor. And mensch, though difficult to be literal, is goodness, kindness, a form of super-duper human being. This Yiddish word is traditionally reserved for males, the good ones. Maybe along with menses, I

131

also had mensch. With hindsight, miraculously restoring twenty-twenty vision, I can see I wasn't such a mess as I thought and maybe between puberty and maturity, I really was a mensch! Hey, it could've happened! Now I'm past menses, past mensch! I made it to mensch and didn't know it and now I'm past it? Yes, that's it! I made it through young, slim, even skinny, smooth, bright. I could have, should have, gone to the beach while I still wore a size 10 maillot. I could have had bigger boobs, been lusty, even promiscuous, worn black lace and bikinis, learned Victoria's secret, flaunted myself. If only I had known those were my mensch years; that they would pass before I got the hang of it. My menschness paused, was put on hold.

I'm well along in this process of life, on my way to really old, ancient. I've passed menopause and it's not a pause in my menses, it's more or less permanent. I say more or less, because in these debates I have with myself and then with my physician, I've been on and off Premarin four times. Partly it's a medical confusion about the benefits, and sometimes it's because I get off schedule, procrastinate refilling the prescription, resent one more form of maintenance. When I'm off the pill there's still the occasional spotting, the moist upper lip, moments of rage, then I talk myself back into the program again, starting at the first of the month, so I can keep track, one through twenty-five.

I also discuss with myself the theory that I have been through all of this before, in reverse. That this is just one more awkward stage in my life, this tilted plateau that slides me toward the big O-L-D. It feels just as confusing as an earlier stage, the no tits, pimply time before I made it to adult woman and iddle age. (iddle age?) Ah, the synchronistic typo works perfectly! Iddle age, addle age, addled-essence. Maybe that's the progression: no tits, addle-escent, menses, mensch, old!

If that's the way it works then I'm an iddle-escent and I suspect it's not much different than that addled time when I was just starting out. The baby fat is back. It's lumpier now and lower than it used to be. Instead of zits my face sprouts hairs. Wiry white ones and straightforward black bristles. Leg hairs are back too, swaddled in jewel-toned sweatpants and slouch top socks. I'm in eyeglasses, again. Back then they were jet black harlequin frames with plain glass lenses. My eyesight was phenomenal but I wanted to look more mature, sophisticated. Now, I reach for the bifocal horn rims as I get out of bed. I need them to read the newspaper and see where to apply new fresh-scent Nair.

In that first awkward time, starting at twelve or thirteen, I worried about my period days. I was convinced everyone knew, the curse being written somehow across my forehead or on the back of my reindeer sweater. I prayed that I would not leak, stain, or smell. I struggled with belts and pads and Kleinert's rubber lined panties. Only hussies would consider Tampax. I begged to stay home from school and certain disaster. Now it's a caution not to laugh too hard or stray too far from a restroom. Coughs and chortles must be subtle or I'll leak, stain, smell and have to stuff wads of toilet tissue in my cotton briefs, just like the old days. June Allyson, still perky, tells me on commercial breaks that I don't have to be embarrassed. Sure!

At 13 or so, there was shame; a "want to die" thing about the body, my body. It was scrawny, knobby and freckled. Covering it became an obsession. It helped to color coordinate, order from the catalogue then remove the brassy trim. I also prayed for early frosts and late springs so I could burrow into mackinaws and overshoes. I prayed my mother's sewing machine would never be repaired and that she would never again shop at second-hand stores.

Nothing seems to have changed in this iddled age except the size and fiber content and the soothing ritual of ironing. I'm still trying to find my true fashion self. Cute no longer works, nor does sophisticated. Mysterious is out. I hope I find it soon, before that last permanent stage; before floral print polyester with three-quarter sleeves, an acrylic shawl and shoes with built-in bunion lumps.

The body is still flawed and there's more of it in that condition, so what I need is something large that makes me look small, youthful but with dignity, color that is lively but not blatant, patterns that have tradition but are unique. I will need to accessorize with a purse large enough for coupons, journal, sewing kit, shopping lists, sale papers, antacids, decaf teabags, diet salad dressing and Butter Buds. It would be nice if it matched my shoes that must be sensible and square enough to fit my widening feet and my custom-made orthotics.

Now, as in my addled youth, I still spend too much time at the mirror. Where I once imagined tiny lines, there are great crevasses. There are still the errant hairline wisps that won't be tamed, only now they are white and crinkly. As my highschool yearbook documents, all that time in front of the mirror only resulted in a young woman who looked uptight and old before her time. Now I question the political correctness of Loreal or foam-in color mousse. Do I hang on a little bit longer to my pigmented hairs? Do it permanently or with a washaway rinse? I go through stages along with the phases of the moon: (1) Let it grow long, grey, and make a bun in preparation for Marmie-hood. (2) Cut it off, get a corkscrew perm, make it orange, screw you, I'll never get old! (3) I'll get old but not gracefully, fuchsia colored spikes, quadruple ear piercing plus a nose ring, scissor carve ERA YES into my nape hairs. (4) None of the above. I could explain I'm in between hairdressers till I find one with no mirror in the shop, or I don't have time for bourgeois concerns and until I run out of green recycled rubber bands or bandannas, I'm boycotting the stylists. I could tell the truth, that some days I just don't give a shit and there's little energy left for style and grace.

When I was young and gangly, all elbows, knees and size nine feet, my grandmother used to poke me in the small of my back. "Stand tall, be proud, keep your knees together when you sit," she'd wag a finger, then demonstrate, "walk toes out, like a lady." All I wanted was to fade into the background, slip by unnoticed. Now, as I fade into my own life and often slip right by family and the general public, I tell myself, in a voice reminiscent of hers, I should not slump or splay. Good posture can look like bravery. It battles gravity, gives a lift to tired feet, eases disintegrating bones.

I'm iddled about a lot of other things, like who would care if I slept in my sweatsuit, didn't make the bed, only celebrated holidays I made up. At the first awkward age, there seemed to be no end of rules to follow in growing up, and no shortage of adults to pronounce the rights and wrongs of my behavior. I comforted myself with books and daydreams and the myths I came to live by. Now, in this second go-round of awkwardness, there are no iron-clads, no absolutes. There's any number of role models, each unique, but none can tell me how it's supposed to be. So from out on my limb, I talk to myself, argue and cajole. Try it one way, then another and hope I settle on a way to be before I slide off into ancientness. The process seems familiar now, as I talk myself through this interlude. Trying out new rules as I try new looks and shades, designing the future me, I remind myself to salvage what I can from my prior states. It may be a long trip if I'm lucky, but I'd like to travel light and this time I hope to get it right.

PROJECTS

Ellen Treen

The afternoon sun brings a hush to the store, time to pick up my knitting, to wonder if I am too old to be so long on my feet. Across the table from me a young woman makes arduous work of a grey scarf. A beginner, her stitches are tight, requiring full concentration, miraculously unimpaired by a head shaved on one side and sprayed magenta on the other. Her eyes never leave the needles, not even a glance at the two women stalled on the threshold, engaged in a comfortable argument. Half in, half out, they repeatedly trip the doorchimes.

I ask if I can be of help and the smaller woman bolts forward, waving me back on my stool. "Don't get up, Honey!" she says. Zippers streak down the ankles of her jeans and over the pockets, drawing attention to the well kept body within. "We came in just to look," she continues, peering through dark sunglasses. A soft hat frames her small face; blond curls cling to the stitched brim reminding me of a child on the beach. "I'm Mitzi," she says, "and this is Della." She points to the taller woman in shapeless pink sweats and greying hair. "I told her I've been wanting to come in here and this is the time to do it. I'm having some surgery. Nothing serious. But I need something to do afterward. Okay if we just look?"

As she speaks she walks around the store, glancing in the other rooms. One is devoted to yarn, the other to rugs, latch hook materials.

"Cute little shop!" she says. "Converted house, right? Where's the needlepoint and embroidery? Do you have that?"

"No," I say.

"How about latch hook? A whole roomful," she says, answering herself. "Dumb question, huh? I'm always asking dumb questions." She smiles and her even features fall into balance above white teeth. "Usually I knit. Simple sweaters with round necks and give them to all my friends. Della's got a whole drawer full of them, right Della?"

Della nods, murmuring how much she likes her sweaters.

"I know, but they're all the same. Plain wool, plain stitch. I'm sick of them. I want to find something different. You have to help me."

Pulling Della with her, Mitzi gravitates to the yarn room. I stay at the table, with my student, supervising her tortuous progress, where I can see and hear the two women, comparing cotton and wool, textures and prices as they move from section to section. They squeeze the skeins and pull out long strands, leave them dripping from the shelves. Finding a mirror tacked between the windows, Mitzi holds contrasting yarns to her face, studies herself. Steadily Della offers suggestions; peevishly Mitzi rejects them, making her search ever more urgent.

"I've only got two more days," she says, stuffing pink yarn in a corner and leaving the room. "Tomorrow I have to get my roots and nails done." Back in the work room she digs into a bin of mohair. "Soft! Pretty! Now this is different!" Gently, she pats a fluffy ball of mint green against her cheek. "Wouldn't this make a lovely sweater?"

"It would," I say. "Except I don't have enough of that color."

"Oh, no. I want this green."

"Come on, Mitzi," Della says. "All these colors are lovely. How about rose? Or pale blue?"

Turning her back on the mohair, Mitzi stands at the table, staring at my beginner, watching her labor through another row of grey stitches. She frowns, then paces between the shelves and the table, her heels clattering on the wood floor. "Help me look, Del," she says.

"Slow down, Mitzi!" Della hoists herself up on a stool and lets her bag drop to the floor. "I get tired just watching you, and we're the same age. You didn't overdo it on the diet pills, did you?"

"After strawberry cheesecake, yesterday, what do you think?"

"Diet pills?" I say, unable to hide my astonishment. Sucking in my tummy I try to sit taller. "You? You look great. Not just your weight but your skin. Everything." Mitzi's jawline is smooth, tight as a well-made bed. I lift my chin, massage under it with my finger.

Mitzi looks me over, then speaks softly, hissing on the s's. "Estrogen, Honey. That's the secret. Lots of estrogen. Twice what the doctor prescribes. Go to two doctors. Two drugstores."

"I took it for hot flashes, after a hysterectomy, but then I quit. I don't know why . . ."

"Just like Del. You have to keep it up, every day. Forever." Conviction powers Mitzi's voice, adds authority to her words. "First, get a good doctor. Then a diet. Exercise. Honey, it's not easy but it works."

"The worst sweating I ever did was month to month, worrying if I was pregnant again!" Della laughs. "What are hot flashes compared to that? Honestly, I was glad to have it over, move on." She shifts her weight and raises her legs. "Now if it would help my feet, I'd take it again."

"And no smoking," Mitzi is saying. "No sun. No booze. No partying. Get lots of sleep." She picks up the green mohair and pets it. "And your skin can be as soft as this yarn, which by the way, is what I still want."

"You always did want what you can't have. Whether it was good grades or someone else's boyfriend," says Della.

"Why is that?" Mitzi asks, her disappointment blooming into a full little girl pout. I can see her at a birthday party demanding all the prizes, the cake on another child's plate, refusing to believe all the slices are the same. "Why shouldn't I have what I want?" She waits but there is no answer. "Well," she sighs, "I have to get a project, want it or not. Let's look at some rug kits." Heading toward the back room, she pauses at a basket of knitting bags and seizes one in each hand.

"Look at these Del! Aren't they pretty? Perfect for my project. I can drag it from room to room. What size do I need? Big or small?"

"What are you going to put in it?" Della has not moved off the stool.

"What do you think, green or dark red?"

"It's your bag."

"Come on Del, help me out here," Mitzi begs.

"Decide on your project first. Then you'll know what size to get."

"Right!" Dropping the bags, Mitzi circles the rug room, looking at kits and patterns. "I could make a rug for my Honey Baby." she says. "Her Mommy could hang it over the crib." She pulls out a small printed canvas. "Here! Look at this. A rainbow. My Honey Baby loves rainbows." She shakes her head. "But not these colors. No blue, no yellow, no pink. Her Mommy hates those colors. It would have to be different colors."

Sensing a final decision, I put down my knitting and go to Mitzi, to show her how to substitute colors, figure out what she needs. Della slides off her stool and calls to us.

"While you do that I'm going to the car and either move it or put money in the meter. We're out of time."

"Wait!" Mitzi says. "You have to help me with the colors! I can't be sure of anything with these glasses."

Della comes back and briskly puts together a color scheme. I gather the yarn packets and take them to the desk.

"Perfect," cries Mitzi. "Plum and peach, apricot and grape."

"Hang it or make a fruit salad," Della says. "I have to get back to the car before we get a ticket."

"You said you'd help me pick out a knitting bag."

Della hauls a large, blue flowered bag out of the basket. "For a rug you need the big size. Blue is your color. I'll meet you at the car."

Taking the bag, Mitzi opens it and hands it to me. "Here you are, Honey. You can put everything right in my new bag. Don't forget to take off the tags." She sighs, smiles with relief. "Now I've got something to do. After the surgery." Her dark glasses are on a level with me; she raises them and I'm surprised to see eyes as dark as the lenses, set deep in a web of fine lines. "I'm having a little plastic, that's all, but there'll be swelling. Believe me, I know what to expect." Placing her fingers on the outside corners she stretches her eyelids, makes the lines disappear. "Plastic, Honey. It's the *real* answer. You should try it."

I hand her the bill and she hands me a credit card, letting the sunglasses fall back in place. "My husband will kill me when he sees this."

"You can't imagine how many women say that," I say, laughing.

She laughs with me, then is quiet while I fill out the charge slip and have her sign it. "He would only kill me if I got old," she says.

Behind her, there is a soft thump, and she turns. The young knitter has jumped from the stool and is heading for the door, waving those few inches of scarf at me. I wave back, at a closing door.

Mitzi shudders. "Why does anyone want to look like that? Imagine, going to so much trouble to look so ugly! At her age she should be pretty all the time!" Suddenly she raises her fists, and shakes them, rattling her rings. "I hate the way things are now. All this flag burning and shit. I hate it. I liked it when things were simple, like it was for *my* grandmother. She had it easy. So easy."

The new bag bulges with her purchases and I hand it to her. She takes it and tucks her purse deep inside then closes it, and smiles, flashing her even white teeth, and thanks me for my help.

When she is gone, I move from room to room, slowly collecting yarn, rewinding the skeins and returning them to their proper places. Passing the mirror, I stop and face myself. The sun, lower now, slants through the side windows, casting long shadows that deepen old lines, and reveal new ones. It highlights patches of silver on the right side of my head, throws a shadow on the left. I pull at my eyelids, stretch and tighten the skin on my face and neck, so absorbed in the possibilities I fail to notice someone has come in until I see Della reflected in my mirror. Startled, I drop my hands, watch my wrinkling relapse.

"Is she still here?" Della asks, almost whispering. "I must have missed her. She probably took a wrong turn. It wouldn't be the first time. I'll find her. I always do."

Both of us smile into the mirror, the same indulgent smile mothers shower on their children.

"Did she tell you about her surgery?"

I nod. "At least she has a new bag and new project to get her through."

"New project?" Della's laugh is short. "She has only one project. I've known her since we were both in third grade and I don't think she has an original part left. Everything from her nose to her fanny, has been nipped and tucked, stitched and reshaped, at least twice."

"So I gathered," I say. "But I think she's tired of it. At least that's the impression I got."

"That would be disastrous," says Della. "Her husband is the doctor. It's his clinic where she goes for repairs. He says keeping her young keeps them both young. Gives them an interest in life."

We stand there, looking in the mirror, at each other, at ourselves. At the same moment, we look away.

"Thanks for your help," Della says and softly shuts the door.

COMMERCIAL MESSAGES

Trudy Riley

It happens again. I am stirring the sauce for the low fat, high fiber, vegetarian enchiladas I am making for dinner when the sensation of warmth starts in the center of my body. "Damn," I mutter, feeling the sweat dampening my shirt. By the most conservative count I'd had at least ten that day. Some had been milder than others but the one coming over me now promises to be a prize winner. I turn off the heat under the sauce and go into the living room to sit near the open patio door.

I think about telephoning Elvera. I hesitate, imagining what my lover will say if she comes in while I'm talking. She can always tell when it's Elvera. "You sound different. Like someone I don't know," she had said once when she walked in on me.

I reach for the phone feeling like an addict fingering the money for the next fix. But what the hell, I think. This is one of those times when talking to another woman my age is the only thing that will comfort me. If my lover walks in I am prepared to take the consequences. They will not be too bad. She will sit down gracefully in all her glowing thirty-five-year-old composure and wait for me to finish. "But why Elvera?" she will ask when I have hung up. "You have nothing in common with her and her politics stink."

I will smile—loving, warm—and try to act like a woman who is in control of her faculties. It will be all right in a few minutes. I have faith. I lift up the phone, dial and settle back in my chair when I hear Elvera's solid "Hello." Within minutes I am deep into a litany of complaints that I know she will understand.

"I can't believe it, Elvera," I say grasping the phone tight to my ear. "These damn hot flashes are getting so much stronger. And embarrassing? Let me tell you about the one I had today. I'm cataloguing some new journals we got in and this medical student comes up and asks me to help him locate an article on premature ejaculation in a recent issue of *Lancet*. There I stand turning beet red from head to toe. Then I start sweating—I mean dripping all over the collar of the only librarian-type looking jacket I own."

Elvera lets out a sympathetic moan. "What a pain in the ass."

"You got that right. I was sure he was standing there thinking he had embarrassed this middle aged lady in her ground gripper shoes with the mere mention of ejaculation, premature or otherwise."

"So what did you do?"

"Nothing, but while I was looking for the article I did imagine some nasty things I wanted to say to him like, 'Don't think you're embarrassing me you little putz. I was experimenting with sex while your mother was still taking you to preschool.' But then I calmed down and realized he was pretty flustered too and I couldn't very well blame him for whatever tango my hormones are dancing this week."

"Christ, Dottie, you should have said it to him anyway."

When Elvera starts her sentences with "Christ Dottie," I know she's into her second martini and in what she calls one of her "old hooker moods," tough, hard and loaded with indignation. I picture her sitting in her condo in West L.A., on her white leather couch, reaching up to run her hand through hair that is bleached and styled to perfection. She is probably wearing something chic. She is the only person I know who dresses up to stay at home.

She was like that in the fifties, when we met pushing strollers in the suburban Chicago neighborhood where we lived. We told our secrets while sitting in overheated kitchens helping one another breathe.

Whenever I stood next to her I felt terminally plain.

Our conversation moves from my hot flashes to hers. "I'm sick of them, and those strange potions mixed up by you and your holistic, lesbian friends haven't helped a bit. I started on estrogen last week and I never felt better."

"Really Elvera?" I say, feeling deserted.

"Yep. You should try it. It's great!"

"Oh, I don't know."

"That's just like you, Dottie—hanging back. The same way you did in the old days. I always had to be the one to get you to try something new. My God if it hadn't been for me you'd still be married to that asshole."

"I know," I answer, picturing her standing in my kitchen and saying, "Let's get the hell out of here." Her children were crying. Mine had caught the tension and joined them. Over the din she had yelled. "You know what that bastard husband of mine has just been caught doing? Seducing one of his fifteen-year-old students at the high school. He's got to leave town. Well I'm leaving too but I'm going in a different direction."

I had barely heard what she had said because I was trying to collect as many inconsolable children as I could. But then she walked over to me and placed fingers with carefully manicured nails on my right cheekbone. "The bruise that fool gave you is fading but if you stick around you'll have another to take its place. Come with me, Dottie. Let's make a life for ourselves."

That day we withdrew all the money from the bank accounts we shared with our husbands, packed kids and clothes in her station wagon and headed for Los Angeles.

By the following year Elvera had remarried and I was working days, taking courses at the University at night and trying not to feel betrayed. It was years before I was able to tell her what her leaving had meant to me.

She telephoned me on the occasion of her divorce from her third husband. I hurried her through the details because I had news of my own.

"At last I've fallen in love. She's wonderful," I said. "We're moving in together next month."

"A woman," Elvera yelled, "Are you crazy?" Then she launched into a ritual bawling out about my lack of good sense.

She calmed down in a couple of weeks and telephoned. "How's it going." she asked.

"Oh Elvera, I'm so glad you called. Some of the other women I told don't seem to want to talk to me now."

"Screw 'em," she said and showed up at my apartment an hour later waving an unwrapped bottle of champagne.

We sat at my kitchen table and after drinking a couple of glasses I confessed how terrible I had felt the year she left me. "I was so depressed."

She leaned across the table and touched my cheek. "You always were one to get attached. Me, I get attached and unattached." Then she raised her glass in a toast. "To your new life adventure," she said in her best, bawdy voice.

"Do you hear what I'm saying, Dot?"

"Sorry, don't yell. I was distracted for a minute."

"I'll bet you were thinking about the past again. That's gone, honey. We got to think about the present. I'm going on a cruise to the Bahamas this summer but before I do I'm going to get me a liposuction."

I gasp.

"Stop it, Dottie. I'm tired of all this sagging, middle-aged flesh."

"Elvera, that's a terrible thing to do to yourself."

"Nonsense. It's exactly what I need. A flat tummy and a new lease on life."

"But it's so dangerous. Why would you want to do a thing like that?"

"Because I'm not going to let old age roll over me like a tank, that's why. You and your feminist friends can go around with your graying hair and your bulging bellies, but not me. I'm fighting back!"

I look down at my own generous belly covered by a rose colored shirt purchased from Imports, Inc. I feel pain. It starts at my navel and spreads outward. "I have to hang up now," I tell her.

"Don't go, Dottie." There is need in her voice.

"I have to, I have something on the stove," I lie, knowing that if I talk to her any longer the distance between us will grow so wide I will lose her.

After I hang up I take off my shoes and lie down on the couch holding my stomach. I picture cuts being made in Elvera's small, white tummy. Worm-like cylinders of fat are being drawn into a tube by a doctor who looks like Peter Lorre.

The pain gets worse. I think of the women I know from the sixties and seventies. Women who would never hurt themselves that way, trying to remain young, but my mind snaps back to Elvera. She is the only friend left from those sad early days.

I hear a distant voice. I have left the TV on. I don't bother to get up and turn it off. I close my eyes. The clipped voice of the newscaster stops. I hear the music that precedes a commercial break. A woman's voice, soft and sultry, praises a night cream. "Oil of Olay melts the years away."

I picture Elvera peering at the television through a martini haze debating whether to add this product to the countless ones on her bathroom shelf. I want to get up and yell, "Leave us alone! Stop promising us things," but I am too tired. Instead I extend my arm off the couch and raise my middle finger toward the television.

FORTY-FIVE

Janet McCann

Why and how vaguely
somewhere in deep
it hurts
because, driving home
with my five-year-old, my last one,
he tells me how beautiful the sun is
going away
and the blue shadows flower
over his upturned face
beside me in the car
in the early chill
as he looks, scarcely breathing
at the red meadow up there
all the way
and there is this ache like a cloud
an old pain
that will not articulate
that will not say itself
& when we walk into the house
hand in hand
my body hangs on me
like an old red dress

EGGS

Gail Koplow

At Thanksgiving, Mama tells me of the miracle she's seen on PBS, that women harbor all their eggs within them when they're born. I'm startled. I've been bleeding for a month, this must be menopause, I say. She nods and stabs a marinated mushroom with a toothpick. How are all the kids, she says. What do I tell her? Does she want the truth? My daughter's sporting wire-rimmed spectacles. She looks just like the teacher she'll become. She might not get her Ph.D. next year. I'll reassure her. There's her sister. Still can't find a job. At twenty-four she sees her face a microscopic net of wrinkles. Baby, you, I'll say, are such a lovely woman and I'll hug her. (Could it be that I too want to be the last to know?) My youngest boy's a feminist. The women's center told him, get your shit together, man, get out of here. So he and I will analyze male privilege till 3 a.m. I'm tired already. There's my oldest, the vice president, still drives his scarlet sports car, but he says he's changed his mind about divorce. Last year I was his Socrates. I tendered question after question, sweating his rebirth. It only took him thirty hours the first time. Well? my mother says. She stirs the gravy. They're all fine, I tell her, carrying the turkey to the dining room.

I lie awake quite often, fiercely pondering my children, and I wonder if my mother ever sits up smoking cigarettes in her pink bedroom. Could it be? She had a hysterectomy the Christmas I turned twelve. My father pointed to the clinic window where she waved. What's wrong with Mama, Daddy? Ah, she's had too many children, he said in his absent, musing way. I wept without a sound, her bitter eldest, while the snow fell on the windshield. Someday I will ask her if she minded, if her heart hurt when they took the eggs. Someday she'll tell me. She's got sixteen grandkids now. She's seventy-three. She stitches quilts all year for them. What happens to a woman's soul when leggy flesh emerges from her own? I want to ask. What knife cuts deeper, tell me, or what sensuality surpasses birth, but she'd say, come let's shop for bathroom carpeting, or she'd say, mostly, you are happy, aren't you? And I'd tell her, Mama, when I spot a two-year-old perched brightly in a grocery cart these days, I'm struck that happy or unhappy's not the thing. It's eggs I've always had a passion for, amazement, yearning, at the tumbling down of eggs, miraculous, I've seen them born, those fabulous haphazard eggs. And maybe then her eyes would fill. She'd take my hand at last and say, not everybody talks.

COMING INTO THE WAR

Patrice Vecchione

My mother was twenty-one when she left home; she moved from a small town in Massachusetts to Washington D.C. in 1943, where she found a secretarial job at the Pentagon. She shared an apartment with three other girls, covered herself with newspapers at night to keep warm. "If you're ever cold use newspaper. It holds your own heat in," she told me. She was a 1940s girl, thin and stylish, strokes of bright red lipstick along her lips. She wore wool tweed suits and heels, she had a government job, lived the big city life. She had an entire future ahead of her, it had a face; it belonged to her.

My mother spoke of handsome men in uniform, of parties for the guys going off to war. "I danced all night long sometimes, and I felt beautiful. I came home when I wanted, no one to answer to. Though there was often not enough food we didn't mind, really. We saved our coupons, we stood in line. I washed my stockings every night by hand, tried to make them last. I could tolerate the cold, anything, because for the first time I was free." There was a unified spirit in the country and she must have touched it. In the photographs she glows, her thin pale hair styled back, away from her plain face.

Throughout my childhood she reminded me of what she would have had if she hadn't married my father. "I would have done things my way, for myself. I would have had a real career, responsibility, choices. Instead, I do things for everybody else." The remorse in her voice made me want to squirm away. That future had been hers. Those twelve life-years before my birth could be held in a glass with everything else she had lost, been deprived of, or given up. And this loss which was always on her face became a part of my life and my guilt.

I remember that when she rocked me to sleep she sang a song she'd made up. It was one line long, and she'd repeat that line over and over, a sweet tune, "I wish I were single again . . . I wish I were single again." Even during my teen years when I'd ask she'd sing that song for me. Her eyes would get glassy, her face would lose its age for the length of the tune. "Pat, it's not that I don't love you, I do . . . you know that, I love your sister and you, but oh, the life I *could* have had!"

My mother always worked as a secretary. But my mother was a smart woman. She had wanted to be more than the office girl who carried out her bosses' wishes. She often resented her employers; this one was a "jerk" and "Dr. R, what a bastard." She held it against her father that he had refused to put her through college. Her two younger sisters had gone with her father's blessing and financial support. She often told my sister and me: "You *will* go to college. You *will* have opportunities." Her life had taken its turn. She married my father, put him through graduate school, had two daughters, continued to work. Something vital had been left behind.

Her life went on, one day and another day, the future's door becoming smaller, fading away with the events of each passing day: two young girls, a move to Chicago and then to California. Until finally it was stuffed at the back of a drawer with her black lace gloves. And future's place was taken by alcohol that kept the rest of us sad and sober, the bottles I grew up pouring for her.

She didn't talk much with me, her first born daughter, about being a woman, the fact that we shared a female body. When I was thirteen and began to bleed, she explained matter of factly: "I have these things in the cupboard for you. You'll have your period every month now, for a *lonnggg* time. It will last about five days each month. You'll have to be careful with boys." I didn't feel as if I entered a shared place, the first tunnel of womanhood, only that I'd wake every month from the forceful pain, throw up, stay home from school. "Mom, tell me about when you first started bleeding." "I don't remember; it was long ago." "Did you have cramps? Do you still have cramps?" "Cramps? Yes, maybe at first." "Mom, the blood smells. Will anybody know I have my period?" "Don't let anyone that close." She'd answer my questions, politely, but there was an invisible curtain between us. I stopped asking. When one box of pads was empty a new one mysteriously replaced it on the high shelf.

Then my mother stopped bleeding. She never said anything to me about not getting her periods anymore. But she often spoke of a new curse: menopause and its accompanying waves of sudden heat. Perhaps somewhere inside her she truly believed the drinking would slow it down. But it only sped up the course of her life.

When the hot flashes came, she'd sit down in the closest chair, move her hands like fans about her face. "Here it comes again. This is hell. My head is exploding." She'd call out to God, lift her arm toward the sky. "Why are *you* doing this to me?" She'd reach for a tissue, take off her glasses and mop her face. She'd call for one of us to bring her a glass of wine, "quicklyyyy," her voice fed up. She'd hold my hand tightly through the heat wave. Sweat beaded on her forehead, the blood rising. She said, "The floor is tilting in all directions." It was during this time she told me, "I will die when I'm sixty-five."

I was becoming a new woman and my mother was becoming an old woman. I wanted make-up which she wouldn't let me wear yet. I wanted skirts, short as possible. I wanted boys. I would stand in front of the mirror looking at my little breasts. "Mom, I want a bra." "We'd never find one to fit! You have nothing to put inside one," was her retort. We did go looking though, and she was right. But she bought a pink stretch-lace camisole to appease me.

Actually, my mother wasn't old. She was in her late forties. But she began to appear old, her double chin falling lower, a cigarette always in hand, and the light that once played in her grey eyes began to dim. She and my father now rarely danced together on the kitchen floor.

And she left him. When I was in the midst of high school she'd repeatedly say to me, "When *you've* had enough, I'll leave your father." It was as though her strength had diminished. "What do you mean?" I would ask, "when *I'm* ready for you to leave my father?" But I knew what she meant.

My father's anger drove through our house, the tanker on automatic pilot. My mother's drinking coupled with the violent mood swings of menopause propelled her away from him and into a painful self-righteousness. We packed bags and moved a few blocks away. "I don't love him," she said, "I don't know how I could have ever loved him. And all men are the same. Beware."

The heat waves came regularly, at any time of day. They'd stop her, no matter what she was doing. Often late at night when I'd wake up to pee she'd be sitting beside an open window, drinking a glass of wine, more ice than wine. And the expressions on her face were part dream, part nightmare. She'd look at me intently. "I don't know Pat, I just don't know. But this sadness, this weight ties knots around my heart." And she'd cry.

Mom spent many evenings after dinner ironing until long after my sister and I went to bed. She'd iron not only our school and work clothes, but sheets, pillowcases, and towels. She even took in ironing for friends. She'd stand there in the hallway ironing, where she'd hum to herself, "Yes Sir, that's my baby . . ." or "Daisy, Daisy, give me your answer true . . ." For hours she would iron, hum, and cry.

Menopause took whatever final hopes remained. She couldn't see ahead. She couldn't see grandchildren in her future, or returning to school to finally get that college education (though she tried a class in chair caning, and lasted maybe two weeks). To her, retirement would be a long series of days with no beginning or end.

The walls inside her head were on fire, a blaze burning out of control. There was only the next glass, the next bottle. My mother was near fifty then. And I don't think menopause ever passed through her. It never left her body so she could come to another side. It just added to life's misfortunes.

At sixty-five she died. Just as she said she would.

THE WOMEN WE HAVE BECOME

Penelope Scambly Schott

1
We see in the old photos
the women we have become

even before the bones
fused, we practiced these faces

a child scowls into the Brownie
creasing, briefly, her forehead

2
After years of indifference
we recommence the count:

bleeding excessively or not
at all, or late enough

that the flicker of wonder
stuns us

3
We are become an embarrassment
to our children: too female

for our large sons, smelling
as we do, of the waters of life,

while our fierce daughters
(yes, even you) exact from us

nothing
we can spare

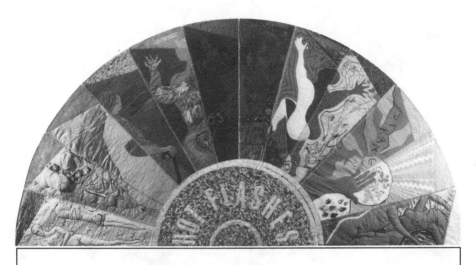

PANDORA'S BOX

The 'dangerous age' is marked by certain organic disturbances, but what lends them their importance is their symbolic significance.

—Simone de Beauvoir

At menopause life can turn into one long pre-menstrual experience. Hormones slap you up against the doors of your unfinished business.

—Maura Kelsea

IN TRANSIT:
NOTES FROM THE BORDER

Audrey Borenstein

These journal entries are culled from hundreds of pages of my journals from May 1981 to November 1982, the year and one-half during which I experienced menopause. At that time, I was readying my manuscripts for *Older Women in 20th-Century America: A Selected Annotated Bibliography* and *Chimes of Change and Hours: Views of Older Women in 20th-Century America* for publication.

In these passages from my journals I find intimations of the decision I finally was able to make in 1986, when I left academia to devote my full time to creative work. In looking back at this formative period, I see that I was becoming ever more fully conscious of an imperative to change direction. It was extremely difficult for me to sever the bond with the academic world that I had sacrificed and labored for many years to establish. Yet, as Willa Cather once wrote, a major work of art demands of the artist that she give herself completely to the material. The fictional works I contemplated writing demanded no less than this from me. That this formative period coincided with my menopause does not seem to me now to have been accidental. In my own case, at least, the desire to complete myself as woman and as artist was all-consuming. "In Transit: Notes from the Border" is an offering to give courage to those who, for whatever reason, were unable to give of themselves fully to their calling as an artist until after menopause.

A whole dissertation on the natural history of ambition is writing itself inside my head. I realize why I am paralyzed: I dare not write certain creative works for fear that what I write will come to pass. This is the source of my silences, this awareness of the terrible power of the imagination. My imaginative writing draws from my gift for "seeing-into," for clairvoyance, that is why it often arouses awe when a story is forming itself on my pages. Awe, and a sense of foreboding. There is an understanding that comes to one if one lives long enough, an inexpressible anguish. The burden of life grows heavier with the passage of time. "Carry it high," one's pride and dignity challenge the bearer. But there is more to life than being proud and having dignity. I think of the beautiful, anointed ones struck down in their youth—the creating-fields burn whom they elect.

* * *

Yesterday, all day, a deep depression. To live fifty years is to confront inescapable truths about this life—not only its limits, but the utter venality of some souls one encounters along the way.

* * *

S and I saw *Tess* last night. A luxuriantly beautiful film. Reminded me of Hardy's genius, and of the brevity of life, how it all is swept away in an instant. And of the moment of passionate love, how that cannot be equalled by anything. Not by anything.

To lose ambition, all ambition and belief in your work—what remains? Nothing. It is an illusion, but without that illusion there is nothingness. What madness is this, what insanity that seizes you when you write something and you are on fire with it and you think it matters?

A sad dream, of M being my husband, of his knowing me intimately and being very kind to me—and of my feeling that I hadn't been appreciating him enough. In the dream, I proposed we write a work together in our old age. All the while I suggested this, I wondered if I really had faith this could come to pass, although I knew it made both of us happy to plan to do this. M was, of course, last night's dream-representation of my Muse. My animus figure, to put it in Jungian terms. My creative self, my life-companion.

* * *

Mailed the manuscript yesterday. I could not believe I ever would be able to write a coherent piece, but I (stubbornly) persisted because I felt honor-bound to do so. I despaired of putting anything together, and had so many false starts. When will I learn once for all that I never believe, when beginning any writing project, that it's possible to do it at all? It *is* impossible, so you achieve it by going at it over and over and over again until it comes together. No work ever is what you imagined it will be when you began. But without that illusion you wouldn't undertake it.

* * *

Mid-term exams waiting to put out my eyes. This morning, I awakened with the feeling I must resolve the question; I can't keep putting off my confrontation with it. Must write THE work, or I can't meet my death as a woman ought. Shall I write stories—or the epic novel, once for all? I have to decide. Now. I have no right to consign this to oblivion.

* * *

Am working *fiendishly* on this bibliography on older women in 20th-century America. Yesterday, the sky was so soft, grey and rose, beautiful beyond all memory. I long to be free, I long to be free to release my creativity.

When I finish these works, *Chimes of Change and Hours* and the bibliography, will I be given time to write the imaginative works? I can only hope for "the chance for further flight." The works are inside me.

* * *

Mailed the final draft of the tome to the press today. I would get up day after day after day, for an eternity, it seemed, going straight to the work. It dominated me, it consumed me. How I longed to be free of it, to "lay my burden down." I felt I couldn't stand it anymore, the responsibility of it. W agrees that one is never worse than when one is almost finished with the burden of a task. How weary I was of it. I could not see around it, but only doggedly, doggedly went to my desk every morning, working with the thousand interruptions of the day, the accursed phone, and all the rest—the delicate thread of thought snapped over and over again. There scarcely was time to read the newspapers (although this really was merciful). It will take time to recover from this siege of labor, this obsession. When L gave me a haircut, she talked of her pleasure in sledding, and I thought of how many eternities it has been since I had any physical pleasure other than sex. Not even from Tai Chi—I didn't give myself to it; I was too distracted because the manuscript was waiting, always waiting for me. I realized once again that my weakest faculty is sensation. This may be why I stopped writing poetry. Yet I know I have the potential, and I want to dive down and rescue it, bring it up to the light, bring it to full expression. By the only way I know now. By writing fiction. Henceforth, that is my sacred task—to bring the right side of the brain from the shadows.

* * *

Went to the hospital to have the blood work done before surgery . . . In the evening, heard of the tragic air crash in Washington. The pity of it. What after all is one's little life? And why should one expect more from it, when one has been given so much? I have far less apprehension than I had the last time before surgery. I accept my mortality this time; that's it. And I am at last reconciling myself to the flesh, my physical self. When L told me she wanted to ride the snow in one of those metal dishes, I thought how completely out-of-the-body I've become. And resolved to change (if there's time). TV on Thursday night, watched *The Elephant Man* with W and J. We three were deeply moved by the film, but I wasn't as depressed as either of them: it gave me even more perspective. Was completely resigned on the way to the hospital, and very calm. I shall never forget how kind and congenial the nurses were, never. The anaesthesiologist asked me many questions. In retrospect, I am amazed that I forgot to list fish among my allergies, since it's the worst of them. Thought I detected a quiver—distaste is too strong a word—of longsuffering on his part. But in the O.R., starting the I.V., he told me I'm a "professional patient," and I took pride in this nonsense! I remember our small talk, waiting for Dr. J, and then the sweet flow of that stuff, and oblivion. Long wait—and a good cup of coffee—before they let me go home. But I was happily aware my brains hadn't been re-arranged. (I'd told them in the O.R. I wanted "lots of oxygen to the brain." *What* a shmuck I can be!) It all was an adventure to me, and I rather enjoyed it, especially the feeling that after half a century of life I was "getting in touch" with my physical being. So I have a reprieve. And I am grateful. Was reminded again how brief a time we're given. And I know what work I hope to finish, and resolved to put my hand to the plough . . . From the perspective of the history of the human race, every day one lives past the age of forty-five or fifty is lagniappe.

* * *

The bow on my reading glasses broke. I feel bereft. A calamity, I told H when I called her last night. And D, who asked, "Must there be these cosmic meanings for everything that happens to you, even breaking the bow on your readers?" Yes, there must. Dreamed I was going into surgery. I experienced again the sweet poison of the anaesthesia flowing into my veins. Then a heavy sleep. And then I began to fly. I wasn't adept at it at first; I parted the air with my hands and left the ground, and soon was flying around the hospital corridors. But I kept touching down. And I kept trying—and I improved, I was able to keep aloft for a longer period of time. I re-entered the O.R. and saw myself, Eliot's patient etherized. It was me. The doctors and nurses repeatedly called my name. But I was not on the table, I was in the air, hovering nearby. I had the sensation of flying, no doubt about it. What was my dream telling me but that this new lift into which I turned since the surgery—the time when I learned I was being granted a reprieve—was all right, that in time I would learn how to "get about" in it? I must trust myself, be patient . . . I am casting off the old habits with great difficulty, but must persevere in my efforts at entering a new dimension of consciousness. My instincts are to resist the temptation to get out my huge folder on militarism and start another "nonfiction" left-side-of-the-brain exercise. Have been working from that hemisphere for too long . . . We live our lives on many levels; we go up and down through many levels of "Reality."

* * *

I am keeping a number of folders, and every day I ought to work in whichever of them draws my mind. Am still at sea, but drift on in fair spirit, squinting at the horizon . . . Betty Edwards' book on *Drawing on the Right Side of the Brain* is releasing right-hemisphere powers. I am learning (slowly) about that shift in consciousness, and learning (also slowly!) to trust myself. For example, I teach without notes. This is the first semester I am doing this—breaking a habit of a quarter of a century, forcing myself to trust myself. But the truth is, I feel a traitor for being involved with Sociology at all. Read about Blake's utter rejection of categorization last night, and know in my marrow that it is past the time for me to leave the classroom for good . . . "The right side is the master," J said to me last night. And it is true.

* * *

Half the day gone, and these letters to write, and another page on the exam to grade. And I'd like to go to the library. I feel so free, and so grateful for my freedom. Also feel gratified that I bore with the last month patiently, the sterility of it and the lassitude of the spirit. I think I am still rowing towards the other side of consciousness. Where I pray I may begin to live the rest of whatever hours I'm granted on this earth.

* * *

How delicate a thing, the slender thread of higher consciousness that breaks off at a breath, and I must begin all over again with it. Yesterday morning, my mind was diamond-clear, and I wrote a letter to J. An hour and a half of illumination, and I wove it into a letter. I was "centered." So I know I arrive at the place for beginning anew, and with this trust one can go forward . . . Wandered through the Village. Went to the library, and read much of June Goodfield's book. Am thinking about what the scientist wrote at the end about our putting people in "drawers"—the young here, the old there, women here, men there. This is the social scientific mode one must resist, once one has mastered it. She wrote that all of us are engaged in one enterprise, the human enterprise—the woman in the lab who empties wastebaskets, each does her or his part.

* * *

Am blocked in my writing because I must descend into my soul and perform an exorcism if I'm to get on with it. At fifty-one, I can't run away from my responsibility any longer. Am tempted to write another informational book rather than confront the inner censor.

* * *

Yesterday, all morning long, went through the folders of "material" for the novel, and decided I must work on this first. What happened was that Monday, I spent the entire day going through my files, and I felt overwhelmed by the life I have lived—an inveterate, incorrigible, incurable "scribbler." I must now, in the weeks ahead, tear up and throw away huge mountains of paper. Beginning with all the *Redeeming the Sin* papers—galleys, page proofs, retyped pages . . . boxes and boxes of paper. Are you saving all this for a display or an exhibit of how the book came to be? W asked. It seems an impossible task, but I must get to it. Then on to all the teaching materials—literally, hundreds of old exams and papers and clippings (ah, those clippings!) and pages of course notes. I could write a meditation just on that collection. Then, on to the old drafts of chapters for *Chimes*. And etc., etc., ad nauseam. Make light, make light; the journey is almost over. I think the most amazing thing that is happening to me in this "turn of life" is my breaking away from the Work Ethic. I am becoming truly lazy and unsystematic in the way I go about my work! W spoke yesterday of the pervasive feeling of hopelessness about society, and I acknowledged I have been feeling this very keenly. Zeitgeist. It is all around us. Physical intimations of mortality. My head has been congested for days. Lay in bed this morning wondering if all this is depression, if I still am recovering from the long siege of scholarship. And then I thought the anaesthesia ruined me for the creative work, undid that part of me. I have never to my recollection been like this before— unable to hold on to an idea, unable to complete a section of a work, even three pages, and to continue.

* * *

On the way to New Jersey, my mind was agile, clear. It's beginning again, the demiurge. My creative writing self is coming to life again, and I'm going to be torn apart by these terrible energies once again. I *must* write the novel. This became apparent to me on Friday. I was writing about Margaret, and then about Sara, and Sara came to life on the page, Sara wrote herself. Sara has a will-to-power, and I am only a medium. This happened with the character in my story "Blue Sunday" in the same way. I pray I will find the strength to carry the work through. I have a novel to write, and nothing must interfere with it.

* * *

Deep inside my head, I am writing about Margaret and Ellie. No straight stretch of time to write the novel. I am learning to accept this, this anarchy among my selves and my work.

* * *

Dream: I was in the back yard of the Hs', hanging up clothes. Some women students were there, and I talked and laughed with them, but did not offer to have them come in and visit. The theme here was my decision not to be hospitable in that way, not to give of myself to them. But there was a much larger theme, and it left me deeply troubled all day. There was a beautiful baby girl inside the house—my daughter—and I locked her inside while I went away for a while, and was anxiety-ridden about having left her. I knew, when I returned, she would be gone. Knew, even as I prayed otherwise. Her stroller was not outside. I turned the key, went in, and saw that her crib was gone. There were crumbs on the floor in the large space where she had been. I pleaded with the next door neighbors to tell me if they'd seen anyone go in the house. Their reaction (they were strangers) was indifferent. They even implied that they didn't know if *I* belonged in that house. But I don't remember that part of the dream (the ending) clearly. What the dream said to me was that I had neglected my Work, and therefore it had been taken—kidnapped—from me. What it told me was that I must put my hand to the plough again. How I ached for and mourned the abduction of that child. How I rebuked myself for having left her untended.

* * *

The novel takes shape in the mind and writes part of itself there, no matter what I happen to be doing at the time.

* * *

Thursday night, before teaching, I had the "elevator incident." Thought I was in the basement when I was on the third floor, and rode up and down. It was Kafkaesque; I felt I'd been in a time warp. Afterwards, I worried about the implications for my mind—the presence of my mind—and memory. That night, I also wrote "megopolis" on the board instead of "megalopolis" (Ms. M pointed this out very kindly). Then, Saturday, when R was here, I said "County Cook" instead of "Cook County" (R was quick to correct me). And on Sunday, I said to W, "Put the lamp near your chair or you'll catch cold." And when I dialed D's area code, I dialed the numbers in reverse order three times (mercifully, it was busy) before I caught myself. Wakeful, as usual, at three or four a.m., worrying about these lapses, asking W what the symptoms of Alzheimer's are. The reply was, "I could have predicted that question. I'm constantly amazed at all the words I have to look up in the dictionary lately. I can't spell anymore. Isn't this something to worry about, too? I've much worse symptoms than you, never mind what they are." (Probably said all this to console me—and it worked.) This morning, meditated on Memory—and it gave me an idea for the novel. One has to try to turn experience—even dread experience—into Art, or it will master one's life. I am lecturing myself about not getting uptight when I don't get to my work, about the possibility that my brain's circuits are being over-loaded, and that these lapses are a way it has of telling me to change course. Also, the artist in me may work this way—causing me to experience what it wants to express in literature, experience it so painfully that I have to pay attention. Finally, I do think my mind is in revolution against my teaching Sociology. As for the fear—I'll have to accept that. You live this long—and it is a privilege—then you must expect to have to pay some kind of price for it.

* * *

Last night, about half-past one, awakened with nausea again, and wan-dered through the house. Gorsuches and Watts? Or Worse? I was very moved by the account in the local papers yesterday of G's interview with the terminally ill minister just hours before he died; he lamented his neglect of simply enjoying being alive. Yes, that's what one regrets at the end. The sun in the willows yesterday . . . I ought to learn how just to be, before it's too late. Most people commit the same sin, but that doesn't make the sin any the less grievous.

* * *

Received the story back; I didn't win the Prize, but was a Finalist. How little I care just now. All this industry of the past quarter of a century has brought me more grief than I, when young, would have believed it possible to feel. If I could give my life as a cautionary tale to a young person, then it would have been worth living for its usefulness to another. But, as J has taught me, the young want to discover everything for themselves, want to go through the fires themselves, don't want to be saved by the "elders." So we "elders" are left to exchange our fragments of wisdom with one another. Yes, this is what the novel should be "about."

The abstinence from writing, the silences these summer days. The writer must find space, work-space, solitude, for putting one word after another. The soul sickens, and creativity turns upon itself and becomes destructive if one is denied expression.

* * *

In writing these letters, I realized all over again the immensity of my one small life—how far-flung and unbelievably rich it has been to this moment. I have lived enough for one hundred women—love, family, friendships, work. All my sins, errors, my most serious mistakes are part of the whole and do not, when my thought is so huge, cancel out the other emotions—of love, and above all else, of gratitude for having been born at all.

* * *

During wakeful periods in the middle of the night, I think about the characters in the novel. They still are unclear. I want to give them life, to serve as their midwife. It's as though I'm asking them to present themselves to me as they are. To disentangle themselves from one another, and come out and stand.

* * *

I am trying to make use of this sadness and of these reflections in my art. One ought to strive to transform experience into an offering to others if they weigh on one so heavily, so insistently.

* * *

When you have lived this many years, and are "educated" enough to know how hard a struggle life has been for 99 and 9/10ths of the human race, you know that you have responsibilities. This is the right moment to set these words down again, on my birthday. Yesterday, I was "all out at the eyes," yet I managed to unearth some of the sources of this character, Margaret. It's going to be a very long pull, this work of fiction. Years. I am beginning to accept this. And the acceptance ought to bring me some measure of inner peace.

* * *

Dream: A has brain cancer and is dying, and in the dream I held him, knowing he was doomed. The dream-scene was a Pietà composition. I said in the dream that a nuclear holocaust is imminent. Awakened in the darkness and pondered the meaning, and thought, since our initials are the same, that I am the one who is dying. That I do not have much time left. And the time I spend on teaching and preparation for teaching—the largest portion of my work-week—

devours the time I ought to be devoting to the novel. I remembered the elevator incident months ago, and my flying dream after the surgery. I do not know what to do. I feel cannibalized by my teaching responsibilities—just thinking about the material eclipses the right hemisphere. One night after class, my brain kept repeating my lecture to me as I lay awake trying to shut it off; I realize how like a computer the brain is. Part of me says I'll never finish the novel, that I don't have it in me—the energy, the intellectual alacrity diminishes. But I know I'll persevere in whatever time I have left. And I know the teaching is my chief antagonist in the struggle to do the creative work.

* * *

These past few days, I've felt—physically—a real change. I have much more energy; I feel lighter, somehow. Is it possible I've been through a major shift, a chemical change that at last has run its course, so that now I've reached a new equilibrium? I can't help but notice the difference in how I feel—not haunted anymore, not worn down with the old lassitude and anguish. I wonder if this will hold? "I feel I have been released from the grasp of a furious monster"— the paraphrase of the philosopher praising old age for its deliverance from the sex drive. But for me, it's not the sex drive I feel released from, it's the angst, the anguish. Well, if it's a genuine release, then I've undergone this sea change without any nostrums. And if it *isn't* going to last, at least I have this reprieve. The light in the sky Monday was exquisite—mauve, with dark fish-shapes of clouds, and a lilac staining that became fainter and fainter, and turned to silver on the tree limbs and mountains and in the water of Roundout Creek. What pleasure I had, drinking in this beauty. For years and years, my aesthetic hunger went unappeased. I am famished for this. I pray that this part of me is coming into its own, now, coming into ascendancy.

AM I THERE YET?

Marjory Nelson

Is it finished? Has the blood finally stopped? Like a child on a long journey, over and over I ask myself, am I there? How much longer? How many more months will it take? It's been two months, now four, let it be done, now, please. Six months.

Before my blood started, Mother would say what's your hurry, you have your whole life ahead of you, be thankful not to have the mess. But all the other girls have their day off from gym, when will I? When will I start? When will I become a woman? Let it be here, please, please, let it be soon.

It should have started last week, that familiar rush that feels like my bottom falling out; trips to the bathroom, a fast wipe with tissue, with my finger, looking for that rusty, muddy splash, let it be here, please, please; I can't be pregnant.

Counting days and taking my temperature, I want a child, please, please, let me be pregnant. The blood has stopped. I am.

Is this really a hot flash? This gush of blood, these thick clots, a sense of my whole self sinking into some mucky bottom, am I there yet? This cramping, the pain in my belly? Will it soon be over? Please?

Am I bleeding too much?

Is this normal?

Can I stand the pain?

Am I there?

It took twelve years, from the first hot flash to the last drop of blood. In the beginning which became an ending, my chest exploded into a thousand white hot needles blasting heat in all directions through my body.

It is 1973, and I am standing in front of a classroom in the University of New York at Buffalo, lecturing on reciprocal roles, explaining how teachers need students and nurses need patients: Sociology 101, a required course for nursing students. Primed with facts and figures, for I have spent the preceding two years teaching Women's Studies, I am explaining how women are oppressed, how that affects their roles as nurses. Most of them don't want to hear it. They are offended by my feminism.

Sweat pours off my head and neck, from my armpits and between my breasts. It makes a big wet patch on the back of my green and white dashiki and soddens the crotch of my jeans. I teach about racism and class issues, but never mention ageism. I don't tell them I'm 45 years old, a graduate student; that I have left everything but my typewriter and guitar with my ex-husband in a comfortable house outside of Akron, Ohio.

I feel so isolated. Isn't there anybody else my age doing what I'm doing? The feminists I meet are all younger; most despise motherhood. I am the woman they decry. They don't want to hear about my children, or my guilt over leaving them behind. Married 26 years, it was as a suburban housewife and mother of three that I developed my concepts of responsibility and sexuality, and learned to function as an adult. Angry at my own repressive conditioning, I feel that I have to prove myself.

I'm trying to create a new identity as a feminist within the left wing of academia. Didn't I get arrested sitting with my former students from Antioch in front of Wright Patterson Air Force Base, protesting the war in Vietnam? Wasn't I fired for supporting poor and Black students in their strike against the college? The students waged a successful struggle to have us reinstated. I will make my way as a teacher. I must.

I look at the faces of my students, and in their critical eyes, see my mother reflected, mopping her dripping red face, limp hair glued to her head. Although I'd vowed never to look like that, here I am in her image, helpless in my body. The more I sweat, the more I feel fat, stupid, out of control; no longer the radical feminist professor, but a babbling middle aged housewife.

How did she get in here? I cringe with self hatred. I will not succumb. So what if I'm getting old, I don't have to look different. Let my body go through its changes, at least I won't be fat.

While still in my thirties, before the women's movement was visible, as I'd worked out my own feminist philosophy, I decided that diets were anti-woman. I didn't realize then what we now know about dieting and "set-points"; that one's body grows accustomed to living on less food. When I stopped dieting, I piled on weight. Ten or even forty pounds for liberation seemed okay, but not a hundred. With no understanding of the problems of dieting, by the time I started menopause, I was using drastic methods to try to keep my weight under 200 pounds.

I meet with my consciousness raising group. That all the women are younger than I doesn't seem important, for we are discussing racism in the prison at nearby Attica. We will demonstrate. We are talking about sexism in the university gym. We will take over the weights room one evening a week. I feel healthy and strong. I'm walking and jogging daily, riding my bicycle, and swimming. We talk about a new diet which allows meat, fat and plenty of water, but no carbohydrates. They encourage me. I do not tell them that I have learned to stick my finger down my throat to vomit my evening meal.

After the meeting, I sit alone thinking about my hot flash, a lifetime of weight problems. I remember a woman doctor who spoke at a N.O.W. meeting about estrogen. "You don't have to be a victim of your hormones." The doctor had convinced me and probably most of the women in the room that we need not fear sagging skin, wrinkles, osteoporosis or dry vaginas, for modern medicine would give us a pill. I'd filed the information away, and now it seemed pertinent.

That N.O.W. meeting took place in 1970. I was spending a year at the National Woman's Party in Washington, D.C., lobbying with 85-year-old Alice Paul for the Equal Rights Amendment, and gathering data for my dissertation. A leader of the militant suffrage movement many years earlier, Alice had been to jail repeatedly for women's rights. Active to the end of her life, she and Mabel Vernon, another suffragist two years her senior, became my role models for old women. That year I read in the Woman's Party Library and in the Library of Congress, biographies of active, political women like Susan B. Anthony, Elizabeth Cady Stanton, Sojourner Truth and Emma Goldman. Menopause never stopped them. I was determined it wouldn't stop me either.

Calling myself a liberated woman, I adventure with sex. A young woman brings grass; we smoke and drink wine, and then make love. Finally I'm breaking out of the housewife/mother role. The next morning she tells me how much she wishes her mother was like me. I attend a graduate student party and go home with a man I've danced with all evening. When I have had enough sex and tell him I want to stop because I'm getting sore, he rapes me. What are you doing here? he screams at me. I am hurt so badly I can barely walk home, yet am too embarrassed even to go to the student health service. We don't yet have the words, date rape.

I attend governance meetings of the Women's Studies College, participate in panels on women's liberation, demonstrate with various groups. Standing near my comrade, Ed, in sub-zero weather in downtown Buffalo, I speak on behalf of a Black man who's been framed on a rape charge. I am learning to shape words of outrage with my tongue and shoot them into the air like arrows, but I do not talk about menopause or my own rape, or about the ache for my grown children which sometimes leaves me gasping.

A woman doctor I consult about estrogen puts me in the hospital for a week-end of tests. (My university hospitalization will pay for it.) When a nurse pours another patient's urine into the bottle I've been filling, we have to start over. Three days become five, and I leave the hospital with a terrible staphylococcus infection which fills me with so much mucus I can't even pee. The doctor catheterizes me and gives me a powerful drug. A week later, shit and blood are pouring out my ass and I pass out in my bathroom.

Shall I stop here? I wish I could. I get caught in a spiral that keeps me going down and down without sign of relief. Is this menopause, too? An iatrogenic disease created by doctoring? No one asks.

The diarrhea won't stop and now there's a pain in my belly that's become intolerable. No longer dieting, in the next few months I lose fifty pounds. I find a respected doctor of internal medicine who gives me demerol and paregoric, and puts me in the hospital for extensive tests. My support group puts posters on the wall; Mary gives me money; Sue brings her guitar and sings revolutionary songs while a doctor puts his face in mine and demands that I swallow a metal gadget that looks like a space craft on a cord that will travel through my stomach into my intestines. Perhaps my throat has been conditioned by my finger, for I vomit in his face. Later, the tests show that I can't digest milk. Although the condition had no doubt been with me all my life, did menopause activate it? On their rounds, the white doctors only seem concerned about my heritage, since this condition is more common to dark skinned people. I tell them I'm a feminist.

My periods change, growing very heavy one month, and scant the next. On the heavy months, huge clots of blood gush out of my vagina every time I stand up. The doctors still don't discuss menopause. By now they are convinced I have cancer. Exploratory surgery reveals fibroid tumors, and massive scarring on my intestines, but nothing else. They send me home with drugs and admonitions to stay on a milk free diet.

I feel great shame that there doesn't seem to be a name for all this pain. In spite of my public bravado, I feel embarrassed by my weakness and inability to finish my dissertation. I have a job offer teaching Social Theory, and several interesting possibilities in Women's Studies, but must put them all aside. My CR group struggles with me to let go and just get well. Our group expands to take in two women my age. One night after a meeting, I'm so distraught over what's happening to my life, that one of the new members, Polly, stays all night holding me.

Polly has hot flashes, too, and we are filled with our knowing and our not knowing and with each other; with women and the revolution, reclaiming our bodies, and our right to our lives. Polly becomes involved with a group promoting feminist therapy. I move in with her, settle down and finish the dissertation. She types for me.

Polly has a cabin in the country where we and our women friends go to sing and talk and eat good food. It is winter, and snow is piling in deep drifts around the cabin while the wind blows through the pine trees sweeping their soft branches against the roof. I curl into Polly seeking warmth from the cold that penetrates even the pile of blankets on top of our double sleeping bag. She stirs and moves closer to me. The crackling flames in the fireplace in front of us that lulled us to sleep earlier have died down. I am so cold, my bones ache. And then suddenly, as though someone has thrown a switch, the heat begins in my chest and rapidly spreads through my body. I throw back the covers, leap out of bed and rebuild the fire. By the time the hot flash is over, the flames are roaring again. Back in bed we generate more heat.

In our Women's Self Help Group, I take a speculum and mirror and look at my os, that opening where my babies passed through into life. Seeing blood ooze out around the edges, I feel like I am standing on the edge of the os of the universe, laboring my way through tradition, tearing the flesh of centuries of patriarchal prejudice to give birth to myself. I have to live fast and deep, for there's so little time. It took a million years to make a woman like me, but how many years do I have left?

In spite of my physical pain, I am determined to be visible and active in my protests against the oppression of women and Blacks. I am invited to go to North Carolina to work as an organizer for Joann Little's trial. I need a skirt. Standing in the center of Lane Bryant's while a saleswoman shows me a black wrap-around, blood spurts like a geyser down my legs and all over the carpeted floor. I run out into the mall to the bathroom to clean up and when I return to buy the skirt, the saleswoman won't speak to me.

Polly and I discuss menopause constantly. We are determined to prove that age is not a disease, and middle age does not need to be a period of collapse and depression. If life doesn't offer what we need, we will create it. We stop smoking, give up caffeine, and try to eat more vegetables. Through the Women's Health Network we hear about the dangers of estrogen and now seek out holistic relief for our menopausal symptoms. Our Self Help Group holds a Menopause Workshop and I write it up for Marjory Collins' *Prime Time*, the first magazine for "older" women. I co-teach courses on the Politics of Women's Health, and on Patients Rights for the SUNY Colleges and a local Labor School.

Polly and I are dreaming about a movement of middle-aged women, menopausal women, and want to find others like ourselves. We sell everything and move into a motor home to go looking. But although we meet many young lesbians and old women of the Left and become involved with them in our common struggles, we do not find anything like a movement of active middle aged lesbians, until we pull our van up into the driveway at Elizabeth and Elana's place adjoining women's land in Oregon. They are organizing OWN, the Older Women's Network, and welcome us to a conference outside San Francisco. At last! During this period, I struggle with abdominal pain, fast frequently to lose weight and break several bones in my left foot. Is the weakening of the bones due to menopause? To fasting?

We reach San Francisco on January 1, 1978. Verna and Bev are offering a six-week Menopause Workshop out of the San Francisco Women's Health Center. Although hardly the mass movement we'd dreamed of, we join in and also create the Crones' Caucus to discuss issues relevant to midlife women.

Then I get involved as part of the new staff organizing OPTIONS for Women over Forty at the Women's Center. Polly is one of the founders of *Broomstick*, originally a newsletter for OPTIONS, but later to become a national magazine for women over forty which publishes excellent material about menopause. We're becoming visible.

My body is still giving me trouble. Now the fibroids are growing, and I'm bleeding streams, getting anemic. Doctors recommend a hysterectomy, which I refuse. I seek out a woman healer who starts me juice fasting, and does acupressure and massage weekly. Mostly, she says that I have to take charge of my own healing. As long as I'm dependent on the doctors to tell me whether I'm okay, I won't be okay. Frightened by the loss of external authority, I struggle with my fears.

I learn to meditate, to go inside to an ancient place I recognize as in a dream. I try homeopathic remedies. Three times a day I sit quietly and visualize a team of dwarfs with pick axes attacking the tumors. Everything helps. After about four months, the fibroids stop growing, then begin to shrink. After about six months, my gut is free of pain for the first time since all this horror began. The diarrhea calms down and I'm gaining back the weight plus more.

Now I have to face up to being fat. I have fasted my way to a set point of 300 calories a day. Any more than that and I gain weight. I feel desperate. At OPTIONS I organize a group we call Fat Female and Forty where we try to support each other. I also meet with courageous women of the Fat Underground who say that dieting is making us fat. Although I'm beginning to accept my increasing size, it's still difficult to believe that I can be both fat and healthy. Isn't it somehow different for midlife women? I don't know, and write about my questions for an anthology by fat women, *Shadow on a Tightrope*.

Polly and I separate but remain loving friends. I meet other women in whom I delight. By this time, I'm in my fifties, working in the peace movement, with the Women's Building, with OPTIONS. In an unpublished piece I write: "This world cannot restrain me. My mouth is a time bomb set to go off in public places."

I become a tax resister, try to support myself as a free-lance writer, and finally give up both to go work in the women's bookstore where one of my jobs is paying the federal taxes.

It's May of 1985. I've been without a period for a year and my body is a mess. My blood pressure soars, I'm allergic to newsprint and slick bookcovers, my left foot is in such pain I'm forced to walk with a cane, and now I have chronic back pain.

The younger women in the store have no tolerance for my disabilities. Unable to keep up the healing regime, I'm depressed about my limitations and feel that my life is over. I write: "I'm freefalling into the center of the os, its bloody walls a fiery rim scorching my hands when I try to grab hold."

When my ex-husband dies 2,000 miles away, without being told, I know the moment of his death. My womb bleeds for seven days, and when the blood stops, I know it will never return. My mourning body shows me what my mind had refused to accept: a major part of my life is finished. After twelve years of stretching and pushing, the os has changed the shape and condition of my body and delivered me to a new land where nothing works the same anymore, not even my radical ideas. But where am I?

The beginning of my menopause coincided historically with the upheaval of the big social protest movements of the seventies. Through my involvement with them, I created a new identity that replaced the one I'd left in suburbia. I believed this identity, which challenged woman's traditional roles, would support me through menopause and into old age. That it doesn't, creates a terrible sense of confusion and loss. I try to tell myself that all the movements are dying, but this doesn't explain what's happened to me. Somewhere along the way, as my body changed and I focused more on the issues relevant to my own life, and as my disabilities kept me from being more active in the community, I crossed a boundary and became invisible, even to myself.

I must find a way to live, find support for who I am, not who I wished to be.

I fall and break my foot again, leave the store with disability insurance, then live on credit cards. I start swimming, use self-hypnosis to control my blood pressure. I go into therapy, take more training and hang out my shingle as a hypnotherapist. Now the struggles of my life become my best resource. I paint pictures of fat old women, draw cartoons, and write fiction about a fat middle-aged woman, her plush bear, and her aging cronies. I join a writing group that helps me find my voice.

Now they tell us fat creates estrogen. Perhaps post-menopausal women need fat to be healthy. At sixty-one, I'm calmer, steadier, and have plenty of energy. My cycles are neither months nor years, but weeks and hours, with weekends of painting, gardening, and friends, weekdays of work, and the daily discipline of exercise, meditation and writing. I'm learning to live in the spaces in between, the narrow passageways that suddenly appear where no door existed. Polly and I have a deep and abiding trust that carries both of us through rough times. And although this fat, disabled, and often pain-filled body restricts me in where I go and how active I can be, I feel better about myself than ever before. I see the changes I experienced during menopause as preparation for the most creative period of my live.

I am whole.

WOM(B)-O-PAUSE

zimyá a. toms-trend

I formally entered midlife on Wednesday, July 29, 1987 at 3:47 p.m. Pacific Standard Time. The word "menopause" directly translated from the Greek is "menos" (month) + "pauein" (to cause to cease). Webster's *New World Dictionary of the American Language* (1960) defines men-o-pause as the permanent cessation of menstruation, normally between the ages of 45 and 50, or the period during which this occurs; female climacteric, or change of life.

I was 45 1/2 years old when my rite of passage was expedited at San Francisco General Hospital by Elizabeth Livingston, M.D. and Susan Reed, M.D. The same dictionary defines hys-ter-ec-to-my as the surgical removal of the uterus or part of the uterus. Technically, I said good-bye to "my youth" and hello to mid-life with the procedure total abdominal hysterectomy and bilateral salpingo-oophorectomy.

Hysterectomy has proven to be more beneficial than I could ever fathom: how can you strive to save the planet, unless you yourself can boast of *optimal* physical, psychological, spiritual and emotional health? That's exactly the state that I've become accustomed to since this operation.

Emotionally, I had prepared myself for a hysterectomy as a teenager, when I first learned of the procedure and how it could free me from what I truly considered "physical dis-ability for almost one-third of the entire month." My periods began when I was ten years old. I didn't tell my mother about them for six months by which time the bleeding had become so heavy that the kleenex that I used as a liner could not hide the evidence. The cramps and backaches became unbearable.

I was rewarded with huge napkins that I had to use for 8–10 days per month, a belt whose metal fastener jabbed into my coccyx hour after hour, and words to the effect "now you can become pregnant, my eldest daughter." My menses never became lighter and I thus termed it "Red River Valley." For the second and third day of my period, I stayed home from school lying on the couch with a rubber pad underneath my mid-section. I wore a double layer of napkins, bent my knees, and in this position strove to read, study and keep abreast of my school work.

Since the mid 1960s, I had known that I had fibroid tumors. I always attributed the pain of sexual intercourse to internal contact with these fibroids. I was the ultimate in heterosexual promiscuity in my teens and twenties (I don't know if the fibroids existed then—I doubt it since I believe that birth control pills, the IUD, and my few bouts with gonorrhea birthed these tumors).

The beginning of the end came in 1971, when I was 30 years old. My male gynecologist and his male resident-in-training had me in stirrups on the table. "Will you look at all those fibroid tumors," he told his resident. "Call in Dr. Roanoke and his resident. They've just gotta see this." There I was, bare feet in cold metal stirrups, legs spread-eagled under the paper sheet, and four men speaking about my uterine growths as if I didn't exist. "Thank you Ms. Trend for providing us with such a learning experience," said my gynecologist. Little did he realize that I had been provided with a learning experience also. It was the straw that broke the camel's back.

In 1971, after one year of begging my male gynecologist for a tubal ligation, I was finally granted this wish. I wanted the end result of this operation to allow me to continue to relate emotionally, physically, psychologically, politically as a heterosexual radical feminist—without the monthly agonies that seemed to be part of womanhood.

Never had I wanted motherhood—not surprising since I was the eldest of eight children in an urban Catholic family. On my 16th birthday, I had birthed a boy-child, but not wishing to marry my much older lover, I allowed Catholic Charities to provide a good home for this baby. Despite this birth and two much later abortions, my gynecologist was *still* reluctant to perform the tubal ligation.

The physician forced me to obtain the signature of my second husband on the medical form *before* I could obtain the operation. It did not matter that I was at this time separated from my liberated husband (who, like me, could not fathom *why* the medicos needed *his* signature for an operation on *my* body).

When I was still unable to convince my *white* male gynecologist to perform the laparoscopy, I used the reverse-racism tactic.

"Dr. Monroe, there are two reasons why you or some other physician will provide me with this operation: one, my husband from whom I am separated is a black man, and two, I am a white woman. Were I black, native American, Asian or Latina, you'd not only give me the operation that I requested, but you'd likely give me a hysterectomy which is the operation that I really want. And you would perform this operation without my knowledge, as the medicos have done to so many women of color." Those fighting-back words empowered me. They did the trick!

In the early 1970s there were no women doctors trained in this surgical procedure, so after rejecting two other male gynecologists I settled for the most innocuous male surgeon. He, however, was the last male gynecologist, physician or dentist that I ever utilized. From then on, it was womanpower *all the way* allopathically and sexually. I had evolved from my bisexual mode to exclusive lesbianism—though unlike other women I knew in the same boat, I resisted the temptation of separatism. My political and social comrades remained both men and women.

The laparoscopy reduced my periods from ten to seven days, reduced cramping and bleeding, and made my menses-times chronologically predictable. There were still physical activities that I forsook and/or declined during menses, but generally I was very thankful.

I was practicing radical feminism in ways beyond mere theory. I had wrested control of my own body from the male allopaths. I became politically and socially active after a long seclusive hiatus and wove this into a new lifestyle combining my politics with art: I learned ceramics and weaving and started a woman's pottery collective in June 1971. We five women took turns selling our collective wares at Pike Place Market in Seattle.

Never before had I felt so positive about my own self-image. It spurred me on to accomplish more and more, cutting a wider swath than any conscious self-images that ever existed. Naturally, I wanted to share my new-found power. Years of living in Seattle and Anchorage as a counselor/therapist, made me wish for even more change in my life. In Alaska, I joined a women's spirituality group and got beyond my fear of technology to produce public radio programs. My own pyramid of power was finally established: political, artistic, spiritual networks were fused permanently.

In 1984, to test the waters, I spent five months in Central America, most of the time in Nicaragua. Always one to question authority, I analyzed my government's policies for myself. I picked cotton with 150 other North American internationalists near the Gulf of Fonseca, where the contras bombed a communication depot only ten kilometers from my hacienda, travelled the breadth of this country from the Pacific to the Caribbean Sea and donated blood to our Nicaraguan brothers and sisters (this to compensate in small part for lost Nicaraguan lives, thanks to *our* CIA and *our* contras).

I'd had it with the boys and their toys and decided I was now ready for the next step of my empowerment. I left Alaska in January 1985 to seek a Master of Fine Arts in the Cinema Production Department of San Francisco State University. The only way to win was to beat them at their own media game and I hoped that this education would give me the tools.

Since the 1950s, hysterectomy had been totally abused by the medical profession, but now in the 1980s there was a dearth of potential hysterectomy patients for the women who were becoming doctors. By 1987, my fibroid tumors (although not malignant) had grown from the size of grapes to grapefruits. I convinced Dr. Livingston, chief resident in gynecology at the county hospital, that I truly needed the hysterectomy. Two weeks before the Harmonic

Convergence (celebrated world-wide on August 16, 1987), I left San Francisco General Hospital Gynecology Ward as what Dr. Livingston and Dr. Reed termed their star patient.

Mentally I had been prepared for this operation for years. Besides being politically, socially, artistically active, my physical regimen consisted of jogging a few times per week and aerobics classes thrice weekly. I quit smoking cigarettes (just before my mother died of cervical cancer), ate healthy foods and drank alcohol very moderately. I was still addicted to killer white sugar, but strove to restrict my intake, not always successfully.

Since my fortieth year, I'd had annual mammograms. I was high risk for breast cancer since my mother and her mother had mastectomies and both died of cancer. I also had Pap smears and rectal exams to check for cervical and/or uterine cancer. Leading an over-active and somewhat workaholic lifestyle, I sometimes let old bad habits of eating sugar and lack of exercise creep into my regimen, but I would compensate for these habits when time permitted.

I was almost lucky enough to have a new laser procedure used by my doctors, but the luck of the draw in this double-blind test was not with me. My total abdominal hysterectomy and bilateral salpingo-oophorectomy procedure removed my uterus, cervix, fallopian tubes and ovaries through a 5–7 inch incision in my lower abdomen. AMEN.

Within 12 hours of my hysterectomy, I insisted on walking to the restroom instead of using a bedpan. The nurses on the midnight shift looked askance at me, walking and dragging a lamp pole apparatus along with me. That is, until they realized that I'd had a total hysterectomy one-half day previously. They were too busy to attend to me, so I constructively utilized my time in the hospital.

The young medical student working with my two doctors was also very supportive—and surprised at my energy. Chris Munoz grew up in a similar situation to mine (eldest daughter of Irish-Hispanic Catholic family from Boston) except Chris had chosen a career that I was totally uninterested in—allopathic medicine. Both Chris, Elizabeth and Susan would sit on my bed and chat with me just like "normal" women—not medical personnel. It was truly wonderful.

When Chris knew that I wanted to leave the hospital on Friday, July 31st—the pagan holiday LAMMAS that I wished to celebrate at my home—she put in a good word with my doctors. "You know, zimyá, that you can leave AMA (against medical advice) don't you?" She took my response in stride: "Yes, Chris, I know, but I've such a respect for you, my docs and the nurses, that I want to be kosher about leaving. I wanna leave with the blessings of my docs—okay?"

My housemate picked me up and took me home on Friday, the 31st, as I had wished. On my way out of the door, I gave Chris the crystal that I had worn around my neck when I entered the hospital. "You will be a wonderful physician some day—just like Elizabeth and Susan," I said as I finished shaking hands with my doctors. I placed the crystal over her head, smiled and said, "This may be of some help . . . at least you can remember me."

Since August 16th—the day of the Harmonic Convergence, my organs sit in a Mason jar filled with formaldehyde on my altar. No, I am not glorifying my internal womanness but just thinking of how far I've come since my first bloods, when I didn't know up from down. Since that time, many wonderful things have happened, some the product of my own hard work, but most attributable to my very powerful self-image which is forever pasted on the inside of my brain.

My health continues to surprise me. I rarely get sick because I treat my body as a temple and prevent dis-ease. Besides cholesterol testing, I've had the entire gamut of blood tests. I wanted to know exactly what my baseline was/is after my operation, and I daresay it has improved. At times when over-work has crept into my routine, I feel like I'm 90 instead of 49, but fortunately that's a rare occurrence.

In 1987 I joined one of the oldest affinity groups in the San Francisco Bay Area. Mother Courage Affinity Group began with sisters who participated in the Livermore Action Group in 1980–81. These women did everything together—including going to jail for opposition to nuclear energy and testing. Just prior to my hysterectomy, I was accepted as a member of this sisterhood.

I have been arrested for non-violent civil resistance at the Concord Naval Weapons Station, at the Nevada Nuclear Test Site (many times), in San Francisco and at the Livermore National Weapons Laboratory. I've participated in anti-nuclear actions at Rocky Flats, Colorado; Los Alamos, New Mexico; and was a participant for the three-week international peace walk in Kazakhstan, USSR, in September 1990.

In January 1991, I represented American Peace Test in global anti-nuclear meetings in New York City, and demonstrated at the United Nations in New York City with hundreds of thousands of American and international global activists. Our aim was to pressure the U.S. government to adopt the Comprehensive Nuclear Test Ban which 118 other nations, including the USSR, wished to ratify.

The U.S. boycotted ratification even though the Cold War has been over since 1989. Since this makes moot the peace dividend that we've been hearing about, I expect that my/our global peace work will continue with renewed vigor.

On spring equinox 1989, I registered my own business with the City of San Francisco. As a writer/filmmaker/consultant, Mother Courage Productions represents exactly where I am spiritually and philosophically at this time in my life. I have two 16mm films in production. *Older=Bolder: Active Anarchists* will be completed in spring 1991, while *If I Can't Dance, I Won't Join Your Revolution* (about my favorite role model, Emma Goldman) will be completed in spring 1992. The latter film completes my work for the M.F.A. in Cinema Production from San Francisco State University.

I envision living in Moscow in 1993 producing my own films and expanding Mother Courage Productions into Mother Courage Health Club. I remain optimistic about the power of the grass roots and citizen diplomacy (ourselves) to change this planet so that Gaia can become an ecologically-safe haven for humans, other animals, plants—all life. The Kazakh people, who in October 1990 permanently shut down their Polygon test site near Semipalatinsk, Kazakhstan, are my grass roots mentors.

As Susan B. Anthony, my first role model, said in 1912, "Failure Is Impossible." As long as I *fully* utilize this axiom, how can I/we fail in this most important task?

POEM TO MY UTERUS

Lucille Clifton

you, uterus,
you have been patient
as a sock
while i have slippered into you
my dead and living children.
now
they want to cut you out
stocking i will not need
where i am going
where i am going
old girl
without you
uterus
my bloody print
my estrogen kitchen
my black bag of desire
where can i go
barefoot
without you?
where can you go
without me?

TRAUMATIC MENOPAUSE: FROM THE FRYING PAN TO DEAD ZONE

Karen Ohm

In September, 1985, I was given a one percent chance to live. My oncologist was brutally frank about the statistics of surviving stage III ovarian cancer. I was barely conscious after the anaesthesia, but had no trouble comprehending the stark bedside manner of this man who had lost his own wife to cancer one year before. My cancer was found during what was to be a routine hysterectomy. I had been pleading with my gynecologist for a year to do at least a laparoscopy because I knew my body, I was not even close to menopause and all the symptoms of ovarian cancer were present. Finally, when the iscites (an enormous collection of water generated by tumor masses in the belly) became obvious he agreed to do something surgically.

The surgery took place when I was 45 years old. I went into the operating room knowing in my heart that I had a late stage cancer. Psychologically, I wasn't really prepared despite having had premonitions for at least a year. It's exactly like when you are told that a close family member has a terminal illness. You prepare yourself intellectually for that death, but when the actual event occurs, the emotional blow is overwhelming.

After my surgery, which included a total hysterectomy plus what reduction of my metastatic tumor could be done, the oncologist informed me that as soon as my belly had healed enough so I could vomit without tearing out the stitches, he would order chemotherapy. I asked him to give me some idea of what to expect, but nothing was forthcoming. I asked the night nurse if she knew what drugs I would be getting. She, though ignorant herself, called the floor oncology nurse to explain the situation to me. She gave me a list of the drugs and brief description of what each one was supposed to do, then left. I was still not enlightened. I am the sort of person who always does my homework before submitting to any sort of medical procedure. I called a friend who had just received his M.D. to request that he find me the latest editions of the *Oncology Journal*. He brought them the next night and I read them with horror. Doctors writing for other doctors don't mince words, and descriptions of the side effects of even one of the drugs, let alone five of them, were enough to send my nervous system straight into shock. I was so terrified that I immediately demanded release from the hospital on the fifth day, rather than the tenth day, because I knew that I had a lot of reading to do to try to find myself some sort of protection. Since I was only given three months to live without the drugs, I knew that I was trapped into taking them until I could figure another way of trying to demolish this monster.

The first thing that I did was to make an appointment with a naturopathic doctor, a homeopathic doctor, and a leading scientist specializing in developing chemotherapy treatments for ovarian cancer. I read extensively in the fields of nutrition and homeopathic medicine. I knew just one thing for certain, that I had better become an expert in these fields very quickly if I wanted to be able to beat the odds. I spent virtually 14 hours a day reading and learning, then began to implement many of the suggestions for coping with cancer. My diet was not quite macrobiotic, but it consisted primarily of grains, vegetables and fruits. I spent four 20-minute sessions per day imaging (visualizing my abdomen as healthy and pink), I learned biofeedback for the pain and practiced mega-vitamin and enzyme therapy. In all, I made a total commitment to healing myself. I spent much of my time meditating and praying. There was no time to give myself a break, because letting down my vigilance hands an advantage to the enemy.

When the chemotherapy was in full swing, I experienced so many negative side effects that I added one five day fun trip a month. Usually, on the tenth day after any chemotherapy treatment one is out of much risk of septic infection for that treatment interval. Having this firmly in mind, I took a luxurious trip to a guest ranch in Tucson, Arizona. While still in the air, I noticed that I had a high fever and was losing strength with every degree it escalated. I told my friend at the airport that I was ill and suspected it was a septicemic blood infection. A few hours later, I was in an emergency room. I spent nine days in the hospital having intravenous antibiotics, then back to Boulder for treatment number three.

After each chemotherapy, I developed sporadic blindness, rapidly falling red and white blood counts, faintness and fatigue so profound that it was an effort even to think. I just kept reminding myself that this treatment could only go on for a total of eight times, when my body indexes would be saturated, making no more chemotherapy possible. Each day after I performed my healing rituals, I forced myself to complete my nutritional requirements, and rested numerous times. I rewarded myself with some little thing that I had always coveted but couldn't have due to monetary restrictions. These were little, simple things, but they gave me great pleasure. They included hardback books for my very own, fancy soaps, dinner out at a fine restaurant with a friend, renting video cassette tapes, and allowing myself the luxury of a $5.00 in-house movie rather than its $3.00 matinee counterpart. I figured that if I did live through this, I could always pay the bill later. Having something to look forward to when times were so bad gave me great incentive. I also had several local acquaintances (including one dear neighbor) who called on me frequently for short intervals to disseminate courage and cheer.

During the entire time of the surgery and chemotherapy, my husband was off consoling himself in the bed of his supposed secret girlfriend. When I dared confront him about his lack of support and lack of care about my condition, he barked back with, "What do I need with a wife who isn't a woman anymore!" Well, that was the end of my seventeen year attempt at loving and trying to communicate with this man. In every case, his response to almost everything was to abuse me viciously and use me shamelessly. He was a professional wrestler in his earlier life and still had the "killer instinct" when confronted with anything. He was also blind, which probably stimulated my need to nurture because I, too, am a handicapped person. Somehow, cancer makes everything more urgent in one's life and I had known for years that I should divorce him, but somehow I always found an excuse not to do it. I had no trouble going through with the divorce and was surprised at how profoundly relieved I was at not having his threatening presence around anymore. I hadn't really realized how many years that I gave to this abusive, cruel tyrant. Now, I really had no excuses left because my very existence was at risk. I was free, and this freedom from being chained to that evil beast profoundly changed my life. Formerly, I could have no friends, now I have many with whom I share.

In 1985, many cancer patients developed AIDS as a result of blood transfusions given in conjunction with their chemotherapy. At one point, during the final half of my treatments, my blood counts became alarmingly low. The doctors threatened me with blood transfusions, but I steadfastly refused. Exactly one day after my fifth treatment, I read in the newspaper that 122 cancer patients were contaminated with the AIDS virus during their intravenous therapy. I have learned over my many years of being a medical victim that you have to protect yourself from your doctor and his professional "wisdom."

After my treatments were finished, I set to work in earnest with a naturopathic doctor. His regimen for me included a combination of controlled fasts, even more vitamin, enzyme and mineral supplementation, prescribed foods and beverages at various times of the day, and Bach Flower Remedies for easing emotional stress.

Since I had an estrogen bound cancer, there was no hope of having hormone replacement therapy, so the hot flashes continued for the next year until my body was thoroughly adjusted to menopause. I think that the most unpleasant side effect of traumatic menopause was the continual, crushing headaches which seemed to be a result of the estrogen withdrawal.

About this time, I added blue/green algae to my diet in the form of dried spirulina. This did more to raise my white and red blood counts than anything, including the naturopathic line of hemogenics that I took for months prior to adding the spirulina. I began to gain strength and appetite very rapidly and was soon attempting my three mile a day walking regimen that I had worked at assiduously while having the drug therapy.

Happily, my body has now adjusted to its lack of estrogen. I don't have hot flashes anymore, but there is one thing that I will have for a long time to come. Without estrogen, I have no erotic impulses or sexual feelings. These I miss grievously. I am doing all I can to restore these feelings, such as reading erotica, watching erotic videos, fantasizing various sexual and erotic situations, attempts at masturbation, which so far have led me nowhere near the pleasure of orgasm. There really aren't any resources, such as support groups, or appropriate literature to address this problem. In this respect, I feel alone and in a very subtle way, less of a woman than I would like to feel. However, in every other way I am ecstatic to be in menopause. Prior to menopause, I had severe endometriosis, which caused excruciating pain during ovulation and menstruation. It was such a force during my years as a menstruating woman that I feel like I have been handed the ultimate liberation. Also, I don't regret having to always carry tampons and pads everywhere because I never knew when my flow might start. Since I was a young woman, I had many embarrassing incidents related to flooding in the most inconvenient places. Being menopausal is also wonderful for me because now I can seriously consider what's ahead for me in life, as I no longer feel like I have to be with a man.

Prior to menopause, I had a small but voluptuous body with large, firm breasts and just enough curves to cause men to take an extra look. In menopause, I now have small breasts and have thinned overall to the size and appearance of a pre-teen boy. In this age of androgyny, such a body is acceptable, but I feel men don't even sense my presence. I seem to have become a neuter who gives off no pheromones.

As a woman who's never accepted the words "can't" and "won't" or "it will never be," I'm determined to find a way to circumvent the death of my erotic life—the sudden and traumatic cessation of the sense of myself as a complete woman. Since I am blocked from taking hormone replacement, I've begun experimenting with barley and wheat grass teas because they both contain small amounts of naturally produced plant estrogen. I'm also taking animal glandulars to see if they will have any effect on my problem. Having come through near death from cancer and the fiery torments (not too strong a term) of chemotherapy, I am certainly not prepared to live in the dead zone of being a woman without erotic connection to this world. Time will tell, but I am alive and determined to come *all* the way back.

MEANING MENOPAUSE

Dori Appel

My gynecologist calls it
ovarian failure.
I didn't make this up,
nor did he. He learned it
in medical school,
reads it in journals,
says it casually
to his colleagues,
who say it back to him.
Every day he flunks
his patients with it
and they take it on the chin,
but when he serves it
up to me, something snaps.
How funny he looks,
clenching a speculum
in his gloved hand,
trying to calm me
while I shriek like a fury
and challenge him
to evict me in my paper gown.
His eyes travel furtively
to his watch as he recalls
his waiting room,
now full to overflowing
with women whose
ovaries are failing
even as they turn the pages
of their magazines. Too bad,

I am going to lie right here,
howling and kicking my feet
on the stirrups
until he recants—this man
so certain of his truth,
whose testicles
know nothing but success.

BLOWING THE FUSE

Elaine Goldman Gill

I was surprised by menopause, primarily because the books I got from the library, mostly written by male doctors, assured me that menopause for most women was easy. The assumption, sometimes not explicitly stated, in these books was that if you suffered during menopause, there was something wrong with you—that is, you were neurotic and imagining things. In the past I had been told by many women that the change was no cinch, but, on my assumption that the M.D.s knew what they were talking about, I disregarded these warnings as old wives' tales. I thought, hey, I'm comparatively healthy and functional—why worry?

There is, incidentally, an interesting correlation between male doctors' assumptions about menopause and menstruation—their belief that if you had difficulties menstruating the problem lay in your head. It is also interesting to note here that, just as bleeding is a taboo in our society (we don't talk about it), menopause, the cessation of bleeding, is also a taboo. Women simply don't talk about menopausal difficulties, whether it is heavy bleeding, hot flashes or vaginal dryness. Anything connected with the bleeding, the starting and the stopping, is taboo. There's an additional taboo. If a woman admits she is in menopause or post-menopausal, she is reassessed by other people; she will be considered somehow unattractive. It is an admission that she is no longer there as a woman with sexual feelings. She is over the hill, invisible. On the other hand, though young girls call the bleeding the curse, they compare notes and celebrate it, though silently.

There are no statistics about menopause that I know of. How many women are troubled, how much are they troubled, how many are not troubled? I'd be interested to know. What I do know from my history and that of my friends is that frequently there is trouble. I believe, just as the onset of bleeding is a difficult time, so is menopause. At the beginning of menstruation everything changes in our bodies. We grow hair in odd places, we no longer feel the same, we no longer smell the same. We sense our sexuality emerging but don't know where it will lead. It's a very tough time. I remember my adolescence with a kind of horror, feeling I was going through a dark tunnel, with no security that I would ever get out to the light. I remember when I was a 15-year-old walking through Scollay Square in Boston, staring longingly at sailors but not knowing exactly what I was doing. Incidentally, most people I know, men and women, swear that, of all the periods of their lives, adolescence is the one they absolutely would not choose to relive.

I argue that menopause is similarly threatening. The body undergoes changes we do not understand. There may be heavy bleeding, so heavy it seems you are hemorrhaging. The body feels strange. You smell different. You don't know what's happening, what will be happening to you. And of course in our culture you don't even admit you are going through it. The first time I had to say I was going through menopause, I had to force the utterance. It actually took courage. The one advantage I can see, and it is enormous, is that you don't have to use contraceptives, a great blessing for spontaneous sex.

After that preamble, I will say that I believe the old wives' tales now. What was the content of those tales? The women told me that sometimes their friends went nuts, during and after menopause. They told me that the change, and they put caps on the phrase, was indeed a change, THE CHANGE—that it marked an important state in a woman's life, that she would not be the same afterward, and that frequently strange things happened to her.

All true, I now think. For corroboration, here is my own experience. I had no serious problems, but it wasn't easy. I first noticed I couldn't control my eating habits. Then I noticed I was becoming increasingly nervous, particularly when I sat in the passenger seat of a car. I'd grow alarmed, fearful of potential accidents. What I didn't figure out is that my immune system was being drained because of the hormonal changes I was going through. My adrenals were overfunctioning and therefore were becoming weaker and weaker. I didn't heed any of these warning signals. I continued as before, worked as I had before, and lived a pretty full, busy life. Because I had never been asthmatic as a child, I volunteered to varnish a pressed wood floor in our bedroom. Unknown to me, when varnished with a Tung-Seal varnish, it formed a chemical reaction, probably producing formaldehyde. I will admit I'm a sloppy painter. I got the varnish all over me, palms, feet, any exposed part of my body. And I slept in that bedroom for three nights. On the fourth day, I was amused to find myself breathing like a harmonica. You could hear four tones at once every time I breathed in and out. Within a month I had a five percent oxygen supply and couldn't climb a flight of stairs. My husband slept in the same room but had no reaction. I was going through menopause and he wasn't.

The point of this story? I urge all women to take particular care of themselves for a few years before they expect to go through menopause. I'd say from age 45 on. That means proper diet, supplementary vitamins, sufficient exercise, and I'd add, avoidance of chemical pollutants. This kind of care is very important, because, I believe, if you have a fuse to blow, a weak link in your body, you'll blow that fuse in menopause.

As for the other physical effects of menopause, the flashes, the sweats, never bothered me. They seemed like sexual rushes to me, but maybe other women have longer, higher flashes. Who is to know? Vitamin E may have helped me with these flashes. The only thing that troubled me and continues to trouble me is vaginal dryness. Some women have told me that they remained juicy. They are lucky.

KY Jelly seems to help; you can use as much as you need. Some women use oral estrogen, some use local estrogen applied to the opening of the vagina. These probably work, keeping the vagina fluid. I don't know. I haven't tried either one. I am troubled about the invisible side effects, even of locally applied estrogen. I imagine anything you put anywhere on your body must eventually enter the blood stream. But on the other hand a locally administered product is nowhere as dangerous as something you swallow or inject. I really worry about taking hormones. Our bodies are so intricately balanced, I am afraid of upsetting that balance. Moreover, having worked in the pharmaceutical industry I have become radicalized. I have seen too many clinical tests, funded by the pharmaceutical companies, with predictable results.

So there's KY Jelly, and there's local estrogen. A nurse I know warned that in the case of vaginal dryness, there's a great chance of tearing the vaginal wall, making it possible for viruses, including AIDS, to enter the blood stream. If you don't know your partner you'd better insist on a condom. In this case, understand that petroleum jellies (not KY Jelly) and other oils can destroy the condom.

Then there's oral intercourse. There's no trouble here at all, except to learn, if you have to, new patterns of loving.

I haven't mentioned another great reward in menopause, besides the impossibility of conception. I think if you get through the door of menopause and continue to face life as a fascinating, though frequently troubling, journey, and trust in that journey, your post-menopausal life will be extraordinary in the amount of energy you will have to do whatever you have to do, in the sexual energy you will have, in the serenity you can achieve. It's a marvelous time, one of the best times of my life. In a crazy way, it's something to look forward to. I feel more centered now, more so than at any time in my life.

Bon voyage to all of you out there who do not know what to expect. My advice in a nutshell is to take care of yourself in the best way you know how, to take it kind of easy while you're going through that door, and that, once through that door, to have a good time.

WHAT IS WAS, WAS MENOPAUSE

Vickie C. Posey

In the early spring of 1989, I had a case of what I and my doctors thought was depression. I felt low, had no appetite, cried much of the time, and felt disoriented. One of the most disconcerting problems was pressure in my head which made me feel like I had a brain tumor. When I described this feeling to my sister, she said she had experienced the same thing during her periods lately. I heard about others my age, with symptoms like mine, who had discovered their problems were hormonal. But when I suggested to my doctor that my problems could be hormonal, she dismissed the idea casually. Saying there was no reason to have the costly hormone tests, she instead prescribed an anti-depressant and psychological counseling. For the pressure in my head, she suggested a decongestant and ordered a brain scan (much more expensive than the hormone tests).

Six months later, I was to find out that I had experienced what my mother always referred to as the change of life. As I was only 39, the news came as quite a shock. Although I had thought my problems might be hormonal, I never once thought they were due to menopause. The worst part is that my doctor failed to recognize menopause.

Though I had pushed to have the hormone tests, I was not prepared to be told I was post-menopausal. Menopause, I thought, happened to women much older or less healthy than I. Just the word itself conjured up images in my mind of craziness, wrinkles, and gray hair. As with other losses, I went through a period of questioning and denial. I thought of my first anxiously-awaited period. I thought of my mother at age 35, who almost died giving birth to a stillborn son while also suffering what I considered an equally devastating loss, a complete hysterectomy. Not only did she lose her last child, her only son, but she lost any hope for ever having another. I was only twelve at the time, and eagerly anticipated my own womanhood. I remember thinking that it must be the saddest thing when a woman can no longer have children.

And here I was at age 39, going through this saddest thing. Ironically, for the last four or five years I had desperately wanted to have another child. Equally ironic, one of my very best friends, a woman from my home town with whom I'd grown up and graduated from high school, was pregnant at the same time that I was going through menopause. Had I not gone through some major changes in my life, I would never have been able to accept these ironies.

During my journey through menopause, I went through a period of self-questioning and self-revelation. The emotional struggle and subsequent counseling forced me to rethink my relationships with my parents, my husband, my children, and my own inner self.

My questions focused on patterns in my life. Why did I have periodic depressions and anxieties and why did I always have the feeling of being stuck? I promised myself not to come out of this depression until I had some answers. My first realization was that I had never learned to trust myself but looked to others for approval. Philosopher Joseph Campbell says, "The world is full of people who have stopped listening to themselves, or have listened to their neighbors to learn what they ought to do, how they ought to behave, and what the values are that they should be living for." I definitely was one of these people and began to see the root of my problem when I recognized dysfunctional and addictive behaviors in my family and in myself.

Changes came when I realized that my feelings and desires are legitimate and should be respected. I learned that taking care of one's self is not selfish, but necessary for emotional health. In fact, taking care of yourself is the best thing you can do for everyone around you. For women, this idea is usually difficult to understand because we are so used to thinking we should take care of everyone else. I learned that when I began to truly take care of myself, others began to take care of themselves, and I felt less resentful and smothered. In every area of my life, my relationships began to change, sometimes slowly, sometimes painfully, but ultimately for the better.

One change that I made was to get a room of my own, a tiny, windowless space I rented in an office building (one that was cheap because no one else wanted it). Although I had dreamed of having a space where I could write, have a darkroom, and do other projects, I always thought it was impossible. I told myself that we couldn't afford it, that my husband and children would think it was a silly thing to do, that my mother would think it was extravagant, that people wouldn't understand why I needed an office when I didn't even have a business.

This room of my own is really a symbol of changes that came from my bout with menopause. I have the space, not because I need it to make money, not because someone else gave me permission to have it, but simply because I want it. I made a choice to pay for an office rather than buy new clothes or go out to eat. Although I can't explain why, I know my room is important. I sometimes have nightmares about its being taken away from me.

After months of struggle, I did finally come to terms with my menopause. Still there are questions. Why did I go through premature menopause when most women go through it at 49 or 50? (Premature menopause occurs before age 40. Only about one percent of women experience this.) Most sources agree that heredity is the main factor that determines when a woman will experience menopause. In researching my menopausal heritage, I came away with little information. Both my mother and older sister, who had complete hysterectomies during their thirties, couldn't tell me when they had gone through menopause. My aunts also did not know exactly how old they were when they went through it. I soon realized that the women in my family, like so many other women, are generally uninformed and even reluctant to talk about this important part of their lives.

Another question is, could I have pushed myself into early menopause by exercise and diet? In 1989 I was thinner than I had been in ages, first of all by choice and later because of depression. By running and working out with weights, I had lowered my body fat considerably. I was turning 40 soon and wanted to keep myself looking young and fit.

This is akin to the old question, "Which came first, the chicken or the egg?" But this time there is a third component. Did my weight loss cause the menopause and thus the depression? Or did the depression cause further weight loss which resulted in menopause? Or, did the menopause cause the depression and thus the weight loss? Most doctors dismiss these theories, but other snippets of information lead me to believe that they have some validity. For instance, we all know of runners with low body fat whose periods cease. Also, I have heard of women body builders who experience premature menopause.

If we, in fact, can push ourselves into early menopause, what an irony life is. When we try to stay healthy through diet and exercise, we then become menopausal. We are forced to choose between taking daily hormone therapy, which increases our risk of breast and uterine cancer, or taking no therapy which increases our risk of heart disease, osteoporosis, and degeneration of the sexual organs.

The last question is why was my doctor so reluctant to associate my symptoms with menopause? In retrospect, I realize that the changes accompanying the process were changes that needed to happen, but I do think the struggle would have been a bit easier if early on someone had suggested that menopause might be the cause of my problems.

All in all menopause is a complex matter; for most it is much more than a physical change. Still women hesitate to discuss it among themselves, with a counselor, or with their physicians. Every day, new information surfaces, new remedies and theories are developed. As women of the twentieth century, we are living longer than ever before. To ensure that our long lives will be healthy and happy, we must stay abreast of medical developments and share our experiences. Most of all, we need to take responsibility for our own health, reading, taking advantage of medical expertise, but always listening to our own bodies and intuition and not being afraid to ask for help.

OPENING PANDORA'S BOX

Geeta Dardick

I have always been afraid of taking a close look at my inner self. I thought that it would be like opening Pandora's box. Not aware of the true symbolism of Pandora (as curiosity which can lead to positive changes), I didn't trust the idea of opening up, because I was certain that it might unleash emotions I couldn't control.

As a spiritually-oriented, back-to-the-land farmer, wife, and mother of three children, I glided through the 1970s with calm and equanimity. I grew all my own food here on the San Juan Ridge in Nevada County, California, and became best of friends with Mother Nature. It was an idyllic existence, and a marvelous way to raise a family. After a turbulent, difficult experience in the 1960s, my life-style was finally stabilized, and I didn't really want it to change.

But then, in the 1980s, the children grew up and I encouraged them to leave home, because I truly felt that personal independence would be important for them. Since there was no more need for so much food or mothering, I took up free-lance writing with great vigor, selling articles to mainstream publications across the country and teaching local residents how to market their writing as well. Now in my late forties, I felt a strong need to identify myself as a professional working woman. I had started my writing career with no electricity and no telephone, plunking away at an old manual typewriter under the pale glow of a kerosene lamp. Now I modernized, joined the twentieth century, and put my connections with spirit and nature on the back burner.

Around that same time, my husband Sam Dardick, who had been my constant companion on the farm, became Executive Director of FREED, the new disability program in Nevada County. I didn't consciously feel abandoned by my husband and children; after all, I had wanted all of them to move forward, as I also wished to do. But I often felt extremely lonely, as I spent long days at my computer, the only human presence on a 34-acre piece of land. I fought my loneliness by deciding to make more money, thus extending the growing list of writing credits behind my name.

Try to picture me, during November and December of 1989, slaving over an assignment for *Reader's Digest*. The *Digest* pays over $3,000 for articles, so you can imagine that I was stressing over this particular story. My editor was tormenting me so unmercifully (the "rewrite this, rewrite that" routine that *Reader's Digest* is famous for), that I ended up working about 12 hours a day, and barely eating or exercising. By the time I mailed the article to him on the day before Christmas, my digestive tract felt like it was on fire.

After Christmas I went down to the Oakland Coliseum to go to a Grateful Dead concert with Sam and our eldest son Caleb. At such concerts, old sixties hippies like myself are supposed to have some semblance of fun, but I experienced an intense anger like I had never felt before.

The problem was the seating arrangements. My husband is a wheelchair user, and before we headed for the area where wheelchair people sit, I noted that there were no chairs for non-disabled people like myself. So I picked up a folding chair that I found, and started to carry it to the disabled seating area. And suddenly, a burly guard stopped me, and rudely took my chair from me. He would not listen to reason. Of course, you might feel that it was normal for me to become angry with such unfair treatment. But my anger wouldn't leave me. I finally found another chair, but throughout the entire concert, negative thoughts bubbled inside of me like a poisonous fluid. For three hours I fumed, suddenly repulsed by the smoke-filled concert hall, the blaring music, and the zombie-like nature of the audience. Yet I had thoroughly enjoyed a Grateful Dead concert a few summers before. What was happening to me?

When I returned home from the concert, I tried to make airline reservations for Sam's and my upcoming research project in Costa Rica, to study disability issues there. But despite the fact that this would be a worthwhile adventure in a fabulous climate, I was unable to decide when to fly because I felt certain that whatever plane I chose, it would crash. A sense of personal danger was omnipresent.

Then, on Monday morning January 8th, 1990, a new woman entered my universe, an encounter which precipitated a tumultuous explosion within my body and mind. She was rather beautiful, at least a decade older than I, and she traveled about the west in a small van. She called herself a shaman, a term which piqued my interest. "Exactly what do you do?" I asked her.

She told me that she put clients into a trance, cleaned their chakras, and then helped them look at their previous incarnations. She then said that she felt like I was a person carrying lots of heavy past energies with me. She thought her therapy might help me. And without a second thought, I agreed to give it a try.

Monday afternoon, inside her gypsy van, the shaman-woman led me into a trance, in which she cleaned my chakras with colored light (including black), and put crystals (and some other stones) on each chakra and even in my hands, but my eyes were closed, so I have no idea what stones were used. She had many. I do recall I had a diamond at my crown or third eye.

After deep breathing exercises, she had me build an imaginary pyramid around myself. It had four sides, and I was lying down on the fifth side. (I was lying down for all this.) She also said that nothing would come that I couldn't handle, and that this would be a healing that would take place on all seven levels of my being, not just the physical.

Then she asked me to pick the chakra that had seemed most problematic as they had been cleaned. I chose the third, because of my intense abdominal pain there, which was still really bothering me. And then, in the safety of my pyramid, I started doing what she told me to do. She said to look into the pain in the third chakra. What did it feel like?

"Metal."

"What kind of metal?"

"A funnel." And then, out of the funnel came two dolls, a puppet named Pinocchio and a clown. First, I saw myself as a puppet controlled by my parents. And then I started seeing myself as a little girl, playing with Pinocchio in my playroom all alone.

"How do you feel now?" said the shaman-woman.

"Well, I feel okay. But all alone." And then, within my mind, I went down into the basement of my childhood home, and my mother was yelling at me from the top of the stairs that I was a rude and obnoxious chid, and I felt a deep sense of shame over that.

As I told the shaman about these feelings and images, she kept asking more questions. "What do you really see there?" she would query, constantly pushing me deeper and deeper.

The memories that came to me that rainy winter afternoon were primarily unhappy, painful ones. One time, the pain was a pimple about to burst, and I lived inside that pimple, alone again, swimming in guk. And then I put my husband and three children inside there with me, and they all had to swim in guk, and that's when I cried aloud because I knew I would never, ever want my family to endure the pain and aloneness I was feeling.

My final image was of a purple marble with a white line in it. And then it turned into a ball of flesh. And I said, "Oh my god, I have a tumor."

And she said, "No that's not it. That's just a symbol for something else." But I was stopped there, by that image. She said we weren't finished. That I should come back in two days. And then we broke the trance and started talking. It was late. We had been doing this work from 12:30 to 3:00 p.m. I paid her $65.00 and left.

But when I got home, the experience continued. More and more memories flooded over me. I sat on the couch, alone, crying, as I watched the images tumbling into my mind: personal losses, embarrassing sexual escapades, feelings of unbearable darkness. And then, the purple marble turned into an egg, and I realized my deeply buried grief over the 1982 abortion of the baby who would have been Sam's and my fourth child—the baby who would have continued my role as mother. I went out onto my back deck and shrieked loudly into the chilly sky with an anguish I had never felt before.

The experience of being confronted by all of my repressed memories and emotions was so overwhelming, that from Monday night January 8th through Thursday night January 11th, I was unable to sleep. Besides becoming extremely anxiety-ridden from sleep deprivation, my stomach ached and my bowels wouldn't move. On Wednesday, I got hold of some mild tranquilizers, and I started taking them, to try to come down. They'd work for an hour or two, and then I would be in a state of panic again. By Thursday, when I went to my friend Donna Lee Brown for a massage, she had to spend most of the two hour session holding my feet, trying to keep me in my body. I just couldn't relax. By Thursday night (the full moon of January 11th, 1990) I felt completely insane. Pandora's box was wide open and a battle between good and evil, life and death, was taking place inside my mind and body.

At 3:00 a.m. I called on Sam for help because I couldn't breathe. Throughout the rest of the night, he held me tightly in his arms, constantly reminding me to inhale and exhale while I continued my struggle to remain conscious. At daybreak I called our family doctor. I felt I needed professional care.

"Ha," said the doctor, upon completion of a five minute exam, "you are manic depressive. Just take lithium." For a few moments, I felt relieved. "Yes," I thought, "that explains everything about my life, about all my confusing memories. I am manic depressive." But by the end of the day, I decided not to take lithium, and opted for ultra-strong tranquilizers instead, which knocked me out for the next 72 hours. Whenever I awoke, I'd try to eat, but I was very weak and my bowels ached. I was sure that I was going to die.

On the following Wednesday, January 17th, I visited a gynecologist for the first time in eight years. He was concerned when he felt a lump in my abdomen. He scoped me with ultrasound, and the lump we saw on the screen looked just like the marble I had seen with the shaman-woman.

The gynecologist suspected that the lump might be able to move through my bowels, so he sent me home with an enema (to clean me out). When he reexamined me on Friday, the lump had disappeared, but now he wanted blood tests done for hormone levels. "I don't think you are in menopause," he said, "but I want to check, just in case."

Saturday the 20th of January I had my first acupuncture treatment (needle to the bowel). By then my heart was fluttering so, it felt like a heart attack. In fact, I had a very difficult time driving to the acupuncturist's office. I felt like I would surely die of heart failure on the way. I prayed for help because I wasn't ready to leave my body.

For the next ten days, my physical and mental condition remained completely unstable. During that time, I experienced the symptoms of numerous well-known diseases. I couldn't sleep without tranquilizers, and even worse, six people I knew happened to die during that period. I was certain that I would be the next to go. The results from the blood tests finally came back. My hormone levels were elevated. The gynecologist said that I was definitely in the midst of menopause. I felt a ripple of relief. Menopause. Perhaps I wasn't crazy after all. I was menopausal.

When the gynecologist told me I was in menopause, he said that he doubted that I would ever ovulate again. And then he asked me if I would like to try hormone replacement therapy (HRT). He thought it might make me feel better.

As a long-time natural health advocate, I was intellectually opposed to the idea of HRT. But I quickly agreed to try it, because I knew my health was in jeopardy. I needed a magic pill that would help me become balanced again. How I wanted to return to my old self, to become normal.

But normal didn't come so easily.

Eleven full moons have passed since I opened Pandora's box with the shaman-woman. Throughout every month, even on HRT, I have encountered physical and mental difficulties, some quite severe. On good days I return to my office, to continue working at my writing career. On others, the monumental task of eating three meals a day and doing some exercise fills all my waking hours.

I continued with the acupuncturist, and in August started seeing a therapist as well. Slowly, I began to process the memories and emotions that were released that day in the gypsy wagon. It is a challenging and difficult process, that is extremely exhausting. But I have no choice. I opened the box, and now I must examine the contents. All of them.

I am committed to calling my experience menopause, although for a long time I was sure that it had to be some other, "more serious" problem, a life-threatening disease or a hex from the shaman-woman. I now realize that my menopause is extremely serious business for me, and because it is my menopause, it is flamboyant and unique, as I am. It has opened the doors to Pandora's box, and brought me to the threshold of a higher consciousness and increased self-understanding. Like Pinocchio, I am in the process of becoming more real, more human than ever before.

I am the birdwoman, free to fly out of the cage now, but not completely sure where I am headed. Perhaps my wings are still clipped. But they will grow soon. That is the law of nature.

I think I am healing. When I fall apart, my acupuncturist likes to remind me how sick I was when we first met, and how much progress I have made toward full recovery. Unfortunately, I still have unstable mental and physical health, but I rebound a bit faster. I think I may be seeing a small light at the end of the tunnel. I crawl toward it on all fours.

A SPLIT ATOM

Clara E. Wood

Gynecologists can tell you what they learned in medical school and what they think about menopause, but I'm here to tell you the way it really is; what can happen and what did happen to me before I started and since I've been on hormone therapy. I'm proof that menopause can be devastating, with or without hormone therapy. I had turned 50 in January, 1988. I really had not thought much about menopause until May of that year when the symptoms started creeping into my life.

I was at work doing what I had been doing for a number of years, being a good secretary. At one point during the day I felt weepy. I didn't know why but thought PMS had come a little early. Not so! Before the end of the day I had two crying jags—I don't mean weepy or gentle sobbing but hysterical crying.

When the crying was over I felt better but puzzled as to why this had happened. I hadn't been upset about anything and my life was, well, not bad. That night while discussing my problem with a friend, I remembered that on several occasions in the past few weeks I had been frightened by palpitations and panic attacks and had felt more anxious than usual.

In May of 1988 I had a blood test and my gynecologist told me that I was going through menopause. I was having mood swings—laughing and feeling good and suddenly crying and having fearful thoughts. Thoughts of dying, thoughts and fear of growing old. Then came the change in my periods. Sometimes heavy flow, other times very little. At night I would have cold sweats and would jump out of bed and sit in front of a floor fan while wiping the perspiration from my body. I had itchy skin and hives, upset stomach, diarrhea, frequent urination, rapid heart beat, palpitations and weight gain. My fingernails became soft and I was very sensitive to the heat. I had panic attacks and was afraid of being alone. I refused to drive my car and my sex drive was nil. The fatigue was overwhelming. There were times when my upper body would crumble as though it had no bones and I would lie across the desk or go to the back office and lay flat on my back on the floor.

But the worst, absolute worst feeling of all was the loss of memory. I sat in front of my computer one day in October of '88—that's all I did—just sat in front of the computer. Suddenly I was frightened, terrified! I couldn't remember what keys to hit to get into the computer. I had taken computer classes and taught the other secretaries and now I couldn't remember anything about the computer. I didn't want to tell anyone for fear they would think I was going crazy and, in fact, this is what I thought. I got up and walked around the office for a while and sat down again. I finally played around with the keys until I was in the main menu but then I couldn't remember what to do next. I jumped up and went to the back office and cried and cried—and cried. I had such severe palpitations that I had to be taken to the hospital emergency room. Tests were negative. I was sent home to "rest."

How could I rest? How could I rest when I couldn't remember how to "work." I couldn't concentrate long enough to read one column in the newspaper. How could I rest when these weird things were happening to me? What could I do—who could I talk to? I felt as though my life was falling apart all around me and there was nothing I could do about it. I was losing control. The feeling of loss of control is devastating. All of these terrible things had happened to me within six months. It was at this point that I realized that menopause had hit me like a "mack truck." It was holding back nothing—I was getting it full force. My hormones were going crazy and trying to take me with them.

I heard voices inside my head telling me that I would be better off dead. I would answer those voices—aloud—and say NO—I want to live and live without all the problems I was having. I called my doctor and told him that I felt I was going crazy. He said that he was sorry I was "having so many problems," but he didn't think my symptoms had anything to do with menopause. He sent me to a psychiatrist who wanted to go back to my childhood days and find out why I was having such a terrible time with menopause. I told her that I wanted her to help me through the problems I was having at the present. Unfortunately, she and I didn't agree. I went home. Home to cry, home to take the estrogen that was prescribed, home to try and find someone who could tell me what was happening to me—someone to help me.

By the beginning of 1989 I was in a terrible state of mind. My fiance was depressed and upset because he didn't understand what was going on and didn't know what to do to help me. How could he understand when I didn't understand myself. So, he did the only thing he could—he held me each time I had a bad "attack." He would drive to my job and get me when I felt I could not stay in the office another minute. He took me to the hospital when I felt that I was having a heart attack and he drove me to my therapist. He stayed with me throughout the bad times. Finally, at the end of January, 1989, my supervisor and I decided that it would be best if I took some time off. In early February I started going for massage therapy and it helped my aching muscles and the tension throughout my body. My massage therapist suggested I see a hypnotherapist who had helped her in the past. I called him immediately and as soon as he asked how he could help me I started crying. He set up an appointment for the same day. I spent three hours with him. When I left his office I felt better than I had in nine months. I started seeing him twice a week—two to three hours each session.

While I was at home, away from the office, and during some of my *sane* moments, I called around looking for a support group for women going through menopause. I checked with all organizations that I thought may have some idea of where I could find such a group. I called organizations in Maryland, Virginia, and Washington, D.C. No one knew of a support group. I was shocked and angry but most of all I was afraid. Was I the only woman going through such terrible menopause? I became more paranoid, more afraid, and more angry. I was angry at everyone and it seemed as though no one could help me. This was when I decided that I would find one woman, several women or many women who, like me, were going through what could be described as one of the most devastating times of one's life.

I called a local newspaper and put an ad in the Health Section. The ad read, "Starting Support Group for Women in Menopause. Please Call" (and gave my telephone number). Within one week I had a call from a woman who was going through a terrible ordeal. We talked several evenings a week for a couple of weeks. The following month I ran another ad and within three months I had a Support Group Meeting with 12 women in attendance. It was GREAT! There was a sharing of experiences, an atmosphere of mutual respect, positive feedback, warmth, honesty, humor and most important, understanding. More critically, was the evidence gained by our shared experiences that we were not unique and that in spite of the nonchalant attitude of our medical professionals, our experiences were commonplace. The attitude of the medical profession caused us to discontinue discussions of our continuing symptoms with them. Their lack of sympathy, accuracy and concern would have caused additional frustration. (Although I feel this way, I cannot emphasize enough the importance of having a good medical doctor. We need our Pap, mammogram and examination each year. And some of us do need the hormone therapy.)

By this time I was back at my job. It felt good to be back in the working place. I had some bad days but many more good ones. There were times when I would cry, feel sick physically and emotionally. But, I was seeing my therapist and I had a Support Group with loving women who cared and understood what I was going through. I was promoted to Office Manager with an excellent pay raise. I was extremely pleased but afraid that I would become unable to handle the job. My therapist helped me with those unhealthy thoughts and through hypnosis I learned to cope with the bad days. I also learned self-hypnosis and used it many times—sometimes two and three times a day. I had tapes that I listened to each night and once during the day. I did a lot of praying during this time in my life; I was raised in a religious home so prayer was not new to me.

Without my fiance, my therapist, my Support Group and the spiritual guidance I received, I don't think I would be where I am today.

In October of 1990 I received another promotion to Administrative Assistant to the Vice President. The Support Group has grown in the past year. We, who have been there since the beginning, though still having problems, are helping other women. They in turn are helping us.

Our group reads every book, magazine and newspaper article we can find on menopause. Copies are given to everyone. We have speakers as often as we can—acupuncturists, hypnotherapists, gynecologists—whoever will come. We attend seminars on breast cancer, hysterectomies, and osteoporosis. We've learned a lot since we began meeting and we're still learning.

I'm not the person that I was three years ago. Menopause took that person and made her a hysterical, moody, angry, anxious, tired, forgetful, and depressed "person." Before, I was a together woman, juggling all life had to offer. Then, Menopause. I felt like a split atom—no longer in control.

Today, I am much better. Occasionally I cry, fatigue takes over my body and panic steps in. My sex life is not what it used to be. But—I'm okay—that's the most important statement I can make—I'm really okay. It's not over yet but I know when I get on the other side of menopause I'll be more understanding and considerate, and I'll be able to say to some woman, somewhere, "I made it through and so will you."

I stumbled, I fumbled, I struggled, I cried, I screamed—and finally, I was heard.

IN THE CREVICES OF NIGHT

Gloria Vando

There's a man in my dream
a man with a hatchet
ransacking my bureau
hacking at the doll asleep
in the bottom drawer.

A bloodless ritual.

He calls himself a surgeon, says
he's up on the latest laser beam
techniques. I know better.
I know the jig's up.
Youth is waning and the end
is closing in on the beginning—
a telescopic fantasy focused
on dismembered limbs, a glass eye
rolling across the parquet floor,
tiny fingernails scattered
in my underwear scratching
at the obscenity of early death.
But not a drop of blood. Not a cry.

I turn from the dream, reaching
for you across the thin ice of night
and pressing my body to yours
long, foolishly, to bear your child.

MIGRAINE

Greta Hofmann Nemiroff

Lying in my bedroom in a dense fog of pain. A thick point of pain drills deeply into the corner between my eye and nose. One side of my face is stiff and aching; any movement at all hurts. My scalp on that side is sensitive even to the pressure of my hair crushed beneath it on the pillow. I have taken medication to dull the throbbing, but it has not worked and it makes me nauseous.

In the distance I can hear my children arguing, their voices getting shriller by the moment; I cannot intervene. My favorite cat, a marmalade fluff, is sleeping warmly against my legs, but he brings me no comfort. Worst of all is the complete boredom. I can do nothing . . . not even listen to music; all sound is an irritant. This boredom and the impatience for life to resume is immersed in a bath of panic. I have things to do. As I lie there, I scan my commitments for the next day . . . the next week. Will I ever be able to deliver my promises to others and to myself?

Waves of panic constrict their way up my chest into my throat. I can't stop them even though I know they will probably exacerbate my situation. Usually I am able to enjoy immense energy and speed; I have no patience with my own helplessness. "Perhaps I should take up Yoga," I distractedly tell myself, forgetting that I already have and hated it.

I have had these migraines for six years, since I turned 42. It took a while for me to realize that they came punctually when I had my periods: one two days before and the other on the second day into the period. Then I was surprised to learn from a doctor that this was a common menopausal syndrome. Surely such things only happened to people over 50? Lately, at the age of 48, I have my answer: along with the migraines I now have the addendum of hot flashes. I have fewer periods, but the migraines have not stopped.

I used to think that menopause, with its intimations of mortality, would not worry me . . . that aging could not affect me the way it might a woman obsessed with youth. At 35, I had accepted my greying hair with aplomb, never feeling any need to dye or tint it. The fact is, though, that I hate other things about it: slowing down, having to think whether or not I will have a good day, trying to schedule future events around anticipated migraines.

Always hovering around my consciousness is fear of the first tell-tale stab behind my eye, the throbbing in my skull. I worry about becoming consigned to the kind of sick room I remember from my childhood, where aging women languished in unexplained and mysterious weakness in shaded rooms, smelling of cologne and slightly rancid medication. My pain, somehow, puts me with them, on the shelf, out of the flow and excitement of daily life. To me, this isolation epitomizes the distancing of society from post-menopausal women, closing the distance only to make us the butts of mother-in-law jokes. I don't think there is a woman who lives to the age of menopause who doesn't experience that moment of realization that in the eyes of many people she has become invisible, the undifferentiated middle-aged woman in the crowd. I guess this has its value for the self-effacing, or perhaps for those who would like to commit the perfect crime.

So I lie in my bed in a dark room, throbbing and intermittently sweating. Waves of panic engulf me. As I finally drop into troubled sleep, I fear this pain will never go away and that I will never accomplish all those myriad tasks I have set myself for the duration. I forget at these times that when the migraine fades, in its wake I always feel a rush of euphoric energy and not only get it all done, but usually get more done than I had thought possible.

Right now, though, lying in my bed with household noises sounding much further off than they really are, I can't remember life without this pain. Suspended in the middle of pain and panic, I am sure that I am experiencing a kind of dying. It both bores and frightens me.

CLIMACTERIUM

Chris Karras

I'm fifty-one and looking good;
I could feel better—wish I would!
My sleep is poor; my heart beats fast;
my nightmares are a special ghast.

The curse is off its beaten track;
the migraines worse; depression's back.
I'm tired and keep dropping stuff.
I'm less inclined to take much guff.

Few people know of my distress;
but, privately, I am a mess.
I bluff my way through most of it
at home, at work—won't dump my shit.

It's Dr. Smart I went to see
the day I sneezed and lost my pee.
I'd been quite anxious lately, too.
My mood's been glum; the color blue.

He took my B.P. and Pap Smear,
and all the time he called me "dear."
"Trust me" he said, "I'm Dr. Smart."
(To me he seemed like one big fart.)

He glanced at me through rings of smoke;
a pregnant pause—and then he spoke:
"You wanna know what is the cause?
The cause, my dear, is menopause!"

His look said I will shrivel up,
no longer need a bra C-cup.
My hips will break, I'll get a rump,
and higher up my back will hump.

"Don't worry, dear, we'll fix you up.
Put this in your daily cup:
a little hormone, estrogen,
will keep the hairgrowth off your chin.

"You'll keep on looking young and fit
and none of it will hurt a bit.
Perhaps some cancer near the end;
that's treatable, you understand?

"Now take this valium here, my dear;
anxieties will disappear.
We'll have you soon as good as new
and keep your hubby happy too.

"We can, of course, do surgery"
he said with phoney sympathy.
"We open up, clean out, then zip;
while there, we'll fix that bladder-drip."

I left his place in quiet rage;
my soul tells me I've come of age.
You keep your pills and surgery.
I'm planning diff'rent therapy.

I have a plan for management;
a strictly private settlement:
I won't turn this into a fight;
It's vitamins and dolomite.

My nightmares I shall analyze;
there goes my psyche in disguise.
To be aware is my main theme
of highs and lows in my life's scheme.

I'll practice yoga as before;
unfractured time, I need much more.
My partner may not understand
all of my latest inner bend.

No chauvinist, no macho-man,
he's stretched himself as best he can.
But one thing I don't want to hear:
the query: "what's the matter, dear?"

Puberty, post-partum blues,
the monthly mess, I paid my dues.
And the climacterium!
A time for growth, not valium.

Depression, yes, discomforts, too.
for most of us, it's nothing new.
A crisis, this, equal to none,
for there's a hint of peace to come.

A new beginning? dare I say?
to get there, take it day by day.
More time to Be, to Do, to Think.
Well, yes, there IS the kitchen sink.

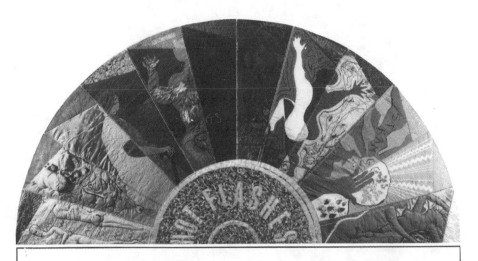

MEETING THE TIGER

It is widely believed that a post-menopausal woman loses her ability to respond sexually...this is nothing more than a cultural fallacy.

—Masters and Johnson

The most creative force in the world is the menopausal woman with zest.

—Margaret Mead

Thank you for asking me to contribute to your anthology on menopause, but I really don't have anything to say about it. I sailed through it without really paying any attention as I was in love at the time.

—Carolyn Kizer

AUTUMN ALCHEMY

Heather

My body simmers like a kettle,
round and steamy;
the elemental brew is changing
in my blood.
I'm percolating in a tropic time,
slow and humid;
the damp leaf compost of my fall
is heating up.

In shadows cast by lowering sun
the dark things gather force,
primordial in my bones.
The earth reclaims me,
cell by cell,
the mystic bond grows tighter
every day.

Hey dark lady
with the fertile breath,
I dance with autumn's colors now;
I blaze!
Watch me—I'll dazzle you
before I come to bed.

NO MORE MONTHLY MESSAGES FROM MAMA

Erica Lann Clark

Mama. An ancient Peruvian fertility goddess. Also, one of the names of *Nin-khur' sag*, the great Sumerian Mother Goddess, worshipped under several names, as *Aruru, Mama* and *Nintu*, throughout ancient Mesopotamia. *Nin-khur' sag* is from the Sumerian word *nin-khar' sag*, which literally translated means, *the lady of the great mountain.* From *Webster's International Dictionary,* 2nd edition, unabridged.

I woke up with sticky fingers. My fingernails felt funny, like dirt under them. Pulling the covers back, I saw the dark red stains all over the sheet. My pyjamas had blood on the crotch, too, and my fingernails were black and crusted with it. "Mama?" I called, but she'd gone downstairs to join the other guests in the resort. What would the resort owner say when she saw what I had done! I put on my bathrobe and slunk down the corridors to the dining room. There she was, surrounded by people as usual, and, as usual, of course she didn't see me until all of them turned to look at me. I hung my head and wished I could disappear into the ground. "Mama, I need you," I implored. Finally, she came over to me.

"Something terrible has happened!" We raced up the stairs. The room played innocent, as if nothing had occurred, but I pulled the covers on my bed back and exposed the truth—the dark, almost black blot on the clean white sheet. She laughed! Laughed and caught me to her, held me in her arms a moment, stroked my cheek. Not angry? Not sad? Not upset with my mess? Even a purr of pride? "But I don't want them to see the stains, Mama," I pleaded. "Don't worry. We'll rub the blood out with cold water." She understood. We put the sheets in the bathtub to soak, and with the vaguely familiar echo of a diaper, Mama helped me put my first Kotex napkin between my legs. I went out to play, and while I was gone, the bloodstained sheets disappeared.

That first message from the Lady of the Great Mountain was a shock; like a rocket, it catapulted me into breasts and boyfriends, birth and babies, and an unspoken, secret understanding with all women, everywhere, regardless of race, creed, color or culture. It was blood and bleeding that bound us to each other, made us mercy-full. Unlike men, who only bled when they were harmed, our blood ran free, a crazy blessing that we called a curse.

And I loved to make love when I was coming on my period. It would well up in me without warning, a demonic, inspired horniness, an ecstatic urge. Or, I'd become a cruel crank, sullen and stubborn. But whenever that monthly Curse of Eve finally arrived, and I was full of blood, I was alive! That heavy feeling in my groin, the weight of me pushing down, dribbling dark truths on my thighs. Life was a red thread and I carried it. I was Her Apostle and I knew it! In the cathedral of Her redwood trees, on secluded beaches and in moonlit cornfields, I practiced Her horny rituals.

In truth, no matter whatever I said in my bitching and moaning about the cramps and the curse, I loved the fact that I bled. Blood belonged to women. It took no talent, no effort, no homework. It just happened and made me one of "them." Then, when I had my children and proved I was fertile, that did it; now it was certain, I belonged. And all through the blood; my power as a human being came to me through my red thread.

Then they began, the thready little bleedings that hardly spotted my panties and disappeared after a day or two. I wasn't the menohemorrhagic type, so my red thread just faded away. But I looked aside, pretending I would be like biblical Sarah, fertile at 90, a medical miracle.

Finally, the Grand Climacteric couldn't be denied. But what a misnomer! No climax here. There was nothing. No more monthly messages from Mama, no red thread, only a pause. A long, long pause. I was scared and sad and angry. No more eggs? How can you be a woman and not be fertile? How be fertile and not bleed? Life had passed me by without giving me enough babies. I never even had my daughter and now it was too late, the source of my power had gone dry.

It filled me with dread thinking how my skin would shrivel and sag. Who'd want me then? Menopause, an apt name, a warning inherent in it: O ye men, o pause! And pause they would when they saw me, the hag, the aging crone. It was terrifying to have lost my quintessential power to make life. Now I had nothing to make me bigger or more potent than a man. Nothing of importance. I'd become invisible: shorter and fatter and greyer and sexless.

I went into mourning; menopause was going to be the death of me. Accustomed to defining myself in terms of my fertility, the fact that the Lady of the Great Mountain was stripping me down to my bare humanness, did, in fact, mean the end of me. How so? Why, I had never doubted my ability to attract a man, if I were drawn to him. Everywhere I went, I always met at least one man who, given the time and attention, would show an interest in me, and there was usually a little sexual something in an unconscious undertone to most conversations with men; and then came the day when I told an attractive man that I was attracted to him and to my deep embarrassment (and maybe even shame), saw a look of horror in his eyes, and he made quick to tell me I had better shift for my likes elsewhere. Another message from Mama?

So, I took off my high heels (they hurt my feet anyway), let my hair go grey and replaced sex with food (a more consistent source of love with absolutely no threat of rejection or abandonment). And thus I became shorter and greyer and fatter and sexless. Now, did mountain Mama take pity on me? Of course not! Mood swings I'd never dreamed possible happened regularly as hormones ebbed to all time lows, nightsweats left me drenched and raging in the middle of the night, and the only red left in my life was in my cheeks—the high color of yet another hot flash.

Acupuncture treatments and Chinese herbs that I boiled and drank smoothed the worst of times. I endured, struggling to find a sense of self-worth. The nightmare was coming true; contrary to all popular media, I was becoming what I had dreaded, an Older Woman. Out of desperation, I glanced at the monthly newsletter from a local hospital. There was a course in menopause! Why not? There we were, a few weeks later, ten of us, bitching and moaning, revealing shared fears, expressing our anger about being aging women in ageist America. But there were discoveries, too—startling new ideas. We learned that in Native American tradition you only become *fully grown up* at 51. The first 50 years are needed to finish making your major mistakes, the ones that grow you up. On the other side of the world, in India, you are *free to follow your bliss* after you finish your householder duties of raising children and managing a family. Once that's over, which often coincides with menopause, you are a free agent. You can dissolve your marriage and start a new life. In our culture, Margaret Mead experienced a new vitality when she reached menopause, and in a hot flash of humor, named it Post Menopausal Zest, or PMZ.

Now, four years later, I see that life's a giveaway, or, as they say in A.A., the only way to keep it is to give it away. Being older means there's a limit to my time, so I don't have to be bothered with stuff that doesn't mean much to me. Like high heels—I can be comfortable out in the world and wear my walking shoes to the Gala Events. Because, you see, the point has changed. The point is no longer earning a buck or building a career, or how much glamour I can score. Now the point is how much satisfaction, purpose, meaning I can glean from the mystery of experiencing life. So, something entered, did it, when the red thread left? Ahh. The darkness. Death Herself.

The first 50 years I used climbing up—up and out of the tunnel of my mother's vagina into the air! Seeing, tasting, hearing, feeling life. Finding food, sitting up, rolling over, crawling, making words, walking, wearing my generation's equivalent of The Right shirt, skirt and shoes. Pleasing my parents, pleasing the teachers, pleasing my friends, finding my freedoms. Feeling foxy, discovering despair, aching to love, dying to be on my own—and getting there. Where? Adulthood. The first apartment, car, set of dishes, vacuum cleaner, solo flight, performance, degree, big love, orgasm, pregnancy, childbirth, marriage, mortgage.

There was always tomorrow. There was always a rush when I thought of the future. It was getting bigger and better and brighter and more. And then, subtly and imperceptibly, things began to change. Seen one vacuum cleaner, not so exciting to buy the second. By the third child, you know what to expect, even though there's always the chance it won't turn out the way you think. Gone through the same arguments with the same people so many times you could recite them in your sleep. And they never change, and it doesn't rile you as much as it used to, and making up isn't as glorious, either.

Where's the sharp, biting edge? Gone. Worn down. Where's the newness, innocence, excitement? Feels like treading water, working like a dog just to keep your chin above the proverbial #*!X! Not going anywhere, flat, flat, flat. The further you climb up, the closer you get to the top, the bigger the view. But what is there to see? A spirit trapped in an aging body becoming decrepit and eventually a corpse—just like all the others who went before. Mortality a fair trade for fertility?

So how is it, now, here on the downhill side, in this downside slide, where I can look toward Death and see She lies waiting for me at the end of even a very long road, like a period at the end of a very long sentence? O, the structure may be delightful and syntactically astounding, with clauses within clauses, which may go on interminably unwinding themselves like a maze of fables, but one thing is certain—ready or not—I will come to my death as terminally as I entered my birth. And that's the madness and the gift. When I look ahead and see the end's in sight, how sweet each breath becomes. Hummingbird, so brief, pauses to drink from the flower. But must move on. Must drop in the end to rest on the ground, a fallen fruit.

Here's a magic big as birth, darker than the red thread, but just as fertile. I shall become an ancestor. My grandchildren are urgently sacred; they will bear what they can remember and some things they cannot remember. Just as I have done! I wish we all lived on one piece of land and that I could be buried and plowed under the fields to feed the family.

Vital desire, compelling priority, life is primary. It's not capricious, full of vagaries and minced words. No, it's direct, necessary, pressing and draining. It drains all your juices, takes everything you've got.

Living closer and closer to the edge now, there's a growing excitement; this really is a life and death situation. It really is about coming and going, and how am I going to do that? How will I prepare to be a crone, to be croned from the flock? Without the worldly stuff, what's left? Is there anything I can take with me as I leave? If it isn't the red thread, then what is it? Where do I find it? Inside me? What happens when I die? Do I liberate the mystery? Who am I? What an adventure—sounds like PMZ to me!

INITIATIONS

Kathy M. White

Mother of torch ginger and bamboo,
you embrace the young boy with flowers,
slender threads of orchid and plumeria
encircle his neck.

Watching the sky with his brown eyes,
you remember a time when he would stalk
wild nene with his slingshot.

Now, he chooses you for his teacher,
brings you blue kapa cloth and bread fruit.
Under red blossoms of lehua trees,
you accept, laying the cloth on misted grass.

Time after time, he sinks deeply within you.
As clouds hide the polynesian sea, he learns
the pleasures of your tattooed body.

Note: In Polynesia, women after menopause became sexual initiators, providing formal instruction to young boys entering puberty. Nene are island geese.

MEETING THE TIGER

Sandy Boucher

A tiny paw print left by a spirit animal. To remind me.

The inflammation burned at first. I lay with legs spread, fanning my fiery vulva.

In a buddhist nunnery. In Sri Lanka.

The flame was ignited, so they said, by bacteria. Little creatures having found this warm moist place to chew away at flesh.

Now the bacteria are long gone. The red print remains. On my vulva, a redness inside my inner lips, around and above my urethra.

At first, here at home, I consulted a string of allopathic doctors—gynecologists and experts in tropical medicine—who performed tests (even a biopsy!) to discover: nothing. Acupuncture and herbs, psychic healing, visualization soothe or irritate this blotch of red, but do not explain it or make it go away.

My women friends bring their most precious, secret, witchy salves. All these potions only inflame it.

"No, no," I say. "I can't put that on. It's like an open wound."

A wound. A sexual wound. A reminder.

For a year, because of this little patch of anger, I have had to focus on my vulva. To pay attention to it, to humor it with baking soda baths, to calm it with slippery elm at night.

Anger, and power.

I look at a photograph of a carving from a temple in India. The woman's thighs are open. From her yoni emerges a serpent. At first the thing extending from her genitals looks like a penis to me (we are so conditioned!). Then I am able to shift my perspective and recognize it as a snake coiling out. I stare. I have never seen anything like this! There is something coming out of that woman's vagina and it's not a baby!

For three years now I have not menstruated. I am a changing woman, consolidating my power. And I am angry not only at how we are treated in this twentieth century North America but at what has been stolen from us. Searching for my strength, I follow the path leading through the thicket of words in the

Women's Encyclopedia of Myths and Secrets, beginning at cunt. Yoni . . . vulva . . . kunda-lini . . . kaure . . . karuna . . . farther and farther back, to the female power, tenderness, mother love, enlightenment and sex that was the foundation of all the religions of the world. The power of the serpent coiling from the yoni.

My body speaks to me now: not with the monthly gush of blood that used to be its language, but with that mark upon my vulva, that slight discomfort all the time. Look here, it says, be here, give your attention and care.

Paw print of the animal I am. Lying in a circle of women, guided by a healer, I took a journey. We filled my body with light, and then that light-body stood up out of this flesh and went for a walk. After a number of passages and encounters I climbed a tree and ascended from its topmost branches. Up, up, infinitely light. Then, above me was a sky cave, an arch of blue. Inside it I waited, naked, for what would come.

From a narrow side cavern sounded a thudding of paws—the arrival of a being, furred and beclawed. I felt it fully—a tiger, but much larger and heavier than an ordinary big cat. Huge, muscular, it padded stealthily toward me where I sat. So big, and something strange about it. I was not so much seeing as sensing it. Something ancient. The long fangs at either side of its mouth. And I am not afraid, even though I am naked and alone here with it. I am not afraid because the tiger is me. I walk slowly, my haunches rolling from side to side. I lie down and stretch and lick my chops.

In this being there is no uncertainty.

I feel my consciousness dissolving down into every cell of my body. I am fully alive in my loins, in my legs and paws, in my tail that twitches and then curls about my body.

My genitals have changed. The hair sparser. The outer lips smaller. A friend said, "Menopause is adolescence in reverse. Remember when we got our first pubic hair, when our genitals began to develop, and our breasts?" In a sense it's like that: adolescence preparing our bodies for the sexual round, the life force throbbing in us. Menopause preparing us for independent strength, friendship with death, wisdom.

Sometimes now I watch younger people cruising and making out, and I remember the great engine of lust that used to propel me. And the many ways I used sex—with partners male and female—over the years. To express love and tenderness, for entertainment, in order to relax, to avoid something that was bothering me, to be reassured, to prove to myself that I was desirable, to make a conquest, i.e., to get someone to pay attention to me, open to me, "surrender" to me. I had sex in bedrooms, living rooms, kitchens, bathrooms, and out on the porch; on cliffs, beaches, hillsides; in boats, cars, buses. I even made passionate love to my female lover on the concrete floor of the print shop where my first book of stories was being printed. Once, in a period between "serious" partners, I had nine lovers in three months, sometimes three at a time.

Now the dust has settled. Some women experience enhanced sexual desire during menopause and after. For me, at least for the moment, the desire has cooled. And my responses have changed. I am slower to excite, and my orgasm when it comes is not that great clap of thunder that I used to experience, but a series of summer squalls that follow each other, more intense each time, as if I could go on coming forever.

Because we are obsessed with sex (we being all of us as well as American society in general), we think it unfortunate when someone is not "doing it." For myself it is a great relief not to be so motivated by lust. When I was making love a great deal, I did not ask myself about the significance of sex in my life, about how I used it, how I might go about it differently. If I felt desire, I did everything possible to satisfy that desire—without hesitation or reflection, and without regret.

The female power of the serpent curling out of the womb has everything to do with sex and nothing to do with it. It is the symbol of the material world—that which can be touched—infused with spirit, embodying spirit as the ocean is permeated by salt. It is the symbol of procreation—creation—the power to make, make new—the primordial rising up of life once more, and yet again, in all settings and against all odds. It speaks of the coming-together and the falling-apart that make our life/death, light/dark, hope/despair—essential misconceptions, for it is a continuous round of creation—its only urge: to *be*.

"Like an open wound," I had said to my friends. I dab the salve someone has brought me on my vulva, and my skin catches fire. This substance will not soothe it.

Perhaps nothing can, for it knows how little women in my time of life are appreciated, how we are denigrated and trivialized and dismissed on every side. I remember one young acquaintance who always jokingly reminds me I am "over the hill," thinking I will find this funny. I remember parties where while others, younger people, danced, I was not asked. The images in the medical magazines: wrinkled worried faces—depressed women who must be sedated; the images in the movies of bitchy controlling mothers or helpless neurotics. Everywhere the touting of youth and anorexic thinness.

Perhaps nothing can calm it for it carries in its scarlet contours the imprint of the experiences that should have brought me gently, joyfully to womanhood and instead propelled me into a certain disillusioned opting-out of life.

Surely it remembers the first clumsy making-love. In the fifties most of us did not have sex until we were twenty or more. I waited until I was 21, and then did it with a boyfriend who had been trying to seduce me for a year, and whom

I liked in a sisterly way. On the appointed afternoon we went to the apartment of a friend of his. And all the way there he told me how experienced he was. But when we had taken off our clothes and assumed the missionary position, he could not get his cock to become hard. He had a cold, he told me; this always happened to him when he had a cold. Embarrassed, he gingerly fingered his penis (I beginning to wonder *what* I was doing there!), and finally he was hard enough to enter me and after a few thrusts, to ejaculate, and sink in relief onto me. Lying under his inert body, I felt sore, and disappointed.

When we had put on our clothes, he fixed me with suddenly timid eyes and said, "I have something to tell you. Actually it was the first time for me too."

Now I laugh when I think of that. But my 21-year-old self did not laugh.

Was I mad at him for lying to me? he asked. I said no, withdrawing back into a place in myself where it did not matter.

Now I am so angry that I didn't know I deserved better than that! I replay the scene, leaping from the bed to yell at him, running from the room and going somewhere—beneath a tree—to sob out my grief at this botched initiation. (And only now can I imagine a different scenario, in which he is honest with me and we slowly explore each other, admitting our shared innocence, until desire grows in us and coitus comes from our care-ful-ness with each other.)

A few years later, there was the older male lover who turned out to be married, who drove me to motels and banged away at me, rarely taking the time to excite me sufficiently first. This one I loved, and he said he loved me. But he was always *at* me; I had no space in which to experience my feelings for him and express them. How embarrassing to admit I chose him because he was as self-centered, as demanding as my father. And I was ashamed of our liaisons in the motels, cringing before the eyes of the desk clerks. Some months of this left me empty and scared.

It is a rainy cold day in the mountains. I lie in a motel bed, a 23-year-old woman, staring at the door that has just slammed behind this man. Because I wasn't ready for sex, because I needed to touch and talk first, he threw on his clothes and went storming out into the rain, saying I do not love him. The scent of wet leaves enters to fill the room. Rain taps at the window. I am so alone here, and so empty.

Now as my 52-year-old self I enter the doorway through which he has left. Without judgment, I offer my comfort. Can this young self let me hold her, let me honor her worth, let me soothe her? She is too tightly pulled back into herself to trust me. I see this will take work: my steady caring, my returning to offer what comfort I can. But eventually she will heal, for somewhere in her she knew all along that he was full of shit. She *let* it happen to her, she fought him by withdrawing, she told herself he was the love of her life. (For this short time she married her daddy, just to see how it would feel.) And she was puzzled by how he treated her, as if she didn't matter. But in some deep secret part of herself she knew that he was wrong about her, that she was a loving, sexual being who deserved to be respected. When he left she suffered terribly, but she only briefly considered following him, for she knew to do so would be to choose death.

A week ago I had my fingerprints taken. The prints came out light and blurred. And the man taking them asked me, "Do you work with paper?" I answered yes, and he explained that what binds the wood pulp of paper together is clay, and that prolonged rubbing with clay smooths off the ridges on our skin. Writers, printers, potters—we are physically changed by our trades.

I liked that. It felt honest to me—the wearing down of the body by what we do. And the smoothing out of that mark of uniqueness. Perhaps one day, if I live long enough, my finger pads will have no roughness, like the rubbery flesh of a sea creature.

As we become more deeply ourselves, some of our persona, our individuality, falls away. I feel I am burning up the dross now. We begin by knowing who we are, then very early the institutions of patriarchy—the nuclear family, the schools, the media, the church—begin to deny what we know and fill us up with pictures of what we should be: docile industrious student, docile efficient secretary/nurse/waitress/maid, aggressive junior exec who docilely plays the boys' game, docile attractive wife and self-sacrificing mother. We learn to deny our wildness, our sexuality, our truth, as we accumulate whole worlds of experience and knowledge which only weigh us down and obscure the nature of who we are. Now I am burning through that mass of matter to emerge as my true self—the one who knew in her heart that her insensitive lover was full of shit. The one who came finally to loving women, and experienced the healing of passionately reciprocal sex for many years. The one who struggles to know herself wholly.

In the last three-year period I wrote a book about American women's participation in Buddhist practice. In my first draft I was careful, in several places I tempered my words, I held back some things I wished to say. But during that time I became fifty years old. It was a momentous shift—that I marked as joyously as I could—and I understood, Now I must say *exactly* what I mean. No more temporizing, no more holding back. I know important things because I have experienced them and learned from other women in the political and spiritual and personal work we have done together. I do not need to apologize for or soften these truths. I need only state them as clearly as possible—and others can do what they will with them.

So I rewrote the book, burning away all the mealy-mouthing and letting the true voice of what I know ring through.

Not twenty feet away, the waters of the lake sloshed rhythmically against the jungly shore. I sat on the verandah in the afternoon, the tropical heat like a heavy damp blanket on me. Most of the other novice nuns were sleeping, I knew, except Vasantha, the Sri Lankan woman, who was more pious than us Westerners. She sat reading a Buddhist tract on the porch next to mine.

As usual, I was studying. A stack of books lay next to my low wood and wicker chair. A volume of verses by the first Buddhist nuns, *Philosophies of India* by Heinrich Zimmer, a thick statistic-studded tome on the economics of the Third World, other Buddhist volumes, a book of collected short stories just for balance. In the silence and enclosure of the Nuns Island (no electricity, radio, TV, phone), I could spend hours reading and thinking. And gradually it became clear to me that when I returned to the United States I wanted to pursue Buddhist studies, comparative religion and women's spirituality, and to attempt to make some synthesis of them. This study and the book I would write would trace the attitudes to sex in religion and mine the world religions for any remaining practices and ideas which honor the female and the body. I thought particularly of Tantra, of the Gnostic gospels, of the Shekinah in Hebrew lore.

This intention formed itself at the same time as the red paw print began to burn on my vulva. I conceived this next task, and was marked. When I returned to the States, in the midst of the distractions of life in Oakland, I tried to wiggle out of this task I had set myself. I let time pass, I thought of reasons why going to school was not practical. But my lover reminded me of the clarity I had achieved in Sri Lanka, the intimacy with my true desire.

Some themes or threads carry through in our lives whether we notice them or not. Always I have been fascinated by sex. In a college Chaucer class I did a report on Courtly Love, not knowing that in this convention of the Middle Ages poets passed on pre-Christian tales and worshipped the Goddess in women. I only knew the phenomenon drew me powerfully. Some years ago I wrote a story about a woman's encounter with a bear in the Sierras, in which she is attacked by the bear but survives, and lives to remember the bear's being merged with hers. Story of an initiation, wherein death came close. More recently, at the urging of an editor, I wrote an erotic story. It began simply, as a litany of desire, but led unexpectedly to a Buddhist center, where the two female characters make love to each other in a meditation room below the image of a dancing goddess. When I read over this story it seemed to me that what I had done was to place female eroticism in direct challenge to patriarchal religion. Now this mark upon my vulva has brought me to a group of women learning to develop their female energy with a guide who grounds our primal power in the menstrual process.

In the meantime, I have started the masters program at a school of theology which also offers a program in Buddhist studies and the opportunity to work independently with a women's spirituality teacher in the community.

At moments I am amazed, when I look at the woman with the snake coming out of her vagina, to think I have arrived here at the willingness to fully acknowledge my female power. This is taking me deep. Suddenly I encounter my terror that I am not smart enough, articulate enough, to do this intellectual work, that I will be shamed before my fellow students. Crying, listening, I hear my father's voice, his telling me that everything I did was wrong, that I was not competent, intelligent, articulate. His saying that to do really well in school was to indicate that one was socially maladjusted.

Why should this old old voice speak up now! This questioning I thought I had confronted and put to rest long ago, had worked out in years of living, and some intensive therapy, with much accomplishment in writing and publishing and editing, with never any particular mystification of academic people or situations, or any particular fear of them. But here it is!

Now that the crying, the admitting, is over, I see that to begin to acknowledge my power—to act it out in the world—is to rouse the paternal shade, the great NO. He rises up to oppose me. He tells me I am stupid, I cannot talk, I cannot think. He says, You must do well, but you are not capable of doing well. He says, It is not graceful or feminine to be really good at anything. He says, I won't love you if you come fully into yourself. I want you partial. I want you silent.

It is my own voice, adopting the worst of my father. My own demon raging at the gate, defying me to enter! But the paw print there in my most secret recesses reminds me I am a tiger embarked upon this journey of the body and spirit. I'll do whatever I must to go past the demon, to speak my anger, own my sexual wounds, step fully into my old/new self.

GROWING PAINS

Louise Mancuso

Summer of 1988. I couldn't bear to have the sun touch my skin. Me, of Mediterranean Italian-American descent, who lived in Hawaii for seven years, stayed out in the sun all day long as a matter of form, and lived for a time in the California desert. Me, one of the original sun worshippers, and I couldn't stand, even for a few minutes, waiting outside for the bus—the two buses needed each way—to take me back and forth to work. And that, one of the hottest summers on record, was the year the air-conditioning in the buses broke down. That was the year I wondered why there weren't massive nationwide riots; why the newspapers weren't filled with accounts of people—especially menopausal bus-riding women in Madison—who seemed to suddenly go berserk, strangling, bludgeoning, maiming whoever happened to be near them when their, yes, *runaway hormones* took the express elevator up their backs, chests and necks, straight on through to the tops of their heads. Several years before, I had been corresponding with another woman writer who was a little older than myself, and who, between the pages of writing talk, inserted the line, "I feel like the top of my head is coming off." I didn't know what she meant, and when I wrote back and asked about it, I received no answer. I don't blame her. How does one write or talk about these things to those who haven't, or won't ever, experience them?

I think of my mother, raging around the house, pale, wide-eyed, yelling at the top of her lungs at my brother and me. We were used to being yelled at, but not like this. This was something different.

"What's the matter, Ma?" I asked her, totally mystified. "What's wrong?"

She stops, looks at me. "I'm sick," she says, putting her hand to her head. "I don't feel good."

"But what's wrong, Ma? Do you have a cold, the flu? What is it?" She stops her pacing, looks at me, opens her mouth ready to offer an explanation, then shakes her head and goes back into the bedroom. She ended up having a hysterectomy in her late 30s. The rages stopped, but she had some not so pleasant side-effects due to the operation: trouble with her bladder and bowel, and the nagging regret she didn't at least have one more child before the operation made it a definite impossibility.

My periods had always been regular: every 28 days, one day late maybe, every once-in-a-while. No missed periods, ever, no matter how much stress I was under. And it always followed the same pattern: some bloating and irritability the day before, a definite signal my period was imminent; slow-starting bleeding and real bad take-to-my-bed cramps the first day; then a day of heavy flow; slower, less the third day; kept a pad on the fourth day for the last brownish smudgings.

Then, in my late 30s, the pattern switched to every 26 days. This was the first big noticeable change in my menstrual cycle. After that, other changes in my body began to occur more rapidly. I was living in Germany at the time, working on a novel, involved in a relationship with a woman ten years my junior. She had left her previous relationship with a woman two or three years older than myself. "Her body is so hot I can't touch her," she told me.

"Maybe she's in her menopause," I said. "Maybe she's having hot flushes."

"No no," my friend stated. "She is this way all the time."

The first years we were together was a time of passionate love-making. A friend would call in the early afternoon on a Saturday or Sunday, and be surprised to find us in bed, having continued our love-making from where we left off the night before.

"Still?" the friend would say. "It's almost a year, and still it is like this?"

My period was coming every 24 days now, and would keep this up for several months, then not come at all for the next two or three months. At this time, too, after I turned 40, I experienced about a week of aching breasts; I couldn't bear for them to be touched, and couldn't get comfortable in bed. I didn't get concerned about it as I figured it was just one more way my body was changing, and I remembered how the same kind of thing had happened to me as a pre-teen. My immature breasts had begun to ache so much I broke down and told my mother, thinking something must have been terribly wrong. Her reaction was to laugh and say, "Oh those are just growing pains."

"What do you mean growing pains? Am I getting taller?" More cause for merriment.

"It's time for your first bra," she said.

So the aches stopped then, and they stopped this time too. And yes, just as those first aches came as a sign of the impending blossoming of my breasts, these last came as a signal that another change was taking place in them.

"I love the way your breasts are so compact and stand out firm against your body," one of my former lovers used to say. She admired that particular aspect of my body as her own breasts were fuller and heavier, and I suppose it may have been a matter of "the grass is always greener . . ." So my chest muscles have relaxed a little. No big deal. I've gotten no complaints, and it sure doesn't bother me.

When I left Germany—and the relationship—in 1981, after two-and-a-half years, I had a mostly-completed novel in hand, and an appointment with a literary agent in New York City. Arriving by cab in Manhattan, after the long flight from Munich, I rented a room at the YWCA. No sooner had I managed to get my toiletries unpacked, when I felt something dribbling down my legs. I had a super Kotex pad on, since my period had decided to come the day I left Munich—something I certainly could have done without during that emotionally trying time. Never before had one pad not proven sufficient in taking care of even my heaviest flow. I pulled my jeans and underpants down to check on the pad, and oh Lord, the deluge came. Grabbing for another pad, I stuffed the already soaked-through one back in place. I was dripping all over the floor, and knew there was no way I would make it down the hall to the bathroom. Only one thing to do: maneuvering a chair in front of the tiny sink in the room, I climbed up on it. Startled roaches scattered everywhere as I settled my bottom, as gingerly as I could over the sink, and let the red river flow. What a time for such a thing to happen. What a time for me to have an appointment with the Senior Vice-president of one of the top New York literary agencies.

I meet her. We talk. She is open, pleasant. I want out of there. I want to go back to Hawaii, lie out in the sun, think of nothing but blue sky and blessed palm trees swaying in the breeze. I need an emotional, physical, and financial bailout. Thankfully, an aunt wires money for a bus ticket, and I and my boxes of belongings spend three days traveling cross-country to California. The agent will read the manuscript; I will spend the next several months alone at my aunt and uncle's house in the high desert, completing the last three chapters of the book. It is the Thanksgiving and Christmas holiday season, and I am in my glory. Nothing to think about but my writing; no one to keep me company but the three dogs from the next house over, and the TV set.

My stay at the house is up. The chapters have been sent off.

I am now 42, working for room and board and a little money at an Inn, situated on an oasis, in the middle of the desert. I am taking a shower one morning, and my hair comes out by the handful. This happens for several weeks, and I fear I'm going to end up completely bald.

43. I am in Wisconsin, staffing a Women's Center in a small town, part-time; in a relationship with a woman 18 years younger than myself. It is the dead of winter; a cold cold day as I walk to the Center's office, located in a house used by the Lutheran Campus Ministry. They have graciously donated the space. I am bundled in my dark blue, hooded parka, sweater underneath, a red-and-black scarf tied around my neck. I am walking into the wind, my cheeks tingling, my nose and forehead on the brink of freezing. I am suddenly hot. My

back and chest are on fire, perspiration soaking through my tee-shirt and sweater. I undo my scarf, unzip my parka. I continue walking, gasping for breath, then feel cold again, zip up. I have no idea why this happened. Perhaps I am rushing too much, afraid I'm going to be late? I simply got over-heated? I don't think about it any more, until it happens again, and again, and again, on subsequent days.

OK OK. So maybe it's hot flushes. (I like to call them "flushes" rather than "flashes" because my back and chest and face flush red, and, while for me it only lasts for a minute or two—like a "flash"—there are women I know who hardly experience a time when they are not having these red hot flushes.)

44. My lover touches my nipple when we are in bed. I flinch.

"What's the matter?" she asks.

I shake my head. "It's okay. My nipples just feel a little sore." She lies back on her pillow. Next morning I notice my nipples look unusually red and dry. I had been using baby oil as a moisturizer over other parts of my body for some time. Now I make it part of my routine to run oiled hands up my breasts. It seems to help.

Thanksgiving. I feel horrible. My period has come with cramps and achiness and the feeling that my head is coming off. My partner/lover is planning on having her younger sister, and her sister's boyfriend, over for dinner. I want no part of it. I want quiet. I want to be left alone. I will not take part in the doings, I tell her. I will be upstairs in my room.

They come. The radio is turned on. It feels like the walls of the house are reverberating with the sound, though I know the radio's not on that high. I come out of my room, go half-way down the stairs, and ask that the radio be turned down. They comply. I go back to bed. A favorite song must have come on, for the volume seems to have been turned up again a few minutes later. My head is pounding. I go to the stairs, call down. No one hears me. I call louder. Still no one hears. I am frantic. I rage in expletives. The sister comes to the stairs, retreats in horror.

They are quieter. Eat. Go home early. I have mystified and scared them. I am mystified and scared myself. I do not want to behave this way, yet I do not want to see a doctor, do not want to take medication or hormonal replacement; will not even consider a hysterectomy. I choose—as my way of dealing with this turn of events—to stay away from dealing with others as much as possible. I am no longer effective in my work at the Center, no longer have the enthusiasm and energy and patience for it, nor for dealing with an intimate relationship. My time at the Center ends. So does the relationship.

I move to Madison, into a rambling old house with four lesbian-feminist women who accept me as their fifth housemate. I have a large sunny room to myself. There is an ample kitchen, living room, dining room. I tell them I keep mostly to myself; not to worry if they don't happen to see me for days at a time.

I come and go, working part-time for an 80-year-old retired librarian as a companion-aide. She only needs someone to come in three days a week for four hours, to grocery shop, do some light cleaning, help with the laundry, cut the grass in summer, shovel snow in winter. The rest of the time I write, read, listen to the radio, watch TV. I am content to be with myself. Helen, the woman, understands when I tell her I have my "good" days and "bad" days, even though she doesn't ever remember experiencing menopausal symptoms herself. She tells me to call her when I am not feeling up to coming. We can always change the days she tells me. If not today, then tomorrow. We work my schedule around this. I feel blessed knowing her, and being able to work this way. I come to understand now how terribly difficult it must be for menopausal women—experiencing extreme symptoms—having to try and deal with husband/partner, children, job, all the day-to-day situations that constantly demand their attention and energies, leaving them no time to be off on their own to care for themselves, or, dare they hope, have *their* needs recognized and taken into consideration?

After two years, Helen discovers a lump in one of her breasts. Her doctor confirms the finding, and she and her son decide it best to have the entire breast removed. Her limited energy has been on a decline. The surgery in October, and a fall in the garden the following June, when she damaged some vertebrae, does not help. Helen, preparing for death, goes to live with her son and his wife in Oklahoma the latter part of August. The following January we have lost her.

I am 47. Working with the Madison Adult Day Care Centers, I learn more now about the "frail elderly," see myself in them in twenty or thirty more years. I am protective towards them, beginning to feel my own frailties, seeing what it's like to not be able to perform even the most private of physical functions without help. I recognize my limitations, take them into consideration in my day-to-day living. There is no one to please but myself, and I experience joy in bringing some mode of comfort and kindliness to the women and men who come to spend some time at the Center. I see what a hardship it is for spouse, son/daughter, having to care for a loved one who is mentally/physically incapacitated to some degree, and realize what a blessing it is for them to have some respite provided by the Center and its truly caring staff. I see, also, how "burned out" the full-time staff can get, and protect myself from being overwhelmed by gradually cutting down my hours, and finally, quitting altogether, and taking another one-on-one part-time companion-aide job, through an agency, working with Beda, a retired high school History teacher.

49. In talking with Beda during our walks, and while sitting by the lake, I find out she wasn't aware of going through menopause in her 40s and 50s.

"I used to feel hot sometimes," she tells me, "but I thought it was just the stove, or where I was standing in the classroom. I would take my jacket or sweater off when I felt hot, then put it on again when I was cold." At age 88 she still gets the flushes, mostly feeling heat suddenly on her back.

50. It has been three years since my last period, six years since my last relationship. I still have hot flushes, but they have diminished in intensity. And, oh glory, I have been enjoying lying out in the sun again this summer, something I hadn't been able to do for the last couple of years. My skin feels prickly every once-in-a-while, and in the mornings, when I first get up, my bones and muscles ache, my fingers feel sore and stiff. I flex them on rising as I make my way into the bathroom, then the kitchen to put the coffee water on. The stiffness works its way out within minutes, and I take delight in my body's recuperative powers. I am constant in my work with Beda, never having to call in sick or take an extra day off. I attend a five-day conference in June, use that as my vacation. I meet other writers, publishers. I know how to take care of myself when the flushes come. Jacket on, jacket off. Sip of cold water. A piece of hard candy to suck on if I get the kind of flush where I feel my head is coming off. For some reason the candy seems to help this particular symptom, and I have found this especially useful when I am riding the bus.

All in all, I have to say that my body has served me well all these years, and is continuing to do so. I will care for it in the ways I feel are best, and take care to be aware of other women who may be going through the same kinds of things. I marvel at woman's tenacity and endurance, at our patience and self-discipline in this, perhaps the most strenuous of times. I am thankful for being on this earth, and grateful for those who have shared their lives with me, for even the shortest of moments.

ANNUNCIATIONS, OCTOBER

Elisavietta Ritchie

As she waits, she gathers tomatoes,
eggs from the snowy hens,

plums from the tree
she planted at seventeen.

The sea smells of flounder and crab.
Her house smells of basil and yeast.

Spiders have woven together
the corners of rooms,

katydids whirr emerald songs,
crickets sing in the cracks.

The younger man comes down the road
with a basket of peaches and wine.

One string hangs from her mandolin:
he winds it around the peg.

They cross the yard. Leaves spiral,
catch on zinnias, jimson weed.

He bails the old boat in the sand
with the shell of a horseshoe crab.

High tide. They sail from the cove
ignoring the squall and rising bilge.

All day his eyes speak
of desire and regret.

All night in the waves
she dreams: after years

a bright rush of blood,
new songs on the mandolin.

SEX, SIGHS AND MEDIA-HYPE

Jill Jeffery Ginghofer

I

These days I am reluctant to make love, but when I do, everything else—children, money, work, gravity—drifts away. My body draws all of my thoughts, the space between my toes, my mouth, nipples, thighs, into one keen place, trembles there, trills. This is wonderful, I think. I must be mad not to do this every night.

After a while, I become aware that my hip aches. It is, after all, a 54-year-old hip. Gently I initiate the final moves in the familiar ballet. Mind and body turn, listen for the approaching flood, split slowly open . . . coming through, catching and sinking into weight, skin, comforter and sleep.

When I awaken it takes me a moment or two to remember why I feel all is right with the world. That was good, I think, but I won't need to do it again for a decade or two. When I was twenty, thirty, even forty, I always remembered, and with the remembering was ready again, and again.

I come to menopause with a long-term sexual partner, someone with whom I feel comfortable and with whom I have orgasms within intercourse. Perhaps I no longer want sex more often than once a week because of the length of our relationship, though I attribute it to a waning libido, and there is some evidence to support this theory.

In *Menopause: A Complete Medical Report*, Pat Phillips states, "(After menopause) the ovaries . . . produce . . . estrogen in amounts so minute they have little if any physiological effects." A survey by Dr. Niles Newton of Northwestern Medical School reveals 60% of women who had hysterectomy with removal of their ovaries experienced a reduced sex drive and 40% never resumed sexual intercourse. As Florence King says in "Benched," (*Ms.*, May 1989), "At 53, I know I'm supposed to repeat the requisite chant, 'I didn't get older, I got better' but . . . I haven't felt a trace of horniness since completing the menopause." Indications are that most women will have a lower sex drive after menopause than they did at 25, and even less at age 75.

My friends report similar experiences. Divorced at 32 and since involved with many partners, Louise at 51 wrote, "My menopause complete, I haven't wanted sex for months and doubt I shall again. Never again shall I take a man's penis into my mouth, have his shoes under my bed. I cannot tell you the relief, the freedom, the wholeness of being that thought gives me." Louise reneged once in the past six years, and then only after a 90-mile-an-hour hurricane blasted her house. "This event excited me no end. Within five hours I had parted my thighs for Michael who clambered out on the roof and, buffeted by winds, secured the skylight."

Joan, who went through a reasonably easy, natural menopause between the ages of 40 and 45, at 55 can scarcely recognize men as human beings. I watched her recently when an attractive man greeted us at a restaurant table, saw her eye the white shirt, the lock of hair over the eye, listen to the deep voice with wonder, as if she weren't sure what world he came from. (This is the Joan who, years before, when a contractor sent four men to tear out her old bathroom, had gleefully commented, "I'd already slept with three of them—not a bad average!") The man walked away, puzzling over his apparent lack of appeal. Joan is, after all, a very attractive woman. But she was oblivious, already immersed in conversation about cats and our children's future prospects.

Sara is reasonably happily married, but she and her husband are at their most intimate huddled companionably over morning tea planning their day. They have not made love in years, something observation reveals is more prevalent than the media or psychologists ever state. However, women rarely comment on abstinence. I suspect we are inhibited about exposing lack of sexual potency in male partners and in ourselves.

On the other hand, Beverly, a beautiful woman in her late sixties, confides, "I love sex and it gets better the older I get." An audience containing young women always responds, "Beverly, you're wonderful." Who can bear to think, in full youthful hormonal longing, that one's sexuality can diminish? And perhaps Beverly *is* being truthful. I do know that Laura, the mother of a friend, had her first truly sexual relationship at the age of seventy.

There are other reasons why we are less likely to have sexual relationships as we age. It is not always possible for an older woman to have a sexual partner. Husbands die or move on to younger women and many women face the prospect of being either self-sexual or non-sexual. The media, with its emphasis on young, reproductive women, denies us the ability to envisage ourselves as sexually deserving. One of my friends says she will not have a sexual relationship again because she could not bear for anyone to see the dimples in her thighs nor to discover her teeth are no longer real.

There are powerful forces that inhibit confession of loss of interest in sex. In *All About Hysterectomy*, a doctor states, "Women who claim their interest in sex has vanished . . . are subsequently proven by psychologists to have disliked their husbands for years." And another says in *The Castrated Woman*, "Intelligent women don't fantasize depression and loss of sexual drive."

The truth that I observe of all my women friends and many of my male friends, is that we become less sexual as we age. I don't believe this loss entirely negative. When asked by a younger man if he missed being potent, Sophocles replied, "Absolutely not! It's wonderful: like being released from bondage to a raving madman."

Under the influence of the full flush of hormones, many women lose the sense of separate-self. In that vulnerability, boundaries melt between themselves and those they love, and they find themselves giving up personal dreams. For these women, a reduced libido in middle-age can leave room for more creative and individual fulfillment.

For myself, I believe there is a vitality in continuing to be sexually active. However, by insisting that our sex drive need not change as we age, we probably deny reality, and continue to emphasize women as sexual and reproductive, rather than as multi-faceted, human beings.

II

At 37, I tested positive for cervical cancer, the average age of death for reproductive women before the introduction of hysterectomy. My uterus and cervix were removed, my ovaries left in place. The surgeon assured me neither my hormone production nor my sex life would be affected. Lying in bed after surgery, waves of tingling dry heat moved slowly down my body and felt ecstatic. When I told my doctor, he replied, "Those were hot flashes. Sometimes the hormone system is depressed after surgery and you experience menopausal symptoms." He hadn't mentioned this before the operation. Later I discovered my orgasms were different; did not produce so much heat, were not drawn so deeply inside me.

For most of my life I listened, mystified, whenever anyone talked about depression: it was beyond my ken. Four years after surgery I began to feel as if my soul was dragging through mud. On the surface, I cheerfully continued to care for three young children, a household, a husband, but once the children were in bed, I would break down and sob. One morning I discovered the first iris of the season had opened. In the past, the sight of its fluttering blue-purple petals, its erect and exposed organs brushed with orange, its light liquorice fragrance, would fill me with the certainty that all was right with the world. Now it didn't move me at all. I was in deep trouble.

A test revealed my hormone level was low and I decided to risk the side effects and take estrogen. The hormone had an immediate sweetening effect on my life, though I suspect it has only muffled, not assuaged, the anxiety. I've been on low doses of estrogen ever since. Because of this, it's been difficult for me to gauge my journey through menopause.

In my late 40s I started having disturbed nights. At first I thought they were caused by a conflict with one of my teenagers, but they persisted. I would fall asleep naturally and awake anytime after 1:30 a.m., my brain spiralling downward. *What have I done with my life? What will I live on when I'm old? Will the children ever be able to afford housing?* Just as I sank back into sleep, my husband, awakened by my anxious starts, would have to go to the toilet. Our nights became an ordeal, jostling one another on the way to the bathroom muttering "You woke me up," until we solved the problem by sleeping in separate rooms. When I awoke in the night, I could read without disturbing him. No matter how little I slept, the next day I'd go to work, run the household, but without the energy to give life the keen edge of change or surprise.

After three years of sleep loss, I found a nurse practitioner specializing in menopause, who listed insomnia as the second most common symptom. I was amazed. I'd read books on menopause, consulted with doctors, discussed it with any woman willing to talk, but no one had mentioned sleeplessness before. Now I rarely find a menopausal woman who doesn't suffer sleep disturbance. I became aware that I often wo're because I was too hot, learned to keep cool, as well as to use earplugs, the occasional aspirin or over-the-counter sleep tablet, and sometimes masturbation, until gradually I began to sleep more.

Naively, I was not prepared for depression or sleep loss. It's true, our mothers and grandmothers told us they experienced disturbing symptoms, but modern authorities dismissed their stories as old wives' tales. However, the truths they passed down are not to be denied. Women in menopause *do* have mental breakdowns. A childhood friend's mother inexplicably stole a pen from Woolworth's and was placed in a mental asylum. In the early 1960s, Frances, older than I, was sent to psychiatrists—not specialists in menopausal symptoms— and, believing she was crazy, took an overdose of sleeping pills. Recently, Jennie's 15-year-old daughter had to sign her into a mental institution, though Jennie has since come back into the world and, apart form chronic forgetfulness, appears to be all right.

Wistfully, I wish I could have experienced a natural menopause, as current treatments for cervical cancer would allow. I plan to try to wean myself from estrogen replacement therapy at 56, the age most women in my family start menopause, and allow myself to experience whatever happens, perhaps find some of that illusive zest Margaret Mead suggested was the reward for coming out on the other side.

III

Nearly all the books written on menopause by both men and women insist that if we eat well, exercise prodigiously, and keep a positive attitude we will sail through without negative symptoms. *The Menopause Time of Life* (U.S. Department of Health and Human Services, 1986) clearly states, "80% of women experience mild or no signs of menopause . . ." Most of us, I suspect, are jostling for a foothold on the remaining 20% of the island. It's what I call the "Buck up Syndrome" of writing for women. Before I had my first child, I devoured books that assured me that if only I panted correctly, I would experience no pain in childbirth. (At the time I had not seriously considered the size of a baby's head.) Of course, when it hurt I knew it must be my fault. Now, when I awaken in the night burning with dry heat, I know it's because I took up chocolate and not tennis in my 40s.

Magazines continuously encourage us to diet, despite the fact that hormones are stored in fat and the bones of heavier women are not so prone to osteoporosis. Television and films feature only those older women who are thin and youthful-looking. Women who can afford it, especially those working in the media, undergo face lifts, breast and buttock surgery, liposuction, rib removal, lip puffs, and the electronic removal of hair from the top of the forehead to create the extended dome of a young child, all in order to continue being accepted as young and sexual. In a society that chooses to view women primarily as sexual beings, if we do not present ourselves as sexual, then we cannot be seen. In *The Summer Before the Dark,* Doris Lessing's heroine, who suddenly experiences herself as middle-aged, felt "as if all her life she had been held aloft by the notice of other people as a flower is held up by water in its stamen, and now that water had been drained away."

Even *Lear's*, a magazine directed at older women, features beautiful women on the cover and articles that emphasize success. Few women over 45 can sensibly envision taking up acting or dance as a career, nor become successful designers. A friend from Europe recently remarked, "No wonder Americans appear petulant. With the emphasis on youth, beauty, and wealth, your media is designed to make most people feel bad about themselves." Hopefully, the recently-formed organizations that watch the media will one day exert enough influence to allow all of us to be accepted, if not celebrated, in advertising and other media venues.

IV

It's important to acknowledge our absolute uniqueness. Human women are the only creatures on earth who have menopause. In all other species, the female reproduces until she dies. (A recent study indicates the possibility that whales might experience menopause, though this is unconfirmed.) There has to be a reason, some marvelous and ancient necessity, why human females survive their reproductive cycle. Few scientific studies have attempted to find out why this is so and none have reached any conclusion. In many societies outside of the West, the older generation of women and sometimes men take care of children, considering them the gift of old age, thus liberating the adult genera-tion to focus on food production. Perhaps that's why we're needed. I'd like to think it was our wisdom that is sought, though I'm not aware of anyone asking for it, nor of many older women with the self-esteem left to proffer it.

Fortunately, we do not all have the same reaction to menopause. I have two widowed aunts who feel that their lives began after menopause. One had a depressed thyroid that righted itself as her body changed, and at 75 she swims, dances and has bountiful, high spirits. The other was literally ill for two weeks of every menstrual cycle until rescued by menopause. Now, at 84, she's county Scrabble champion. However, we will never understand and cope with menopausal symptoms if the truths of our experience are sacrificed to theories. Menopause has been largely ignored by scientific and cultural researchers. Hopefully this will be rectified and answers found to both the mystery and the complications that can follow in its wake.

My body had done disturbing things in menopause: bled uncontrollably; denied me sleep for years; caused me to cry in a sadness so deep and perplexing that it cannot be articulated. After puberty I seemed to be searching for the young girl who once had felt clear and strong. Now I have to learn to give up the vulnerable, melting self, and hopefully become lusty of mind and will for the journey to come.

TOFU AND TEQUILA

Dena Taylor

My daughters and I had a solstice celebration this past winter, during which we talked about the previous year and what we wanted for the coming one. I said I planned to take it easy, that I was going through some changes and needed to recognize that. The girls reminded me that I had said the same to them when they were going through the beginnings of menstruation. "You don't have to decide the direction of your life right now," I'd tell them. And now I'm saying that to myself.

The girls are very aware of what's going on with my menopause, and they tease me about throwing open the doors and windows, going around in a tank top in the middle of winter, and losing things. Once, when to everyone's amazement I was actually cold, my sixteen-year-old looked at me incredulously and said, "Have a hot flash, Mom!"

She wrote me a poem on my last birthday:

> As we watch you hunt for your keys
> We wonder what the next stage is going to bring
> Will your clothes turn to shades of
> electric pink and green, wild blues and
> yellows, and extravagant colors never before worn?
> Or will your hot flashes heat up
> And we'll soon move to the boonies where
> you can sleep out every night

We laugh about it, but even so, some of the time, it's no fun. I wonder, though, if this is a privileged way of going through menopause? If I were in Central America, the mother of a disappeared child, would I be feeling any menopausal symptoms?

I understand nothing, feel everything. I am wise. I am silly, often teary and goose bumpy over the most amazing things. I want a lover. I want to be alone. I feel strong, yet afraid of death. I don't put up with any crap. I am not sure where I am going. Words from a blues song stick in my mind: "My brain is cloudy and my soul is upside down."

Women often say they are shocked when they look in the mirror, feeling the same as always yet seeing an old woman. But I am not shocked. I expect to see changes. I look at my mother and know I will become like her, and that is fine with me. She is beautiful.

I can't put just anything into my body anymore without feeling its effects. Alcohol, caffeine, and rich foods are likely to result in sweaty sleepless nights. So I decide whether it's worth it, and sometimes it is. I've changed the way I eat (less of the offending items) and exercise (now I do some), and that feels good, but haven't entirely cut out my old pleasures. I now enjoy both tofu and tequila.

And sex. Sometimes I think about it, want it, try to set something up. And then, surprisingly, might lose interest. And then, surprised again, find myself looking at men of all ages!

Once, during what I now realize was the beginning of my menopause, I spent a wonderfully sexy week with a lover. From our porch we watched the ocean's soft and powerful swells, and our bodies matched its rhythm. We drank the local rum, smoked pakalolo, and knew this was the end of our relationship. We would soon be living in different parts of the world. On the last day I had my first menopausal flood. The rushing blood would not stop. I'd no sooner get the bathroom cleaned up when I'd have to start mopping it up again."Are you all right?" We were supposed to be getting the house ready for the next guests.

"Oh yes, I'm just cleaning the bathroom," I cheerfully called out.

"Oh. I've done the rest of the house. We can leave when you're ready."

I left a trail of blood from Maui to San Francisco.

Then followed a long period of celibacy, until I met a young artist. I was definitely ready for sex again. In anticipation, I carefully get together some old roaches and scrapings for a skinny joint, and tear off a foil-wrapped condom from the string of them in the box (it's cheaper to buy in bulk), just in case those last-to-leave eggs are still fertile.

We have some brandy and the joint, he lies down on the rug, does a few yoga stretches, then takes out his penis and plays with it.

Oh my. Well, you get what you ask for, I guess. I snuggle down with him and he says, "I've been wanting to do this with you. Come on top of me and . . ."

"And what?"

"Put me inside you."

So I do it. Or try to. It seems he has already come. I'm rather disappointed but know these things happen, so I say to myself, well, as long as he doesn't go to sleep now. Which he does. I decide it's too damn cold in his room and I really don't want to be there. I dress in the darkness and leave.

When I get home I see that my underpants are backwards and my pants inside out. I laugh. I laugh at myself for taking things seriously. And then I have a hot flash.

THE LAST CYCLE OF THE MOON

Nancy Mathews

When I hear moon cycles and women spoken in the same breath, I think of my history of menses from puberty to menopause. Life after menses continues but I wasn't taught about that in school where we giggled over plain brown covered booklets titled *The Facts About Reproduction* and *Feminine Hygiene*. My mother didn't share with me what life would be like after the child-bearing years were over. And would I have listened? She had a hysterectomy at forty-four and I, at eighteen, thought she was old.

Carrying four children in my belly, over a thirteen-year period, didn't prepare me for this time in my life. I read the articles in *Good Housekeeping* and *Ladies' Home Journal*, but they weren't written for me. I was different and much admired by my younger friends because I didn't have night sweats, debilitating headaches, hysterics. I took my calcium and vitamin E. I practiced yoga and went on long walks in the park.

Friends my age didn't want to talk about "the change," unless they had serious complaints which were diagnosed as menopausal and were the cause of their hysterectomies. I refused to believe the old wives' tales of diminished sex drive, unbearable depression and the end of an active and fruitful life.

I was too immersed in survival. At fifty, I divorced the father of my four children. My husband was between business deals and for the first time found himself with free time to think about what he wanted out of life. He wanted an "open marriage" which was a popular media subject in the seventies. I felt threatened but agreed to give it a try. I didn't meet any eligible men, but he found many women who admired his boyish charm and charismatic personality. My husband proceeded to lie, which was the antithesis of an "open marriage," about his affairs. He told me I was crazy when I confronted him with my doubts and fears. Fortunately having had many years of therapy, I knew my intuitions were correct.

That was the most devastating year of my life. The children, who ranged from twenty-five to twelve years old, didn't think I could survive the pain and humiliation. My one goal was to survive. I had managed to live through my son's experimentation with psychedelics; my oldest daughter's sexual adventures; my middle daughter's dropping out of school at sixteen to raise chickens and train horses; and my rebellious pre-teen daughter who hated her father.

Most of my married life I had stayed home, raising kids, putting on business dinners, doing church and volunteer work. I had never supported myself and felt ill-equipped to do so. I was very fortunate that my husband, feeling guilty, offered me half of all our investments in the dissolution settlement. However, I needed to work to bolster my self-esteem. Based on ten years of being a volunteer instructional aide and taking some extension classes, I earned an Adult Basic Education credential and could substitute, but I wanted to do more, so I went to graduate school.

In 1948, I received an impractical B.A. in General Curriculum from the University of California, Berkeley. Thirty years later I picked my school and program very carefully. I was scared to death that first day of graduate school, as I sat in the Cognitive Learning class with twenty- to thirty-year-olds at St. Mary's College. My days were filled with learning to teach in a way that made sense to me, a way that combined the affective and cognitive modes of learning in a balanced whole, creating confluency. I found much success and many new relationships in school and began to feel better about myself. At the end of two years I had an M.A. in Confluent Education and a job teaching remedial math and English at Holy Names High School. I had more than survived; I was a success.

While writing my thesis and starting a new job, I married a man I met at the Unity Church singles group. My youngest child was in high school, my other three children and my husband's two sons were on their own, so we had fun traveling: Easter at Club Med in Puerto Vallarta, honeymoon in Mexico City, Christmas in Oaxaca. We took long weekends on the Mendocino coast and at Carmel; we flew to the British Isles several times for extended vacations. Life became a romantic adventure; concerns about menopause vanished; I felt relaxed, the fear of pregnancy was over.

My husband was very appreciative of my physical body and I began to feel truly sexy for the first time in my life. He acted as if I were what he had waited for his whole life and I was turned on by his attentiveness. In the beginning he was very romantic and I felt free to exercise some of my fantasies in the bedroom. We drank champagne in bed in the afternoon; we made dates to entertain each other at home by putting on simple dinners, giving massages, making love in the living room. I felt confident about what I wanted sexually and I could ask for it even though my husband did not always remember and I became impatient with him. Nevertheless, my sexuality was more clearly defined and uninhibited. Unfortunately, my husband developed angina and our relationship began to lose its excitement and spontaneity.

After four years of marriage, my husband was forced to take early retirement, without any financial benefits. I quit my teaching job and we moved to an apple farm in Sonoma County to spend our twilight years living off the land. My husband and I had elaborate plans for turning the farm into a profitable business, but he soon lost interest and was content to sit and read and watch television when he wasn't playing golf. There was little that stimulated him.

I felt my husband was giving up living life fully, becoming too old too soon. He refused to diet, cut down on his drinking, or exercise regularly, as his doctor had suggested. His arteries were clogged and he was taking several kinds of medication for his heart. I cooked low cholesterol food for both of us but he seemed to avoid taking responsibility for his own well-being. I felt frustrated and angry when he didn't help himself.

To keep up my enthusiasm and interests, I became involved in Beyond War and led educational evenings to facilitate change in people's thinking about nuclear war and to show them how they could make a difference in our world. I went to church and became a member of the Peacemaker's Committee. The banner I sewed helped wrap the Pentagon when Women Against Nuclear Destruction went to Washington, D.C. for a peaceful demonstration on Hiroshima Day. With the Earthstewards Network, I revisited the Soviet Union (having been there ten years before), and returned to give slide presentations on Citizen Diplomacy in the USSR.

As for the farm and my marriage, I realized too late that I was more suited to country living and had more of an interest in growing apples and vegetables than my husband. Without his active participation, the farm was neglected and I felt let down. I couldn't keep up with the work required, and we could no longer afford to hire someone to do it. We went for counseling to find a way to put new life into our marriage (at least, that's what I went for). He said he didn't want to change anything, that he was ninety percent satisfied with our life together. So I divorced for the second time. I was sixty years old, wondering if my life, make that sex life, was really over now. Although there was the pain of separation, of selling our country home, of starting over, this time with less financial security, the emotional trauma was not as severe as the first time.

I looked in the mirror one morning and saw a woman looking very much like my mother who had died at sixty-nine, had been a widow since her late forties and never showed any interest in men again, because she felt old. I didn't want to spend the rest of my life alone. What if I died at sixty-nine, only nine years from now? Certainly my skin had lost its resilience, lines were etched more deeply around my eyes, my waist line was thicker, but those were external changes. Did I really know what was happening inside my body? I read more articles, none of which gave me the definitive answers I was looking for. I had rejected hormone therapy because I had taken birth control pills from forty to fifty and felt that was a sufficient hormone dose in one lifetime.

At the same time I was frightened by the specter that I would begin to experience all the symptoms I had scoffed at when I was fifty. Vaginal dryness became a problem, hot flashes continued and bothered me now. I was single again and worried that intercourse would be more and more painful. I had tried vaginal hormone cream and found it difficult to regulate the dosage. So off I went to see what medical miracles had been discovered in the past ten years. During a presentation on the facts about menopause, I was impressed by the replica of a menopausal woman's vertebra, showing actual bone loss and hairline cracks, caused by osteoporosis, which could silently steal the calcium from my bones. I wasn't surprised that vitamins and exercise were strongly recommended. I didn't want to believe that hormone therapy was so generally accepted by the medical profession, who, the last time I paid attention, emphasized the dangerous side effects of hormones. I, who bragged about toughing out menopause, agreed to take estrogen and progesterone in order to avoid osteoporosis, cancer of the uterus, hot flashes, vaginal dryness.

After several weeks, I noticed old and almost forgotten body odors. My breasts were tender, and much worse, I started to menstruate regularly because the hormone dosage was twenty-five days on and five days off. When I went to the store the choices of sanitary napkins and tampons were staggering—new shapes, sizes, packaging, something for every contour and occasion. I was actually embarrassed to check out with my purchases, a sampling to experiment with, since I had no idea what was meant by "light, night, liners and maxithins." I chose a pad "with wings," only to have my youngest daughter say, "Mother, what is this?" I trimmed those wings off with the scissors because they stuck to the pubic hair, not the panties as advertised. After ten years without menstruating, I resented the familiar feeling of pressure and tension, not to mention the inconvenience of it all.

In addition, I experienced anxiety attacks and felt lonely. I had trouble going to sleep and the more I tried to breathe deeply and relax, the more my heart would race and my left side was sore. I feared a heart attack or a stroke, like my mother. I imagined the children finding me alone in bed, having died before I could dial 911. There was no one to talk to since I was living alone and my friends were younger and wouldn't understand. Besides, wasn't I an example of an older woman who handled this cycle of the moon so well?

I put up with the inconvenience of menstruation for six months because that was what I was advised to do, before consulting my nurse practitioner again. Now I was told that I had the choice of taking both estrogen and progesterone every day without stopping. If I don't fall into the group of women who spot on this dosage, there will be no more bleeding or the necessity for buying those darn pads.

As I look back over the past year, I admit to being lonely, without a partner. My ex-husband, who was still my friend, died in June, following bypass surgery, and I have been in mourning without giving credence to that reality. I am more gracefully adjusting to my status of being single and in my last cycle of the moon. Having read a well-recommended book, *Menopause Naturally,* by Sadja Greenwood, M.D., my feelings are less panicked and I am seriously considering going off of the hormones.

My summer project is to experiment with not taking any hormones. *Menopause Naturally* has a rating scale of advantages and disadvantages of estrogen replacement therapy which helped me to sort out my feelings about hormones. My biggest concern was osteoporosis. I don't smoke, drink alcohol very often, or have more than one cup of coffee a day, so that's a plus. I am physically active, avoid salt and eat a high carbohydrate rather than a high protein diet, all of which contribute to low risk of brittle bones.

Hot flashes have returned, but only bother me at night. I have never sweated much, but lately the sweat drips down my forehead when I walk and garden, so I wear a headband under my sun hat. My hair and skin seem to be dryer than before. My energy seems about the same, up and down. The real advantage is that I don't have to remember to take the pills every day and it feels good to say, "No, I am not taking any medication." And I can always go back on the hormones when I'm older.

The incredible thing is that inside I still feel eighteen, with the fears and expectations of a young woman. When I look in the mirror I remember that there is inside me a wise crone. The crone says, "You're doing fine." Perhaps I was wrong, no one else could have prepared me for my last cycle of the moon. Or is it my last?

RED

ellen

Our deck is dry, needs linseed.
Sun debilitates, evokes chants.
Flowers beg to be out of constant sun.
I am like the thirsty chrysanthemums.
My make-up has become bolder, my hair limp.

Stones are the color of my face.
There is no joy left in the lines
that track years.
I hold a baby and my body becomes confused,
sends estrogen, bleeds, bleeds.

This is no ordinary cycle.
This is a cycle of ending.
I stand in a pool of my blood.
It stains our bedsheets, mocks our union,
colors you red.
I am not saying this gracefully.

I could get through this as a woman,
but as a married woman, it is impossible.
The New Zealand Christmas trees
flaunt red brushes against gray leaves.
I see only the red that comes between us.

FLOSSIE'S FLASHES

Sally Miller Gearhart

Flossie Yoroba woke for the third time that night with the tingling at her hairline skipping around to the nape of her neck. "Here she comes!" she thought, opening herself to the gathering explosion of pleasure. She grinned in the dark, "It's from the bones tonight."

Always it was one of two sources. She called the first "Volcano." In an increasingly urgent rhythm it would rise from the spot directly behind her navel, erupting in bursts upward to her arms and head, downward to her legs and feet. It moved patiently, irrevocably, relentlessly, inevitably, over muscle and bone, nerve and tendon, capturing layer after layer of forgiving flesh under its flow of molten energy. Then, in its surges toward freedom, it would strike the wall of skin and burst free of its encapsulation through welcoming pores, transforming itself always at that last second into ten thousand rivulets of pure sweat that sang and danced their way up and down her body. Or across and under it, depending on whatever position that body occupied at the moment. Her toes and fingers always got it last, just about the time the sweat on her back was beginning to cool.

The other kind, and the ones she was waking with tonight, rose from a different place, from the geometric center of each part of her body, simultaneously from thigh, elbow, backbone, phalanges, the middle of her head. This kind she called "Hot Seep," oozing as it did from the marrow of each bone outward toward the skin, not in waves but at most in small eddies, all pacing themselves according to the thickness of the flesh they sought to conquer, all carefully timing their emergence from the body to be a synchronized drench, all at once and altogether, over her whole being, top to bottom, back to front, spilling out at precisely the same instant from her big toes and her nipples, her shoulder blades and her waistline, the palms of her hands and the caverns of her ears.

This Seep was seconds short of emergence. She reached for her clitoris, carefully avoiding its tender, aggressive tip. She pressed it gently side-to-side, then up-from-under. Once. Twice. Then with a whoop of joy she flung off the quilt and arched her back into a long stretch of denouement, collapsing at last into inert flesh, drenched and dazzled in the frost-filled air.

A high wind was outflanking the protective eaves of her cabin. It drove a deluge of snow through her window and onto her naked skin. Sweat met flake in a mighty clash of elements. Flake melted. But flake won, cooling the seat in an embrace both familiar and triumphant.

Flossie whooped again. She stretched wide another time and urged more of her undaunted wetness into its stark encounter with the cold. She smiled and shuddered as she sucked a raging winter into her lungs. She felt the air transfer itself from lungs to bones, there to entrap the heat and follow its path, moving on it from behind until now her skin felt downright crisp, crisp and encased in what she knew must be a thin sheath of ice. She whooped a third time and catapulted to the window, drawing it tight against the storm.

Back under her quilt she subsided, giving thanks to Whoever Was that Daaana had decided not to stay over with her tonight. She preferred not to share a bed these days, much less Spoon, what with this waking up four and five times a night to sizzle and freeze, sizzle and freeze.

Though as for that, she thought, marvelling at the completeness with which the quilt encased her, cuddled her—though as for that, Daaana was a great bedpartner for flashes. She actually envied Flossie, and advertised her in public to be better than Solar Central, hottest woman in the Grand Matrix, north-south-east-or-west.

Even from the depths of an early-dawn Spoon Daaana could sometimes feel the moment coming before Flossie knew it herself. Then she would chuckle and cling to Flossie, holding her close in anticipation of the explosion of heat. Flossie, torn between the loving clasp of a good woman and her desire to leap to cold freedom, would throw the covers at least from her own burning flesh and lie only tokenly connected to Daaana by finger or kneecap. That, of course, threatened to deprive Daaana of one of her greatest pleasures: the slick sensuousness of their undulating sweat-bathed bodies. It led, usually, to loud laments as Daaana protected herself from the window's blast and Flossie, naked as a jay to the churlish chiding of the wintry wind, inhaled there like a card-carrying health freak. Sometimes it all led to a tussle that ended in shouts and uncontrolled laughter.

Flossie loved her nights with Daaana and sometimes missed the dreamwalking that Spooning could bring. But right now, these months, these years, she was exhilarated with her changes and often sacrificed the adventures of Spooned sleep for a night of solitary encounter with the elements. Since childhood she had loved the run from the sweat tent to the waterfall, the smell of hard-worked body dripping in pungent clothes and the subsequent dunk into an icy mountain stream. She craved the contrasts, the sudden changes, the jig that her feet danced and the thanks that her heart sang every time she gifted them with those extremes.

Under the cover now she stroked her ample body, drawing her knees to her chest and lying Spoon with a phantom self as she cozed back into sleep. Not only did she get these wild free swings of heat and cold, but several times a night now she got to fall asleep again. Falling asleep, she thought. Sheer contentment, always, even with another Spooned body. But, she mused, there's a special balm to doing it in a wide bed all alone, with the margins of your body quite unbounded . . .

Alien androids were attacking the cabin, rattling the windows and whipping the roof with giant rubber hoses. They were calling her name. "Flossie! Flossie, open up!!" She clamped her legs together. She heaved her extra pillow over her head, dug deeper into the tired old foam that supported her. "Stick it where the sun don't shine," she mumbled, trying for her gentle drop back into dreamland.

"Flossie! Get the bar off this door! I gotta talk to you!" More beating on the non-offending cabin. Flossie turned her face to the foam and smothered her breath. She willed the androids back to their planet of sterile basalt. She held her breath.

"Floss, dammit, it's me, City Lights! I'm freezing my butt off out here! Flossieeeeee!!"

Flossie breathed. No fun to wake up this way, she thought. She hauled her bare feet to the floor, feeling for her nightgown. Where had she left it? More banging. "I'm comin', I'm comin'!" she croaked. The banging stopped. Fighting her way into the warm flannel she reached the door and drew back the bar.

City Lights, No Bigger Than A Minute And Twice As Frail, stomped into the room and kicked the door back into place. She dumped a large patch of snow onto the floor with her jacket and laughed a greeting. Then she made for Flossie's stove. "You still got fire," she warbled. "How about a lamp?"

"City, I'm a gin day short of lacing you good. What you want?" Flossie cut the damper and opened her stove door. She lit a candle from a twig.

City shook possible spiders from some kindling and forced the wood under the smoldering logs. She looked over her shoulder at the flannel-clad figure, its arms akimbo, and got to the point.

"We got to Spoon, Flossie. You and me."

"You and me? City, your peanut butter's slippin' off of your bread. Last we Spooned was five years ago . . ."

"We can do it." The younger woman sank to a stool in front of the fire and held out her hand to Flossie. "I'm not proposin' wild abandoned sex. Only a sweet gentle little Spoon . . ."

"You proposin'—!"

"Not that I wouldn't love it, Floss. In fact . . ."

Flossie let out her breath. "Wait till I get my socks." She threw the quilt from her bed around City's shoulders. Then on her knees she strained to rescue one wool sock from under her bed, another from her boot. She sat on a straight chair by City. "Coldest night in a universe and you got to come knockin' your way into my sleep."

She felt a reassurance, a satisfaction, as the sock stretched itself around her leg. When nothin' else helps, she reminded herself, pull up your socks. It always worked. She cut her eyes toward City. The tiny woman was intent on moving a log to catch the center of a volunteer flame. Still pretty, Flossie thought, the girl's still pretty, else the fire's makin' a lie of her face. Flossie pulled up her second sock and resigned herself to a conversation.

"City, I'm bound to tell you I won't try that flying' again if that's how come you want to Spoon."

City wove her hand up through folds of quilt and held it out to Flossie a second time. "No," she urged, "I just need to dreamwalk. All the demons been visitin' me lately. Like when I go to the lake where Eleeea died. You know?"

Flossie knew. She wanted to reach for her pipe, light it up and stay safe behind a could of smoke. Instead she took City's hand. "Umm-hmmm," she said.

"I just need you to hold me, Floss. You always been the best for walkin' together with me and findin' healin' waters. I can do a new incantation I made up for right after the master chant. It'll take us so deep, so easy." City Lights, No Bigger Than A Minute And Twice As Frail, raised the soft brown openness of her eyes to the soft brown openness of Flossie's. "Will you Spoon with me, Floss?"

There was never any brittleness to be found anywhere in Flossie Yoroba, and at this moment, she was sure, there wasn't even a trace of solid bone or cartilage. She harumphed her way toward a response. "Well, we might be ridin' a lame donkey," she growled. "It's not for certain I can stay down long enough to dreamwalk anywhere."

She was about to say more but at that moment her forehead began to tingle, just around her hairline. Her eyes grew a millimeter bigger. She stood up and wiped her brow. "City," she said, "City, come here to me." She pulled the small woman to her feet. "How come you got on so many clothes?" She turned toward the door, heaving the quilt onto the bed as she slid the bar closed.

City Lights knew when she'd been blessed. Move, girl! she admonished herself. Don't let your coattail touch the ground! She began peeling off her clothes, struggling all the while to meet the swell of primordial earthpower that was emanating from Flossie's body. She was just working her way out of her last pant leg when Flossie flung off the flannel nightgown and stood before her, wet and shiny in the candlelight, exuding wave after wave of unquenched fire.

First it was the warmth, then it was Flossie's arms that encompassed her. As she sank onto the bed, City Lights, No Bigger Than A Minute And Twice As Frail, heard the big woman say, "They's good Spoonin' tonight, girl. But first you got to let me show you what a hot woman is all about."

The candle, outdone in both heat and light, guttered, and then courteously extinguished itself.

ONE WAY

Amber Coverdale Sumrall

I met George on American Airlines Flight #702. I was going east to New York to meet my editor, a man much younger than my 45 years. After months of letters and telephone exchanges our business relationship had taken a decidedly romantic turn. George slid into the seat next to me with an innocuous grin. He could see that I wanted to be alone. I'd lowered the armrest and stretched out with the latest issue of *off our backs*. I was sure that I was going to have the seat to myself because the gay ticket agent had assured me he'd do his best to keep the other seat vacant. "Why in hell are you going to New York in August?" he'd asked. "Don't you know you'll sweat 24 hours a day?" Yes, I know, I'd replied, thinking that I wouldn't be wet only because of the humidity and occasional hot flashes.

So George introduces himself and plops his luggage down as I curl into the window, cracking my gum loudly.

"So, uh, are you going to the City for business or pleasure?" he asks.

"Neither," I reply.

"Me too," he says. "I'm going to get my dog back. My ex-wife thinks she's real clever. Thinks I'm not capable of tracking her down. Getting Max back."

I sneak a sideways look at George. He resembles a retired athletic coach: red-faced, blond crewcut, striped t-shirt, plaid bermuda shorts and the mandatory baseball cap. Women actually marry guys like this, I thought. By the millions. This is a six hour flight. I'll pay the extra $4.00 for headphones immediately.

"Yeah," George continues, spitting the words at me, "she's going through the change. She went nuts, left me for an Italian guy in Brooklyn. He's young enough to be her son. I can't believe it! Mario somebody. A fag hair dresser. He has a white poodle with some kind of French name. I don't mind my old lady getting screwed by a homo, if you know what I mean, but the thought of Max being polluted by a poodle really gets to me. Max is *my* dog, a real stud. She only took him because New York is so full of scum. She needs protection. So she takes up with a fag. Can you understand the reasoning behind that?"

I'm staring at him, unable to speak. Where is my eject button? Where is the ticket attendant who did this to me? I'll have to fax him George's phone number.

He mistakes my shock for attraction. "Say, you look like a woman who might appreciate a guy like me."

"Oh really, whatever led you to that conclusion?"

George laughs and a wad of pink gum drops from his mouth. He doesn't miss a beat. "Well, because you look like one of them natural women—no make-up, jeans, probably your own color hair. Not like Sandy. Bitch!" He heaves himself up in his seat, unfastens his seatbelt and reaches down for the gum. After rolling it in his hands he tosses it back in his mouth. "And I like to think of myself as a natural man and all." He flashes another in a series of grimaces. "Whadda ya say?"

"Well, as a matter of fact, George, I'm going through menopause at the moment and my pussy's as dry as a desert spring. My lover, Francine, recently left me for a younger woman and I've been feeling really crazy lately. And my cat, Flaubert . . ."

He has already vacated his seat. My seat.

MEN OH PAUSE

Maude Meehan

and please take note
I pen this semi-demi
dithyramb
in hope
that I may set
you men struate
That sparse
and very final show
of red
says *only*
that a woman has bled
not that she's dead
or past delight
in those
hot-blooded lusty rites
witch still transpire
on any given night
in grey and white
haired womens beds

LOOKING FOR THE BIG M AND ENCOUNTERING THE BIG N

Carol Pascoe

When was it going to happen? Or had I already been through it, as they say? Ten years before, when I was 39, I had undergone a hysterectomy. Was it possible, I now wondered, that I had breezed through the menopause, unaware and unscathed? When you no longer have a uterus, how *do* you know if you've gone through the menopause?

Hadn't I had hot flashes for six months? Hadn't I paid my dues by sweating diligently into my Baked Alaska at Ernie's while San Francisco's temperature gauge registered 56 degrees? I could speculate no longer. I needed to know *for sure*.

I decided I would try to extract a definitive answer from the gynecologist who had, a decade ago, extracted my beloved uterus. From past experience, I knew that the rather effete Dr. Z was not a man fond of direct answers. I remember when I had approached him after the surgery. "Now," I asked quietly, "How long does the healing process take?" (Four weeks? Six weeks? Nine years?)

"Oh," he replied rotely, "you can't have intercourse for six weeks."

"Sex!" I fairly screamed, thinking of my poor, sore mutilated body. "Good Lord, sex!"

He might as well have told me, "Oh, I'm sorry but the killer bees will not hatch in your bathroom until mid-summer." After I'd convulsed for minutes into fits of hysteria at the mere thought of intercourse, Doctor Z frowned (clearly empathizing with my deprived pillow partner), and said rather sternly, "That's *enough*, now."

Then he took a blue ballpoint pen out of his pocket and, babbling about my non-uterus and my non-cervix, drew a picture of my still-present ovaries on the paper covering the examination table.

Two years later, when I asked him about the pros and cons of estrogen, he took out his blue ballpoint pen and deftly sketched my ovaries while giving another jumbled discourse on female organs.

In fact, he had always drawn a picture of my ovaries whenever I asked him any question at all. Because of his devotion to medical illustration, and his tunnel vision (the inevitable outcome of his occupation), I had never really gotten an answer to *any* question. But this time, I resolved, this time I will look him in the eye and say, "When a woman does not have a uterus, how does a woman know if she *has gone through, is going through,* or *will go through* the menopause?"

I sat on the examination table in my quilted paper robe looking like a pale green hand grenade with legs. When I asked Dr. Z my question, he expertly flipped out his blue ballpoint pen and started to sketch my ovaries—Why mine? Doesn't everybody's look the same?—on the paper covering the examination table.

I reached out and tapped his hand. "Dr. Z," I said, "I can draw my own ovaries. Believe me. I can draw my absent uterus, and the fimbria and the cervix uteri. I can also draw the labium majus, the perineum, the prepuce, even the meatus urinarius," I intoned.

"Oh Carol," he said, turning with dismay toward my chart, "you're a character."

"Well," I said, "am I a character who *is going through the menopause, has gone through* the menopause, or *still has to go through* the menopause?"

He smiled ruefully, "Well, everything looks good. Your vagina looks fine . . . good!" He nodded at my chart. "Young. Pink."

I thought about my cascading chins and the pruney look around my eyes. "Well," I chirped, "I'm glad *one* end is keeping up appearances!"

At this, he wheeled out the door to the next room where another woman waited for the wisdom that would pour forth from his ballpoint pen.

As I drove home, I mulled over what had happened. Let's take this one step backwards, I said to myself. Where did *he* learn about menopause? He learned about it from a textbook. I thought of that old medical text nestled on my studio bookshelf. "Of course!" I cried and careened through the yellow light.

Within minutes I had located the resource which was to render me knowledgeable. The book had been published in the mid-50s, but what the heck I said to myself, remembering the words of my Aunt Myrtle when she told me the facts of life: *"And,"* she had ceremoniously concluded while whacking the head off a fryer hen, "from *then* to *now* there ain't been no change at all in a woman's giblets!"

Now, settled in a cushy chair, book in hand, I set up the ground rules for what was about to come. I told myself, If you have experienced most of the symptoms, then it's safe to assume you have been through *it*. If you have not, then you're still *in* for *it*.

I opened the book and read. Instantly, my skin grew clammy, my mouth dry. My eyes raced along each line in terror. "The menopause is usually accompanied by elevation of blood pressure, hot and cold flashes, feeling of

249

weakness, and, in some cases, marked mental derangements. In plethoric types, symptoms are those of congestion—flushes of heat, rush of blood to face and head, uterine and other hemorrhages, leukorrhea, and even diarrhea. In chlorotic subjects, sallow complexions, semi-chlorotic skin, weak pulse and various other indications of debility. In nervous subjects, the overanxious look, the terror-stricken expression as if apprehensive of seeing some frightful object, the face bedewed with perspiration and a remarkable tendency to hysteria."

The horrors continued: "The unusual development of hair on chin and lip generally coincides with final cessation of menses; so does an unusual power of generating heat, indicated by throwing off clothing and opening doors and windows. There is often rheumatism of shoulders or thighs, or swelling of joints. Often nymphomania is present."

I stopped. I reread the last sentence. I stared hard at the sentence. I closed the book and opened it again. It was still there. What ruthless fiend, I wondered, had inserted the word "Often" into the sentence—*"often* nymphomania is present." How often is often?

Is that why Aunt Myrtle's twin sister, when she turned 50, had shocked the family by quitting her job at the post office, changing her name to Buffy, and getting a clerking position at Fredericks of Hollywood so she could get a sizable discount on black lace teddies?

Well, the big N couldn't happen to me! After all, I had been divorced since I was 23. I had, of necessity, developed my own four-point fail-safe moral code: 1) Never go to bed with a man who has never heard of Virginia Woolf. 2) Never go to bed with a man who, when eating an artichoke, zooms in and consumes the heart before relishing the leaves. 3) Never go to bed with a man who is revered by the members of his basketball team as being the slam 'n' dunk king of the court. And finally, I just have to admit it, that old devil LOVE was the fourth and deciding factor. The kind of love that has to do with voltage, Astaire, and neurons—but I'll get to that in due time. The point is, in twenty-six years, these four rules had eliminated all but three applicants. Now, what was to become of me at the ruthless and indiscriminate hands of Mother Nature?

No sooner had I, a fallen woman, settled into a stupor at the kitchen table, than the object of my monogamy walked through the door. That old familiar electricity started just like it had for years and my neurons slipped into their Fred Astaire routine, creating a distinct shiver along my limbs . . . but I stopped myself. Poor dear man, I silently lamented. What will become of you? Of us? Should I warn him?

He joined me at the table for coffee. My eyes misted over as I gazed at him. "Maybe," I ventured, "maybe you should join a health club."

"Health club? Me? What for?"

"Well," I lamely suggested, "to keep your strength up." Then I added in nearly a whisper, "People change."

"Never felt better," he bellowed, puffing up his chest and ignoring the significant factor mounding on the north side of his belt.

He left, uninformed of my impending obsession. I reread the page, starting at the top and ticking off the symptoms. *Hot flashes?* Yes. *Feeling of weakness?* No. *Mental derangements?* Borderline. *The over-anxious look?* I ran to the mirror. Sure enough. Definitely over-anxious. I ran back to the list. *Hair on chin?* I dashed to the mirror again. Nope, no beard. *Swelling of the joints?* I felt my hip. Impossible to tell the cellulite from the swell. Then there it was again: *Nympho-ma-ni-a.* I slapped the book face down on the table. "Well!" I said aloud, "What do the medical texts know? Weren't they written *by* men and *for* men in a *male*-dominated society?"

I would go to the real source. I would consult the oracles of ovarian wisdom. I would go to women who had been through IT.

First, I visited my friend Lydia, a wispy woman who always dressed in long, flowing garments of pale gray and washed-out lavender, yardage that seemed to move her effortlessly from one room to another. I had never really put much faith in Lydia's introspective or analytic qualities, but she *was* 58.

When I drove up, she was sitting in her window, spinning yarn, her head bent toward her creation. I got right to the question. "Lydia," I said, "I was wondering if you could tell me what it was like to go through the menopause."

"Yes," she said wanly.

"Yes, what?" I asked

"Yes, I could tell you . . ." she sighed dreamily.

"Well, tell me!"

"Oh," she said, pulling the wool with her long fingers. "Ohhh, I neeearly LOST my miiiind." Then she rolled her vague watery eyes around in her head as if to prove her point.

Next, I dropped by the apartment of Jacqueline, my English friend who, it was rumored, had once been the confidante of a prominent member of the House of Commons. She understood the subtleties of *all* personal tragedy. I asked my question. Jacqueline flipped her tea bag neatly into the saucer, rolled her eyes, shook her head and said, "Ohhh, I neeearly *lost* my miiiind." Then she quipped, "Yes, love, nearly *went bats!*"

I left, never having popped the question *behind* the question: "Are you now or have you ever been, a nymphomaniac?" I was wasting my time. What I wanted to know *now* was if I needed to install a turnstile in the doorway to my bedroom.

I decided it would be easier to ask the question long distance. I would simply call my 55-year-old, globe-trotting friend Anna. After calls to Haifa, Barcelona, Huejotzingo, and Liverpool, I caught up with her back in the U.S.— in Bangor, Maine. I hoped the name of the city was no indication of her present obsession.

No sooner was the question out of my mouth, than Anna seethed her answer across the miles, "I detessst sex," she hissed. "I'm never going to have sex again! All men ever think of is what's between . . ."

"Okay," I cut her off. "Sorry. Guess I'm taking this all too seriously," I tried to edge off the line.

"No one needs to have sex!" she screamed. "Sex is outdated! It's ludicrous! Carol, are you *there? Art* is all that's important," she shrieked. "Art. *Aesthetics!*"

I hung up.

Never a quitter, I vowed to tackle the dilemma from a new perspective. I reviewed what I had already done to solve the problem: 1) I had talked to my gynecologist. 2) I had talked to women who had gone through *it*. Suddenly, something clicked and I had a new plan of attack. It was simple. I would *combine* the two methods I had already used. I would talk to a gynecologist who had been through the menopause.

I presented myself in her office and explained the problem. She listened intently, her kind face radiating concern and intelligence. Then she examined me. "Your vagina looks . . ."

I waited. Young and pink? "Nice and normal," she finished.

"It has a will of its own," I explained.

"Well," she said, settling herself on a stool in the corner of the examining room. "Menopause *means* cessation of menstruation and you, of course, don't menstruate, so . . ."

I wanted to cry with glee, "So that means that I have permanently escaped the bordellos of my worst fantasies!"

She smiled at my over-anxious face. "So if you begin to experience any other symptoms—night sweats or so forth—we can talk about estrogen then. No need to prescribe it now."

I searched her face. She took out a blue ballpoint pen and glanced at the paper covering the examination table. "Oh, God," I silently pleaded, "not another drawing of my ovaries."

She looked down at my chart, made a quick mark, and asked, "You're a writer?"

"Yes," I replied.

"What do you write?"

"Mental health books," I confessed.

She gave me a look that said, "It's always the dermatologists who have incurable skin disease, and the psychiatrists who go crazy."

I managed a weak, yeah-I-ought-to-know-better smile.

She stood up. "Is there anything else you'd like to ask?"

I blurted, "When you went through menopause what was the worst thing about it?" I braced myself and set my jaw.

"I don't know about *that*," she said, poised with her hand on the doorknob, "but I'll tell you what the best thing was."

"What?"

"Not having to worry about getting pregnant, and not having to take the pill."

"Aha!" I screamed to myself. What did those male medical writers of the 50s know? In 1955, the pill was not in use. The average female had about 37 years of undaunted fertility during which she worried herself sick. Our "nymphomania" was only a free-at-last syndrome.

I exited the office wearing a bliss-ninny grin and humming to myself, "Who's afraid of the Big M or N." I sauntered across the parking lot in the sweet afternoon sun. "No problem, Pascoe," I said to myself. "Just go with the flow. Or without it, as the case may be."

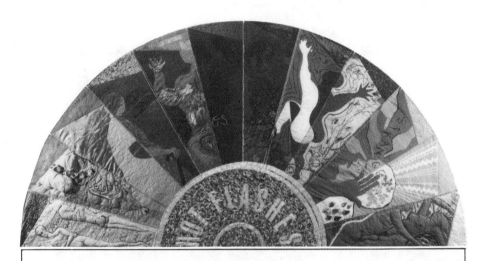

INDIAN SUMMER

Aging is the term for a continuous process of growth through life.

—Maggie Kuhn

The old woman I shall become will be quite different from the woman I am now. Another I is beginning and so far I have not had to complain of her.

—George Sand

After a woman passes menopause she really comes into her time. I feel that. I've never felt so well or had so many images before me.

—Meridel Le Sueur

WYOMING BURNING 1988

Mary Dominick Chivers

As the summer turns
Toward my fiftieth year
I burn with strange, shuddering fires.
Every night between clammy sheets
My blood rushing with mortality,
My skin flames
Against my will.

All July, all August
Into September
In the Wyoming forests
Of my girlhood
Fires have raced through the trees
Running faster than the horses
Through a spring meadow,
Pouring down the hills
Like water.
At night the ravines glow with sparks
Like cities lit for Christmas,
But in the deadly heat
Of the afternoon
The monster rages;
Borne on the back of the rising wind
Its hot breath
Crackles into terrible jaws
Hundreds of histories.

Lovely homeland of the Crow
Where will your spirits live now?

At noon the sun is a red ball
In smokey eclipse.
We walk through a strange yellow haze,
Light filtered as light must be
In the bottom of a murky pond.
But no water here,
No awakening from dream.
Ashes fall instead of rain
Into the dry creek beds
Smearing on the picnic tables
And covering the patient mountains
And trees, which stand
Exhaling resinous breath
Into the hot air
Waiting
Silent and helpless,
The moment of
Immolation.

How could I have known
As a bareback roan rider
Girl of thirteen
Happy following my father's
Palomino, sweat-streaked as
He climbed, switch backing through
The sun-flecked pines,
That all trails would come
To such days of fire?
I rode without thought of
The generations before me
Or the days of their bounty
When the mountain sheep were
More accessible than the deer,
Plentiful as the buffalo.

Now I glimpse the ghosts of the tribes
Gone like a vision in smoke,
Lost into ashes.

I would sing a kaddish,
I would dance in a frenzy!
Black stalks of trees

Speak, pointing like fingers
To forests of losses.

Spirits of the wild,
Spirits of the soil,
Do not desert us!

GRANDMOTHER LODGE

Brooke Medicine Eagle

The Grandmother Lodge is the lodge of the white-haired (wisdom) women—those who have gone beyond the time of giving away the power of their blood, and now hold it for energy to uphold the Law.

When our elders step across the threshold of the Grandmother Lodge, leaving their bleeding behind them, they become the Keepers of the Law. No longer is their attention consumed with the creation and rearing of their own family. In this sense, they have no children, and in our ways those who are not parent to any specific child are parent to ALL CHILDREN. Thus their attention turns to the children of All Our Relations: not just their own children, or the children of their friends, their clan or tribe, but the children of all the hoops: the Two-Leggeds, the Four-Leggeds, the Wingeds, the Finned, the Green-Growing Ones, and all others. Our relationship with this great circle of Life rests ultimately in their hands. They must give-away this responsibility by modeling, teaching, and sharing the living of this law in everyday life—to men, women, children—that all might come into balance.

What this means for women, in very practical terms, is this. When you pass beyond menopause, you have the opportunity for a renewed and deeply powerful experience of yourself. As you drop away from the silliness and fear that has been generated by the "over the hill" cultural trance, and open yourself to the truth that lives within you—body and spirit—you will find an incredible challenge—a challenge for which you are better equipped than any other two-legged. You have the opportunity to sit in council, and using the power of the blood held among you, create a harmonious world around you.

Let me speak for a moment of women's moon-time (menstrual) blood and its power. This blood has been shown to be among the (if not THE) most nurturing, bio-energizing substance on Earth. When placed upon plants, they are deeply nourished. In our native ways, during our ceremonies of planting and nurturing our crops, we had moon-time women (women in the days of their menses) move among the plants and give-away their blood. Always, our women gave-away this wonderful blood in an honoring way. They sat upon the ground and gave-away directly, or bled upon moss and later placed it upon the Earth to nurture and renew. Vicki Noble reminds us that this blood was the first blood offered on the altar—a most blessed gift. Then when women were no longer honored and the power of their life-giving blood was ignored, animal and human sacrifice was used to give blood on the altar.

This is the blood, then, that you hold among you when you no longer bleed in the moon-cycle: you have passed your moontime. Elders, perhaps you have not been aware of the profound responsibility you are now to assume: if you had known you would have had the conscious opportunity to learn and deepen yourself in good relationship through your lifetime, so that you might serve your people and use yourself well in these years. Younger women, you who read this now are conscious and can choose to learn and grow in this way, that you might feel ready when you, too, step into the Grandmother Lodge.

Among many of the tribes the primacy of the Law of Good Relationship was remembered and the Grandmother Lodges, or the societies within it, were known to hold the highest command. If a peace chief was not leading his people across the land in a way that all people and animals had good food, clear water, and sheltering valleys in the time of cold winds, then the Grandmothers asked for someone new to lead; they called someone to step forth for the people who had the probability of doing a better job in his active work to nurture and renew the people. If a war chief was creating such animosity among surrounding tribes that frequent attacks disrupted the life and well-being of the people, he was asked to find productive rather than destructive uses for his energy. Such was the power of the Grandmothers: they took seriously the charge to nurture and renew the people, and took action in line with it.

The Grandmother Lodge was the lodge of all post-menopausal women. Within that, smaller groups formed around their various functions. For some women, it might be the keeping of a sacred basket, for others a certain kind of healing, and for yet others the maintaining of a beauty way (art) among the people. A basket weaver might belong to a basket-makers' society and also to a society that maintained a sacred bundle (these latter often came through family lineages). A woman might belong to a ceremonial Sun Dance society, and as well to a society of herbalists.

As you begin gathering with others now, you will likely have a small and mixed group, and need to determine the common interests, skills, and goals among you. Perhaps you will choose a focus of 1) speaking to children's classes about the Grandmother Lodge; 2) working with the Rainforest Action Group; 3) creating a babysitting service for working mothers; or 4) speaking to men's groups on issues of harmony and good relationship—the possibilities for good are endless. Some of your time together may well be to increase your own learning and understanding—meetings to share skills with each other, to meditate and learn to listen to the Great Voices Within, gatherings to hike upon the Earth or to strengthen and tone your bodies.

Something I am often asked is about those of you who have experienced amenorrhea, early menopause, or hysterectomies. Where do you fit? Although I cannot say I know the exact answers, this is what makes sense to me through my own experience. The first thought I have is that you will very likely want to get a sense of the rhythm of activity/receptivity—worldly action/great Mystery—that is your natural cycle in synchrony with Grandmother Moon, for this cycle still echoes through the waters of your body even though external bleeding does not accompany it. Deepen your experience of the moon's cycle within you, it is very powerful and useful for you and All Your Relations to reach through the veil into the Great Mystery during your bleeding and bring back vision for your people. Secondly, many of us who are younger and don't yet experience ourselves as elders are being called into the Grandmother Lodge because there is an urgent need for the awakening of this function among women. Because of the crushing of the native cultures and the loss of the women's ways, there are few who sit in these Lodges and uphold the nurturing and renewing of the people. So younger, awakened ones of us are being called into the Lodge through many different means. Accept it as an honor.

The final aspect of the Grandmother Lodge I will address is the rite of passage into it. Those of you surrounding a woman who is crossing this threshold will want to honor this special woman and to let her know of your support of her in this time of her great responsibility. There are many ways this can be done and I will suggest only a few: ritual bathing and anointing by her closest friend, then being dressed in a white gown (for wisdom) and a red sash (to represent the blood, or life force, in All Our Relations and the dedication to them) for a circle dance and feasting; an honoring of her by each woman gathered expressing her appreciation for this woman; a special dedication from the honored one can be given. Certainly an invocation of the Goddess, of White Buffalo Woman or the Wise Crone can be done—perhaps in the form of a guided meditation for the elder one to deepen her contact with this source of strength and wisdom. You who know her will know those aspects which have special meaning for her. Always when I do such a ritual, I include as part of the rite, the charging of this woman with the primary responsibility of the nurturing and renewing of All Her Relations—and remind her of Creator's Law of Good Relationship. Among you, one already in her Grandmother Lodge might perform this function.

WOMEN OF THE FOURTEENTH MOON—THE CEREMONY

Eleanor J. Piazza

It's summer. Time to get the invitations in the mail for the annual ceremony to honor women in menopause. Time to organize the feast. Time to confer with this year's spokeswomen, flautists, firekeepers, drummers and singers.

The invitations always begin "Dear Sister, Daughter, Mother and Grandmother, you are invited to participate in a ceremony to honor Women of the Fourteenth Moon." The rest of the invitation is different every year, modified and revised as the ceremony itself evolves.

The name "Woman of the Fourteenth Moon" came to me as I sought an honoring name for menopausal women. Simply, if there are thirteen full moons in a given year, a woman who has not had a period for a year will begin a new phase in her life upon the fourteenth full moon without bleeding. For most women, unless they have had a hysterectomy, there are skips and starts so it can take a long time to achieve this status. It is cause for celebration.

To me, the name "Woman of the Fourteenth Moon" is more empowering than "Crone," or "menopausal." It is empowering because not only the word "woman" is used, but "moon" is in the name, which identifies us with nature. Finally, "Woman of the Fourteenth Moon" names an experience and tells of a phase in a woman's life.

Menopause, or "a pause of the menses," may be etymologically correct, but most of us have lost our sense of connection with the Latin root of that word and so we only know it intellectually. The aspect of "cessation" is not in keeping with the spirit of this celebration. The accent is on regeneration and beginning, not degeneration.

Women tell me they like being referred to as a Woman of the Fourteenth Moon. I think rites of passage deserve titles, linguistic overtures. I wanted the language of the ceremony to reflect a time of grace and dignity in a woman's life.

The idea of this ceremony began in 1987 when a woman I know mentioned it had been a full year since she'd had a period and she hadn't done anything special to acknowledge this rite of passage. I knew instantly that I wanted to have a celebration for her, for other women in the community who were menopausal, and to prepare the way for myself when my time came.

How does one create a contemporary ceremony? I thought about all that was good and rich in the gatherings I had been to through the years.

Twenty years ago I sat in a circle with women for the first time. It was an honoring circle, only we didn't call it that. We called it a Women's Gestalt Workshop. It was in a beautiful natural setting on top of a mountain. The Gestalt therapist had certain guidelines. We had to make "I" statements, for example, to consciously own what we said. We expressed our fear, anger, grief and rage as well as our joy, and it was a healing circle. The therapist, Jay Croley Ben-Lesser, exemplified the creme de la creme as facilitators go: "Don't try to give me your power," she would counsel, "I have my own." Her workshops were rituals of empowerment.

A good ceremony, then, is empowering. The "inner teacher" is brought forth. One learns to trust oneself and not depend on the facilitator. I wanted the ceremony for Women of the Fourteenth Moon to be empowering for all women.

Jay encouraged us to begin circles of our own when we returned to our respective homes. She called what she did "community building." And so I did that. I still see some of these women and they are the nucleus of a very important community of friends for me. We stand by each other at births and weddings, through times of separation, floods and earthquakes.

I wanted the ceremony for Women of the Fourteenth Moon to be a safe place for women in my community to meet; a place where comfort, gentleness and support can be expected. I wanted a sense of continuity from year to year.

The next group of women I was involved with was a Santa Cruz writing collective, "Moonjuice," that evolved out of a writing class with Ellen Bass. This was about fifteen years ago. We met once a week for years and published several volumes of our poems. In our diversity, we found our uniqueness. We found the common threads of our womanness and we bonded. We were open and non-judgmental. We listened lovingly and carefully to the intricacies of each other's visions, ensconced in poems. We learned first hand that if we tell our truth, it has universal application.

I wanted the truth of woman's poetic voice to be heard at the ceremony for Women of the Fourteenth Moon and the diversity of my community to be reflected in those who participate.

Finally, every month for three years, I attended the women's full moon ceremony at a Native American spiritual community where I lived. Every full moon the women would gather on a little hill above the village around the sacred fire, prayerfully and purposefully. That has been almost ten years ago and I can still smell the sage, hear the rattles and see a tongue of flame leap up to accept a corn meal offering. For all those years I lived with an awareness of the cycle of the moon, Grandmother Moon, we called her, and her effect on my own moon cycle, rhythms and moods.

A menstruating woman was referred to as a woman on her moon. A lot of women are on their moon during full moon. This moon time was time each month for a woman to set aside for herself. A time to reconnect with her source in whatever way she does that. It is a time of great power for women.

I wanted to give the gift of Grandmother Moon to menopausal women who may not have had the opportunity to live with the effects of the rhythms of the moon consciously when they were younger. I wanted the ceremony for Women of the Fourteenth Moon to be instructive on these matters.

The community I lived in was intertribal and interracial. I wanted the ceremony for Women of the Fourteenth Moon to be inclusive, with a recognition of the elements of ceremony that are public domain, and come under the heading "natural," as opposed to being specifically African tribal, Neo-Pagan, Native American, Buddhist, Christian or Jewish.

Now I live in an eclectic community near Santa Cruz, California, where we meet in ceremony every year as Women of the Fourteenth Moon. We transcend age differences, religious, political and socio-economic backgrounds, sexual preferences and racial biases. We are united in our desire to connect with our own aging process in a positive way and to honor those who go before us. We are united in our sincere desire to learn from one another about our life changes. In our rich family of women, we have researched and asked Grandmothers in Hong Kong, Honolulu, Guadalajara, Chicago, Marysville, Michigan, Templeton and Atlanta if they could tell us of words or deeds that might have once honored this time of change that all women who live so long do experience.

"Can you tell us about a ceremony, a special name for, or a consideration given to menopausal women?"

"Well, no, not really," comes the reply.

So, we must exalt the symbols of elderhood as we see them and create ceremonies appropriate for our own communities. This is an invitation to each of you to visualize and create a ceremony for yourself and the elders in your village.

Small things emerge. We must seize the symbols. Take sage tea for example. Younger women serve this tea to the Women of the Fourteenth Moon at our ceremony. A younger woman would only drink sage tea to help dry up her milk if she is weaning her child. Only men and menopausal women drank the wild sage tea in the Native American community where I lived. It is an elder woman's privilege to drink this tea.

Throughout the year, if she wants to, a Woman of the Fourteenth Moon can sip sage tea and remember the tingling sensation in her hands as the Talking Stick was passed to her in the ceremony; she can remember the sweet scent of the woodsmoke from our sacred fire, whiffs of cedar, piñon, sage and lavender. Perhaps she remembers the beat of the drums and how her heartbeat synchronized with that ancient sound, lending a deep sense of peace. Did she really see belly dancers twirling in the light of the fire? Well why not? Belly dancing was created by women, for women, as part of the birthing ritual. They were dancing for her, to honor her for her days of childbearing and nurturing. And what was it exactly that woman from Australia said? Something about not being afraid to age now because, as she put it, "for anyone who has eyes to see, elder women are quite beautiful."

Perhaps she pours another cup of tea, our Woman of the Fourteenth Moon, peers out the window to see if Grandmother Moon is up yet. Maybe she closes her eyes and sees the image of an elder in red who opened and closed each part of the ceremony with the sweetest prayers to the creator; words that teach, enlighten, comfort and invoke strength. And late, late into the night, this same woman danced the Dance of the Crone, agile, fluid, surefooted and barefooted on Mother Earth.

Maybe, in this reverie, our Woman of the Fourteenth Moon sees an altar with eagle feathers and a turtle shell, little bowls with earth and water in them, wands of sage and mystery bundles. Maybe, just maybe, she tunes in to ancient visions of her own heritage. When she opens her eyes she could see the Woman's Staff she was given at the ceremony or the pottery bowl she received at the giveaway.

Ceremonies are experiential and unique to each community that creates them. I believe that the essence of ceremony is simplicity. We are fortunate to have the skeleton, the bones, of our ceremony brought to us by such diverse heritages as this community provides. We are black, white, red, yellow and brown. Every year we flesh it out differently, and every year we learn from the ceremony itself. It is an entity unto itself and it teaches us about power and control, about giving and receiving, about humility, self esteem, appreciation, friendship, community and much, much more. Each woman who attends, attends her own unique ceremony.

Surely this is magic.

TO MY LAST PERIOD

Lucille Clifton

well girl goodby,
after thirtyeight years.
thirtyeight years and you
never arrived
splendid in your red dress
without trouble for me
somewhere, somehow.

now it is done,
and i feel just like
the grandmothers who,
after the hussy has gone,
sit holding her photograph
and sighing, *wasn't she
beautiful? wasn't she beautiful?*

BEYOND THE STETHOSCOPE:
A NURSE PRACTITIONER LOOKS AT
MENOPAUSE AND MIDLIFE

Maura Kelsea

Somewhere around age 46, I made my annual trip to a Nurse Practitioner colleague and commented that my periods had become closer together. Now they were every 24 or 25 days instead of 28, and a little lighter, with an occasional heavy one every few months. She smiled and said that was a very common pattern as one approached menopause. Menopause! I was amazed. It was something I had never thought about in any real way. An "out there" event for the distant future. She went on to say that the increased breast tenderness and slight abdominal distention around ovulation, which had suddenly appeared out of nowhere, were further signs of hormonal change. As the ovaries produced less estrogen and progesterone, the pituitary was signalling it to get busy, by producing sudden bursts of FSH (Follicular Stimulating Hormone). This erratic hormonal pattern leads to increased symptoms around ovulation and sometimes the menses as well.

Forty-six was a tough year. My husband changed jobs, leading to financial and emotional upsets. I was teaching half-time and working at the Health Center more than half-time. With class preparation and homework, I worked seven days a week, up at 5 a.m. and to bed late. Concerned about finances, I worked another position on-call. Two friends who also worked there insisted that I should fill in on more holidays. Already overwhelmed, I became furious at their insensitivity. When they decided I should either work more or quit, I quit, unable to comprehend how friends could act in such an uncaring way.

Although it was viewed by others as a misunderstanding, I became obsessed with the quarrel. I wrote letters, cried, felt depressed and unworthy that I had been treated so badly. Eventually, patient friends and husband pointed out although it was natural that I should have some feelings, what I was doing seemed to exceed a reasonable response. The two by now ex-friends accused me of over-reaction and paranoia when I tried, unsuccessfully, to reconcile with them. I struggled to find some deeper meaning in it all.

A client introduced her friend, Connie Batten, who wanted to interview menopausal women for a book she was writing. Connie, noticing her own beginning menopausal changes, couldn't find information about women's experiences and decided to write the book herself. In her article, I found the first clue to the upset.

> The most insistent as well as the most elusive indications for me have been the periods of emotional intensity. The feelings themselves are nothing new, but their strength and persistence are greatly increased. It is not hard to imagine how a woman experiencing such waves of strong, often painful, emotion all by herself, afraid to utter the impolite word, menopause, could go slowly crazy. I believe it is the secrecy, the fear of ostracism, as much as the strong feelings, which cause the craziness. *(Menopause: An Invitation to Open Inward)*

Here was the key. I had heard about the moodswings and emotional ups and downs of menopause, but now I knew what that meant, from the inside out. Now when women came to my office, crying, sometimes nearly hysterical, insisting that their lives were falling apart, I knew what they meant. There is an intensity that feels desperate in the negative, ecstatic when joyful. Fine, having understanding in hindsight was all well and good. What on earth do women do with these feelings? What could I do? How to prevent such happenings? I value friends and am loyal for years. Losing two was painful. I still mourn that loss.

Medical seminars on Menopause and Midlife Care didn't help. The fact that most of the information was assembled and dispensed by male doctors who could not have the internal experience of menopause, merely accentuated the lack of real life-experience information. Most of the emphasis was on the "cure-all," hormone replacement therapy (HRT). Although the literature stayed medically correct by insisting that "emotional disorders" should be treated with psychotropic drugs and counseling, there were constant references to the alleviation of emotional swings by the use of hormones. Dr. Sadja Greenwood's now classic book, *Menopause Naturally,* helped with an outline of good health practices. However, it didn't deal fully with the intricacies of helping women understand and work with the deep emotional happenings of midlife. I began a personal search for more.

In retrospect, it was a relief to know that something predictable and understandable was happening, but I was faced with entering a new stage of life with no preparation. My mother had a hysterectomy at 40. Grandma was 50 the day I was born, and she never talked about such things to me anyway. No sisters. Lived thousands of miles from my aunts. Had no friends who had gone through menopause. Even the medical education as a Family Nurse Practitioner (FNP) hadn't really prepared me. The medical books talked about hormone replacement therapy, but not about *life!*

With the synchronicity life so often provides, when you first become aware of something, suddenly it's everywhere; several women came to the Health Center, asking questions that I couldn't answer. What to do about hot flashes without taking hormones, what to do about moodswings, would they be at increased risk for cancer if they took hormones?

Our medical director asked me to update our clinic protocol (a sort of medical cookbook) on menopausal care. A friend developed a mysterious illness with high fevers at night that went on for months. Antibiotics hadn't helped. But when her practitioner recommended hormones, she felt "so much better." I discovered Dr. Greenwood's book and devoured it, hungry for her kind and common-sense information.

To most of us, menopause refers to a process occurring over several years, as the ovaries slow their production of estrogen and progesterone and the menstrual periods eventually cease. As with most things feminine, it is complex, not merely a physical event, but a great life transition affecting every aspect of us. Our physical body, our emotions, self-image, relationships, work, world-view and more, are all affected by this profound alteration of hormones.

It is no surprise that such a far-reaching experience should have dread, awe and mystery as its inevitable companions. What is surprising, to this generation of women, at least, is how little information there is regarding this transition. Menopause may be the last taboo. A friend said recently, "Now it's okay to talk about divorce, sexual problems or coming out gay at the dinner table, but *nobody* says 'I'm having a hot flash.' I feel shame about that, and I'm tired of feeling ashamed when my body is just doing what it's supposed to. Why can't we talk about it?"

One of the fun things about getting older is the ability to have some history behind us and stories to tell. I would like to "talk about it," to tell you a story which is still evolving, about the development of a unique health care program for Midlife and Menopausal Women. This program is entitled CHANGES, which I initiated in Santa Cruz, California. I work with women from a whole-person perspective, recognizing that body, mind and spirit all need to be acknowledged in health care.

The Women's Health Center has been providing client-centered health care for 16 years. The emphasis is upon maintaining women's sense of power and providing educational health care which encourages informed participation in health care choices. As the clinic scope began changing, serving older women, practitioners were beginning to have to answer tough questions about how to cope with menopause. Personal experience and lots of work with young women prepared us to assist them into maturity, but we had neither qualification for the older women.

For better or worse, most of us will agree that hormones affect the emotions as well as the body. In working with women experiencing Premenstrual Syndrome (PMS), I often ask the rhetorical question, what purpose could nature have for tying the emotions to hormonal cycles? Reframing the problem into a larger perspective of seeing the patterns in human history, has a way of taking it out of the personal and victim picture, into opening up a curiosity about our own complexity.

I reviewed the components I use to help women reframe PMS, in order to see how they could apply to menopause, both in my own life and for those women who come asking for help and information.

Perhaps most important is the recognition that nutrition, exercise, general physical and emotional health, environmental factors, availability of a support system, specific stressors and the ability to cope with them, history of family dysfunctions, and spiritual framework are some of the more vital elements which affect PMS. The large majority of women who learn how these factors interact in their lives and consequently make lifestyle changes are able to cope with the monthly cycles as part of the rhythm of life, rather than as a disabling curse. Women who have been able to make this shift are able to more easily deal with the ups and downs that can happen in menopause.

Anthropological theories are very helpful in enlarging the perspective. I found it fascinating to discover the biweekly increase I had noticed in sexual interest was actually a theory. Peaks around ovulation are clearly related to procreation, but the peak around the onset of menses seems to point to pleasure for its own value. Perhaps this pleasure could play a part in the bonding that occurs between mates, much as the pleasurable sensations of nursing contribute to the bonding between mother and child.

Many traditional cultures view the menses as the time of dreaming, when inspiration can come in during "the dark time" of the cycle. Prehistoric cultures were based on the monthly moon cycles, 13 in a year. It was the custom of some Native American peoples for women to set themselves aside during the menses to pray and receive guidance and inspiration for their work and the community. Women, with their mysterious abilities to bleed without being wounded, and to bear life, were considered closer to the Great Spirit than men, who didn't have such abilities.

Some studies have shown that when life is going well, a woman is most sexually aroused during the two weeks between ovulation and menstruation. This is the time when the so-called "male" hormones are at their highest level. (Both women and men have the same hormones, but in varying amounts.) Is it a coincidence that this is the same period of time that PMS can be experienced? Ancient civilizations regard this half of the cycle as the "yang" time, when energy is highest. If life is not going well, could the extra energy available turn into unpleasant manifestations?

If these stories and speculations have import for a woman during her fertile years, what might be the stories for a woman in midlife and menopause?

There is an awakening of curiosity and seeking of information about the matriarchal, prehistoric cultures. Each year, new books, seminars, articles emerge. Popular fiction such as Jean Auel's *Earth's Children* trilogy and books by Marion Zimmer Bradley foster the mythology. Political activists, labeling themselves feminist, contribute toward a new ideology. It is clear, as we look around the world, that the patriarchal societies of the last 6,000 years have brought us to the brink of global destruction. From this perspective, it isn't surprising that the archetypal feminine would be seen as the answer to the imbalance.

In the same way that both females and males contain the hormones of the opposite gender in their bodies, feminine and masculine archetypes exist in all of us, woman or man. Archetypes are the universal human patterns of the psyche, much as the skeleton and muscles are patterns of the body. We carry within us the archetypes of the Great Mother, the Great Father, the wicked stepmother, the absent father, the Fairy Godmother, the infant princess or prince and so forth. Jung and others, including Joseph Campbell in his popular TV series, have shown that the archetypes are universal to humanity, and similar in all human cultures. The overlap of archetypes, and of the hormones, allow us the experience of relating to the opposite sex from within our own knowing. We see men declaring themselves feminist, and women taking up political leadership. The last thirty years have shown a widespread increased androgyny, which we see in popular entertainers and in clothing styles.

Genia Pauli Haddon, in her remarkable book, *Body Metaphors: Releasing God-Feminine In Us All*, opens up new vistas of the spiritual and feminine. She avoids resurrecting ancient Goddess images. Instead, she enlarges and extends the Jungian point of view, that we humans contain both female and male in our psyches as well as our bodies. She builds her thesis from the human body, using biological studies of embryology to show how female and male chromosomes develop and differentiate. Tracing the biology of the shared female and male hormones in our bodies, she skillfully weaves between body and psyche, female and male.

Postulating that our human concepts of God or Divine Creator are based on our human bodies, she defines the past 5,000 years of culture as patriarchal, with a God who is phallic and yang in nature. This cultural-religious perspective has no equal female divinity. The only role for the feminine is to be submissive mother or wife or servant of the superior masculine God. The feminine physical parts that are valued are the vagina and the breasts, receptive and nurturant, or yin. Using a four-part analysis, Haddon poses two other possibilities to describe the Creator, based on the human genitalia.

Overlooked in our society is the strength of the uterus. Primarily a large network of muscle, the uterus has the capacity for receiving and nurturing, but its work is only completed when it rhythmically and vigorously pushes the child or the unused uterine lining out into the world. This strong exertive force actually initiates the new being or the old (menstrual blood) into a new phase of life. It is a yang feminine power.

One other possibility is left, the yin masculine. That is evident in the testicles. Soft, but sturdy, undergirding, they hold the seeds of life. These four descriptions contain a chart of cultural development as well as a graphic illustration of our innate human procreative possibilities. It is not hard to find examples of the phallic masculine patriarchal and submissive feminine in everyday life. This is how we grew up. Models of the strong, exertive feminine have begun emerging, consciously. Haddon sees the new emphasis on feminine as the balancing force to the over-dominant masculinity of our current culture.

In the "rise of the feminine" that has occurred in the past two decades, women's spiritual groups have formed a grassroots challenge to established religions. Jungians and others have noted that we are in the process of creating a new mythology. Myths are the language of the collective unconscious. Myths are timeless; even new myths have the language and story form of ancient tales.

The current ecological concern for Mother Earth is a beautiful example of the way in which the species-wide shift of consciousness unfolds. The new mythology affirms that before the rise of patriarchal religions, the earth was respected and cared for by its human inhabitants. Food was taken with thanks for the sacrifice of life from the animal or vegetable kingdoms. We contrast that to the devastation and pollution, which everywhere now threaten life. Part of that earlier world view included a recognition that all elements of the cycle are important. Night and day, summer and winter, growing and fallow seasons. Similarly, death was seen as part of a cycle, in contrast to the modern view of death as the end.

Whether these stories are literally true is beside the point. What they provide is a model, an alternative way of approaching problems, problems that have no solution in our masculine-based perspective. In the same light, I view the movement to care for the whole person—body, mind and spirit—as representative of the developing feminine world-view, which values the whole *and* all the parts. This is dramatically different from the prevailing medical model, which sees the body as a complex mechanical device that can be fixed by tinkering with the physical parts. Cut out, suppress or exaggerate with medication, x-ray, kill with chemotherapy; these are the sorts of remedies which we have come to accept as the norm. There is a cry for change, for more information, and with it, valuing *all* the female cycles—not just the reproductive one focused on by patriarchal society.

In Nurse Practitioner training, which is based on conventional western medicine, we learned that 85% of all conditions that bring a person to a practitioner will heal by themselves, whether or not care is sought. We also learned that all new medicines are tested against the placebo effect: 30-40% of people given a medicine will get better from it, whether or not there is an active ingredient. To be considered useful, a medication must be more than 40% effective. The question becomes, what are we really doing for the vast majority of people that are seen daily in a medical practice?

To facilitate healing it is essential to trigger the curative placebo effect. This is one of the reasons that in conventional medicine so many tests are done. Rather than give someone a medication or treatment that isn't indicated, the test has become a way to impart a sense of doing something about the complaint, without actually giving inappropriate care. As we can guess, tests are expensive and often create increased anxiety while awaiting results, but may offer a great sense of relief when the results arrive that nothing serious is wrong.

Whole-person care offers another approach. I frequently tell people that symptoms are a message from the body, mind, spirit. Although we may want to kill the messenger (remove the symptom), it would be useful to at least listen to the message first, so it doesn't have to find another way to try to signal us. This same model applies to Midlife and Menopausal health care.

Asking questions about the current life situation takes time and requires careful listening. Discovering nutritional and exercise habits, work and relationship issues, and stressors, as well as the person's own strong points, will usually provide a context to understand the message. Once this becomes clear, choices open up. For example, a recurrent yeast vaginitis can be recognized as an outcome of stressors, compounded by a diet rich in sugar, caffeine and instant food. Once a woman understands this connection, she has the key to prevention as well as knowing what to do about the current problem.

When the hormonally-based cycles which have dominated a woman's life for 35 years begin their radical alteration, a new woman begins to emerge. She will have a new chemical balance. As she notices the many other physical, emotional and spiritual changes occurring simultaneously, she will need a view of herself as a whole person in order to birth the emerging new being.

Menopause, all too often, is seen as a disease of ovarian failure, a failure of aging. The emotional impact of menopause is strikingly different if it is seen as a necessary transition toward becoming a Wise Woman.

Where, in our culture, do we have the expectation of becoming a Wise Woman? Who are our models? Those of us fortunate enough to have strong women in our families or lives can be grateful. However, with the rapid pace of cultural change, the particular solutions our models have provided may no longer fit. The stay-at-home grandmother who is the family stabilizer becomes increasingly rare. We are having to create solutions at the same time as we experience the necessity for them.

We need to find help for the woman who is experiencing many hot flashes every day; wakeful nights of soaking sheets; moodswings which create a feeling of being out of control, not only of one's destiny, but even of one's own no-longer-familiar body and emotions; and the recognition of turning older that can't be ignored. This is the arena in which the new mythology of the feminine begins to make a difference. Our own mothers may not have viewed "the change" as an opportunity to become a woman of power; however, we do have that choice.

Whole-person health care doesn't force a choice between the medical model or the philosophical self-help model. It recognizes that many options are available; that both approaches may be followed by the same person; that elements of many styles may be adapted to find the unique solution which fits. The major contribution is in the area of education. Giving information, in a way that can be understood, allows each woman to choose her approach to caring for herself.

As in dealing with PMS, I find it helpful to focus on the larger picture, to give a framework of understanding what is happening in menopause. Why would nature create menopause in human beings? In most of the mammal world, females bear young until they die. In fact, many deaths occur from late child-bearing complications.

One of the more common theories is that older women are valuable to the society, even when they can no longer reproduce. Speculations about the value to society are many. Older women have been the midwives, herbalists, healers and teachers in premodern societies, the respected Wise Women. It appears as if nature chose to free women from child-bearing in order to serve the larger community needs. Women are the keepers of emotional bonding, perhaps due to hormonal influences; as they mature, that bonding enlarges from immediate family to the welfare of the tribe or group as a whole.

Genia Haddon points out that as the female hormones decline, the masculine hormones have less suppression, and so become more potent. Male hormones are known to increase libido and assertion in both genders. For many women, menopause signals an increase in "yang-femininity physiologically, emotionally, sexually, behaviorally," allowing the potential to have stronger emotional responses and to express emotions more directly, to become more assertive, to become more sexual.

In regard to menopause, an old medical dictionary states, "Often nymphomania is present." In a nutshell, female sexuality at midlife is succinctly labeled at once pathological and pejorative. Studies have shown that sexuality around the menses is more clitoral-centered, with orgasms of more intensity, while orgasms around ovulation tend to be vaginal-centered. Masters and Johnson were the first to verify the validity of the clitoral orgasm as normal and more intensely pleasureful than the vaginal orgasm. Again, nature can be admired for its wonderful pattern. As the female hormones decrease, leaving the vagina less moistened and able to accommodate penetrative intercourse, an increase in the fiercer clitoral pleasure arises.

I haven't found any typical pattern of sexuality in menopause. Many women find a gradually decreasing desire in the late forties. Some women find intercourse unpleasant due to vaginal changes, thinning of the skin and decreasing lubrication. Others find more intense pleasure and may become multiorgasmic for the first time in their lives. Some women turn to other women at this stage in life. Others embrace voluntary celibacy, turning inward to find the woman becoming, from within. Some relationships fall apart, others are stirred up, and reshape with greater depth and connection.

When estrogen and progesterone levels fall, the pituitary gland in the brain increases the Follicular Stimulating Hormone (FSH) and Luteinizing Hormone (LH) levels. The rapid, erratic releases can affect emotional stability in much the same way that the onset of menstruation led to the emotional ups and downs most of us can recall from adolescence. From my own experience, talking with many women, and reading, I have come to feel that the hormonally-based changes will lead us to confront any unfinished areas in our life with an increased intensity.

Remembering back to my upset with the two friends, I could see that expressing anger was an area of life where I was inadequate. I didn't know how to express strong differences of opinion in the friendship without feeling angry and/or threatened. In retrospect, it felt as if the hormonal shifts slammed me up against my vulnerable areas. The pattern of being forced to confront and deal with areas of emotional unfinished business is not unique to menopause. It happens in each of the stages of development. The elements unique to menopause include the hormonal and chemical changes which compound the physical, social and emotional transformation.

Simply aging doesn't equate with becoming wise. To be wise implies a knowledge of what is true, lasting, important. Wisdom comes from interacting with life in such a way that the experiences increase one's knowledge and capacity. Each of the stages offers new challenges. One of the final stages in adult development is characterized as interindividual, in which a person is able to be autonomous *and* in intimate, inter-dependent relationships. Psychologists often characterize the decade of 50 as an age of mellowing; an ability to see the whole picture more completely and to understand the complexity of events, leading to a more balanced, and at the same time, more powerful stance in the world.

Looking around at the community, I see that women in their fifties are the driving force for many community activities: running Sierra Clubs, leading election campaigns, becoming candidates. Mayor Mardi Wormhoudt of Santa Cruz was a model of the strong, sturdy woman in the days and months after the 1989 Loma Prieta Earthquake. Concerned, collected, able to share her emotions freely, she cried when announcing the death of a woman trapped for several days; and then later appeared on TV, businesslike and official, with President Bush. Women past the stormy hormonal adjustments have a more stable physiology, freeing the emotions from the hormonal roller-coasters that even the best-balanced women have learned to cope with. Margaret Mead's famous observation that there is no force on earth equal to that of women with post-menopausal zest, begins the reframing of aging which is demanded of this time.

Midlife is also the time of Grandmother. The age of Grandmothering begins with releasing concentration on the nuclear family, and developing recognition that the third generation includes others, the community, in which the new generation exists. Women of Grandmother age have a wider perspective which sees beyond the immediate situation with some history and experience in living, allowing more vision, compassion, balance. A friend, upset by the Supreme Court decisions limiting abortion, called in a fury. "I'll take to the streets," she yelled, "What if Tiffany (her 11-month-old granddaughter) needed an abortion and couldn't have one!" This usually quiet and conservative woman who had never had an abortion herself and wasn't sure she approved of them, radically enlarged her point of view when she considered the world her grand-child would inherit.

Work with midlife women coincided with my own need to educate and prepare myself, leading to the development of an educational approach to midlife health care. There are no easy answers to the questions of how to prevent osteoporosis at fifty, when the time for prevention is in the teens, twenties, and thirties. Whether a woman can experience hot flashes without undue stress depends on many factors, such as how severe they are, how often they occur, what kind of environment she lives in, the nature of her relationships, her current emotional balance, and diet. Whether vaginal changes are a problem depends on a woman's hormone levels, the style and frequency of sexual activity, susceptibility to bladder infections and yeast vaginitis, and partner reaction. Increased emotional reactions, often appropriate to the situation, but with an overlay of sudden unexpected intensity, affect many women. It is important to learn how to recognize and deal with volatile emotionality in the moment. Clearly, it is impossible to recommend the same solutions to each person.

After reading Genia Haddon's book, I now experience a dilemma in the use of Hormone Replacement Therapy that has nothing to do with safety or usefulness. I am wondering what will happen to society on a large cultural scale if we interrupt the natural order, which is to go through the menopausal changes and to come out on the other side with a changed and more even hormonal balance—a balance which brings women hormonally closer to men, just as men's declining level of male hormones in their fifties allows their female hormones to become more significant. Will giving artificial hormones to large numbers of women alter that natural development toward increased assertiveness and coming into one's own that is the reward for completing the rigors of menopause? Will putting women back into hormonal cycling interfere with the ancient biological pattern which has fostered Wise Women? What will these hormones do to the potential healers, teachers and communal grandmothers of our society? These are critical questions which are not being addressed by any of the major factions involved. I certainly don't have the answers, but do try to encourage women to look at the larger picture in making decisions about HRT.

Some women are eager to investigate, question, and make their own decisions. Others are overwhelmed and just want someone whom they trust to advise them on a course of action. Many women are troubled by their changing bodies and desperately need to know what is normal and what to expect. Others are delighted at certain benefits of menopause and are philosophical about less desirable changes. Levels of education and sophistication vary. Support systems and role model availability are not predictable.

As a Practitioner, I must be prepared to deal with all these variabilities and many more. Each woman is unique. Each deserves care tailored to her particular needs and style. I usually use two comprehensive appointments to work with these needs. The order varies, but a typical consultation would be:

First appointment:
- Establish rapport, take history, list concerns, problems.
- Do physical exam, including Pap Smear, breast exam.
- Order complete fasting blood screen and/or mammogram if needed.
- Homework in the form of Health Questionnaire and booklet, or books to read. Particular emphasis is given to self-evaluation of osteoporosis risk and self-evaluation of pros and cons of hormone replacement therapy, as well as any particular health concerns that need addressing. Make list of questions.

Second appointment:
- Review blood test and mammogram results (if needed).
- Review questionnaire.
- Answer questions.
- Evaluate need for hormone therapy or alternatives.
- Develop Health Plan, which includes community resource referrals if needed, and follow up as appropriate.

The form of health care will continue to evolve over time and experience. I look forward to creating a network of women, models who will be available to share their life experience and creativity with women entering the passage of menopause. Developing rituals to honor and support ourselves is vital. The nearly universal emergence of spirituality in the climacteric is heartening and provides the container that can hold and give meaning to the rigors of change.

Midlife is the critical time when completing unfinished emotional business, learning to relate more fully to our physical vessel, the body, and anticipating further development set the stage for the Wise Woman to emerge. The storms of menopause may be seen, in retrospect, as the testing ground for the new capacities being birthed. At the critical age of menarche, body and psyche are preparing for physical birthing and mothering. In menopause, the birthing is of a new woman who will mother herself and the greater community.

The ten or so years before, during and after menopause are sometimes called the "climacteric," a term which is especially apt. It refers to climax, which is the point of greatest intensity or culmination. In biology, it is the stage in ecological development or evolution in which the community of organisms becomes stable and begins to perpetuate itself. One can interpret climax as the peak from which everything goes downhill, or see it as the point from which an entirely new level of possibility arises. In looking at the women in our lives, perhaps we can see examples of each point of view and how life is shaped by the perspective of the woman. We, too, have this choice.

It is always important to create one's unique being in the world, and in Midlife, it is imperative. If Nature has prolonged our lives 25–40 years beyond menopause, it is vitally important to create/discover our purpose in the large picture, and to use our living, developing wisdom for the good of ourselves and those with whom we share life.

NATURAL HEALING THERAPIES
Pela Sander

As a child of eleven, my menses suddenly and very unexpectedly became a part of my life. As a woman over fifty, I've had much more knowledge and time to observe the changes that are currently taking place in my body. To me, the cessation of my menstrual flow will be like losing an old and valued friend. Right now this friend seems to be a bit more erratic than it has been in the past but other than the normal changes of age (graying hair, wrinkles, extra weight, and a less than firm body), I have not experienced any menopausal discomforts.

Does this mean I have just been lucky? Or that I have some fortunate inherited pattern? I don't think so. I expect to have few difficulties in passing from one stage of life to another. Why? Several things have shown me that menopause does not need to be a time of difficulty. First, my mother, although she had wide mood swings and great pain prior to and during menopause, seemed to accept her aging and later her dying as a natural process. As I grew older, I came to understand that her moodiness and pain were related to old emotional and physical problems that had never been completely addressed and not related directly or inherently to problems of menopause. Although my mother did have discomfort, she didn't blame her physical or emotional problems on menopause. She has provided a wonderful role model for me to follow. Secondly, since childhood, my mother, godfather, and many others have fostered in me a great interest in natural healing with a special emphasis on nutrition and herbal medicine. I have found that understanding that life is a process and working with the process is a key to a healthy life.

As a practitioner of Traditional Oriental Medicine, I have worked with women in all stages of life. My experience has frequently shown me that problems relating to menstrual cycles including menopausal discomforts can be directly related to general health and well-being and that by improving the health and quality of a woman's life her physical problems are usually greatly reduced.

Several examples of this type of approach come to mind. One case is of an older woman who complained of a lack of energy. After a few treatments, she exclaimed that her night sweats had disappeared. Since she had not complained about night sweats to begin with, the treatment was not meant to deal with them but rather aimed at increasing her energy levels. Another case involved a woman being treated for asthma. As her asthma improved so did her difficulties with hot flashes. Again the main focus of treatment was working with the physical and emotional stresses that caused her asthma attacks, not the hot flashes.

In traditional medicine (that medicine which has been practiced by human beings, particularly women, for thousands of years), all of the discomforts of menopause are seen only as symptoms of an imbalance in the body. Therefore once the particular imbalance is correctly diagnosed and treated, then the symptoms should disappear. In the Wise Woman Tradition, the discomforts are seen as keys to a larger and more vital understanding of ourselves rather than problems that we just want to vanish.

When counseling either myself or others on the use of natural healing therapies, my first rule is to keep it simple. As long as the problem is not acute or life threatening, you have time to work slowly and slow changes are the easiest to make. The first thing I help women to do is to create an over-all health plan of diet, exercise, relaxation, and life style that fits them. I suggest trying only one or two new things at a time and observing what happens. This way we begin to learn who we are and treat ourselves as gently as we would anyone else who is important to us. As we begin to know ourselves, we also begin to trust those inner voices that will lead us to the "right" changes. Thus life can be a wonderful journey of adventure and exploration if we approach it from an attitude of openness and fearlessness even in those moments of deepest doubts.

What I have been doing in my own life to keep me in balance physically, emotionally, and spiritually is a combination of preventative and remedial actions. Preventative action is my daily and seasonal routine; remedial action is called for as problems arise. It is very important for me to discover the source of what I am having difficulty with in order to know if I can handle the situation myself or if I need help. Women have been seriously injured on all levels when their problems are dismissed as simply change of life "irrationality." First and foremost in my health plan are diet and exercise. These two things affect us in so many ways that even when I find myself in the most difficult of times I try to keep as consistent an eating and exercise pattern as possible.

Vitamin & Mineral Therapy

Everyone seems to have their own ideas about vitamins and I'll give you mine. I believe that if you are a reasonably healthy person and eat a large variety of foods in the appropriate season which are grown and harvested under good conditions—i.e., organically grown fruits and vegetables, and animal products (meat, eggs and dairy) raised without the use of hormones, antibiotics, poor food for the animals, and stressful conditions—you will have little or no need for supplements. (However, a person who has any chronic health problems may need supplementations and should work with a qualified practitioner.)

If you do choose to use supplements, please don't over-do them. While most excesses will be excreted through your kidneys, Vitamins A, D and E are fat soluble and can build up in the body causing problems. Vitamin supplements should be taken with meals. Certain vitamins and minerals combine to give better results whereas others should not be used together. If you choose to do supplementing do some research and begin slowly. Observe the changes you experience and begin to trust your own instincts as to what, when, and how much works best for you.

Vitamins

Vitamin E: For some women Vitamin E gives relief from hot flashes, vaginal dryness, and leg cramps. All of the studies quoted by Barbara Seaman in her book *Women and the Crisis in Sex Hormones* indicated while dosages may vary, the consistency of taking a daily dose over a length of time (at least a month) will bring marked relief in about half to two-thirds of all those who are experiencing discomfort. A word of warning is needed here as the resumption of menstruation may occasionally occur after continued Vitamin E supplementation.

Some people are sensitive to Vitamin E and may experience a queasy feeling or gastric problems. In such cases the dry form of E may be more digestible. Anyone who is using E who develops blurred vision should stop taking it at once. A person with diabetes, rheumatic heart condition or high blood pressure should take E only in low or moderate dosages (30–100 International Units daily) unless they are under medical supervision. *It is recommended that dosages over 600 I.U. should not be used.*

Vitamin E with Vitamin A, C, and B complex (especially B_6, B_{12}, and folic acid) helps prevent various forms of anemia. E seems to be more effective when the minerals selenium and manganese are also included. E needs to be taken at the end of a meal which contains fats, particularly polyunsaturated vegetable oils, as it is absorbed from the intestinal tract only in the presence of fats. *It should not be taken at the same time of day as iron.*

Food Sources: Asparagus, broccoli, cabbage, whole grains, wheat germ, safflower oil, peanuts.

Vitamin B Complex: There are nine generally recognized B-Complex vitamins (B_1 [thiamin], B_2[riboflavin], B_3[niacin], B_6[pyridoxine], B_{12}[cobalamin], folic acid, pantothenic acid, biotin, and choline [which doesn't have any RDA]). Three others, inositol, PABA, and B_{15} (pangamic acid) have limited acceptance.

The B Complex is often referred to as the "stress" vitamin because many of the Bs play a role in maintaining a healthy nervous system and they frequently give a person a feeling of well being. They also may help problems of edema, joint pain, and fatigue. In the past some people have taken B_{12} shots for fatigue.

The Bs are not stored well in the body and therefore must be replaced frequently. Many vegetarians who eat no animal products suffer from B_6 and B_{12} deficiencies and may need to take a supplement, bee pollen, or an occasional egg. There are good references that indicate that the B_6 and B_{12} that are contained in plants cannot be utilized by humans. It is better to take a supplement that offers all the Bs at the RDA levels than take mega doses. First of all the vitamins are expensive and since the Bs are water soluble they are rapidly absorbed and excreted. If you take a B complex supplement, you will notice that your urine is a bright yellow color. This is the excess B being excreted.

Food Sources: eggs, wheat germ, whole grains, brewers yeast, organ meats (liver, heart, kidneys), some fish (salmon, sardines, herring), fruits (plums, prunes, raisins), vegetables (broccoli, asparagus), legumes (peas, peanuts, beans), bee pollen.

Vitamin A: Vitamin A is required for the growth and repair of all cell membranes. It is needed for vision and maintains the health of the eyes, skin and reproductive system. It regulates the formation of cartilage and the synthesis of hormones. It also aids in the detoxification of poisons. There is some indication that Vitamin A deficiency is associated with heavy menstrual bleeding.

Food Sources: beef and chicken liver, carrots, yellow squash, sweet potatoes and yams, apricots, cantaloupe, broccoli, kale, chard, parsley, turnips.

Vitamin D: Vitamin D works with the parathyroid to maintain proper balance of calcium and phosphorus in the body. It works with calcium to maintain the hardness of the bones and teeth.

Food Sources: liver oils, egg yolk, fortified milk, sea food (shrimp, salmon, tuna). Also Vitamin D is created by our bodies in response to the ultraviolet light of the sun.

Vitamin C: This is essential to maintaining many functions in the body including regulating amino acid metabolism, strengthening the blood vessel walls, affecting the health of all cell and tissue membranes, maintaining the adrenal glands and ovaries and aiding them in their production of various hormones as well as aiding in body growth, wound healing, and reactions to stress. I eat Vitamin C-rich foods throughout the day. I grow strawberries, tomatoes, and parsley and munch on them frequently as I pass them by going in and out of the house. To prevent diarrhea when taking this vitamin in supplement form, use an ascor*bate* form rather than an ascor*bic*.

Food Sources: citrus fruits (oranges, lemons, etc.), strawberries, guavas, parsley, tomatoes, peppers, broccoli.

<u>Bioflavanoids</u>: Useful as an adjunct to Vitamin C, especially when women bruise easily or have gum problems. They are usually taken in proportion to Vitamin C. Rutin is very valuable to use when there is a problem with hemorrhoids.

Food Sources: the white inner skin of citrus fruits.

Minerals

<u>Calcium</u>: Required almost everywhere in the body. It is as necessary for the nervous system as it is to preserve bone mass. A deficiency of calcium and magnesium can cause foot and leg cramps, muscle tremors, twitching, or weakness as well as irritability. The best form of a supplement of this mineral includes magnesium and is chelated.

Food Sources: dandelion and mustard greens, chickweed, kale, chard, broccoli, milk, cheese, yogurt, sesame butter and seeds. Wild oats and nettles are calcium-rich herbs.

<u>Magnesium</u>: People on magnesium rich diets seem to have fewer heart attacks and less arteriosclerosis. Severe deficiency may produce brain deterioration.

Food Sources: green leafy vegetables, whole grains.

<u>Iron</u>: Needed by the blood for the transportation of oxygen. Vitamin C helps the body to absorb iron. Some women who are not anemic (as defined by laboratory tests) and yet are cold all the time, may find adding iron to their diet helps. Iron can be stored in the body so if your diet is rich in iron, don't use an iron-rich mineral formula.

Food Sources: liver, egg yolk, molasses, wheat germ, brewer's yeast, apricots, beans and peas.

<u>Manganese</u>: Recommended for women who have been on birth control pills or are taking estrogen.

Food Sources: green leafy vegetables, wheat germ, nuts, beans, whole grains, organ meats.

<u>Selenium</u>: Supports Vitamin E and is recommended for women who are either on the pill or have post-pill syndromes, or hot flashes or other menopausal discomforts.

Food Sources: brewer's yeast, garlic, eggs, liver and desiccated liver.

Because many vitamins are destroyed and minerals "washed" away when cooking vegetables, it is recommended that vegetables be lightly steamed using a stainless steel strainer. The liquid collected then is either drunk or saved for soup stocks or stews.

Mineral Formula

2 parts Yellow dock root
1 part Nettles leaf
1 part Parsley root
1 part Dandelion root
1 part Burdock root
1 part Wild Oats (oat straw)
1/2 part Alfalfa leaf
1/2 part Comfrey root
1/4 part Kelp

Weigh out all the herbs desired. (You can make this formula with less iron by taking out the yellow dock root; if you want to increase the calcium add more wild oats. Don't add more kelp.) Use 5 oz. of the herb mixture to 1 quart of water. Pour boiling water over the herbs and simmer at very low heat for 1 to 2 hours (if you have a slow cooker use that). Let the herbs sit overnight. The next morning remove the herbs and press out or drain any remaining liquid from them. Measure the liquid and return it to the pot and slow cook until the liquid is reduced to 1 cup (if you started out with 1 quart of water). You can make larger batches and share with friends or family. While you are cooking the liquid down take a portion of the herbs and reduce them to ash. Stir the ash into the liquid. When the liquid has been reduced to 1 cup stir in an equal amount of black strap molasses. If you desire the liquid to be thick like a jelly, add agar-agar. Pour into glass containers and refrigerate. Take one large tablespoon a day.

Food Therapy

As mentioned before, eating a large variety of foods in an appropriate way for the climate we live in should give us all the nutrients that our bodies need. Many practitioners of natural healing believe that "good" food eaten at the "right" time is all anyone needs for good health. However, every day people, especially women, are literally starving themselves into a state of chronic ill health not because of the lack of food but because food has become an obsession. Food is one of our basic sources of energy and it should be treated as such.

Billions of dollars are spent each year on fad diets and diet aids. While it has been demonstrated that either chronic yo-yo dieting (gaining and losing weight) and/or extreme weight (200–300 pounds above normal weight for a person's height, body type, and profession) can lead to serious health problems, we have yet to completely assess the long-term health effects that our national preoccupation with dieting has done to women. Therefore instead of an attitude of continued deprivation (dieting), let us enjoy an attitude of continued gratitude for the bounty available to us.

If you decide that your diet is not supporting your life in a manner that is fulfilling to you, start making changes by:

1. Keeping a food diary for one month. Truly be honest and record everything you eat and drink, estimate the amounts, and the time at which you are eating, and the reason for eating (e.g., feeling hungry, sad, etc.).
2. After the month is over, sit down with your diary and begin to study your patterns (e.g., do you go all day without eating and then binge in the evening, do you eat to be social, etc.).
3. Without setting up a struggle between you and food, decide what kind of eating patterns would feel good to your body. Don't forget indigenous people have no food problems. When food is available, they eat when they're hungry. They feast when it is appropriate (celebrations, etc.). Food fills more than just an empty space.
4. Seek help with emotional problems that may cause you to take on obsessive eating habits (e.g., not eating, eating too much, throwing up after eating, yo-yo dieting, low self-esteem, loneliness, abuse, etc.).
5. Be loving and gentle with yourself. Develop your own style of nurturing yourself through food. Be like the best mother in the world: offering delicious foods that are well prepared. Know what, when, and how often your "child" likes to eat and offer good food at these times. Give occasional "treats." Making changes of any type can be very difficult and we will change almost anything in our lives before we change our eating habits. So start making changes slowly.
6. Increase your exercise level by doing things you like (more walking, dancing, swimming, etc.). Thirty minutes a day of vigorous "play" will do a lot for your health. Air is another basic source of energy and it is needed to help us metabolize our food.

General Dietary Rules

Because food is literally the foundation of all life, we need to know the rules and principles that will best guide us, but always remember that these are only guides and being too "fussy or finicky" will not serve us well in the long run either. The key always is the middle road, "moderation."

The rules are simple and clear:

1. Food and drink should neither be too cold nor too hot.
2. Food and drink should be taken in moderation, preferably not together.
3. Eat foods that are produced locally and in season and eat as the season dictates. Eat warming foods when it is cold (soups, stews, casseroles, etc.) and cooling foods when it is warm (salads, fruits, juices, cool drinks, etc.).
4. For an adult a balanced meal consists of:

40–60% whole grains, supplemented with beans, seeds, and nuts to form a complete protein

10–20% organic vegetables and fruits

10–15% dairy, eggs and meat

5% seaweeds

5. Eat a wide variety of foods prepared in an appealing manner.
6. Avoid greasy, overly spicy foods.
7. Take your time eating and avoid eating in untranquil conditions.
8. Spring and summer are times for cleansing or eliminating, for eating fresh greens and lighter meals. Fall and winter are times for nourishing or accumulating, when we eat more cooked foods and heartier meals.

Herbal Therapy

When dealing with herbs, it is important to understand that not all herbs are appropriate for every person and that frequently dosages have to be adjusted individually not only by age and body weight but also by body chemistry. Some herbs are very mild and can be safely used on a continuous basis. Others have a much more powerful effect and need to be used in specific amounts for a specific period of time. Some work slowly and need time to show results and others affect us quite rapidly. Tonic herbs such as ginseng, Dong Quai, etc., should not be used during acute stages of illness.

Each herb or herb formula has its own energy, which to be effective for you, needs to be matched to your energy. If you feel cold all the time, you will need warming herbs that increase circulation. If you feel warm or hot, you need cooling herbs. Someone who is affected by dampness will need drying herbs and a person with dry skin will need either herbs that moisten or ones that circulate the moisture. This is a simplified way of looking at what is appropriate but it can be a helpful place to start. Pay very close attention to what your body wants. Frequently, our bodies will tell us what herbs to take, and when to stop taking them.

When taking herbs or herbal formulas for situations that are *not* acute begin slowly. Take a minimum dose (for example, when using whole herbs, take 1/2–1 cup a day) and observe your body's reaction. Usually herbs are taken on an empty stomach either 1/2 hour before eating or two hours after eating. Take the herbs for two weeks and then give your body a rest for three to four days before taking the herbs again. When cooking whole herbs *always* use glass or stainless steel pots (never aluminum). When taking tinctures, heat a half cup of water and add the amount of the tincture recommended on the label. If the tincture is alcohol-based, let the water and tincture stand for five minutes until the alcohol evaporates.

The most common mistakes made in using Herbal Therapy are:

1. Not using the right herb(s).

2. Not taking the herb(s) correctly.
3. Not being patient. Herb Therapy helps our bodies create balance and that takes time.

Herbs come in many forms: whole herbs (fresh, dried, freeze-dried, powdered), tinctures (extracts of herbs in water, alcohol, apple cider vinegar, glycerine), tablets, capsules, or elixirs. Seek out the best sources possible. If anyone is giving you herbal advice, ask what their training or background is. It takes many years of studying and working with herbs to become a knowledgeable herbalist. If you are unsure what a certain herb that you may be interested in looks like, ask a herbalist to identify it for you. There are many cases of substitutions happening.

When doing Herbal Therapy for hormonal changes, I usually ask women to take the herbs for two to three months. The first month, I give the Women's Tonic Tea for the first half of their cycle (from the end of the blood flow up to ovulation) and then use the Mense Ease Tea (or other formula depending on her particular needs) for the second half (after ovulation to the beginning of the blood flow). During the menstrual flow, I ask women to take a rest from the teas. After the first month, I will adjust the Mense Ease Tea according to what the woman has observed (e.g., if she has experienced greater moodiness, I will use less bupleurum and more peony; more constipation, I will add dandelion root; more skin problems, more burdock root, etc.). If a woman no longer has a menstrual cycle, I will work with the moon cycle and give the Women's Tonic Tea during the waxing moon and the Mense Ease Tea during the waning moon and the rest period is the few days during the dark of the moon. After three months, only the Women's Tonic Tea is continued. Then I ask women just to observe the changes in themselves over time. It may be six months to a year before another round of stronger herbs is needed.

Women's Tonic Tea
1 part Red Raspberry leaf
1 part Nettles leaf
1 part Motherwort
1/4–1/2 part Fennel seed

(One part means by weight. Therefore if you want to have 7 oz. of mixed herbs, use 2 oz. each of raspberry leaf, nettles, and motherwort and 1 oz. of fennel seed.) Boil one cup of water. Place one tablespoon of herb mixture in tea ball. Pour boiling water over herbs, cover and steep for 10–15 minutes. Drink 1–3 cups per day.

This tea is delicious and is excellent for women of all ages. It can be drunk year round and is safe to use even when ill. It is nutritious as well as having hormonal regulating properties. A quart of the tea can be made in advance by placing 1 oz. of herb mixture in a pot, pouring one quart of boiling water over herbs, covering and letting the herbs steep overnight. Strain and place in the refrigerator. Warm to drink. If you wish to increase the calcium in this tea, add one part wild oats.

The Mense Ease Tea is mostly Chinese herbs and it is useful when irritability and signs of congestion are present. Some western herbs could possibly be substituted for the Chinese herbs but as the particular Chinese herbs used in the formula are relatively common and inexpensive, I prefer not to make the substitutions. I do however adjust the formula with western herbs more often than with Chinese ones. Just a note, for women who are already experiencing being too warm, I usually remove the ginger from the formula.

Mense Ease Tea

(Xiao Yao San)

6–9   grams Bupleurum chinense
6–9   grams Angelica sinensis
9–12   grams Paeonia lactiflora
6–9   grams Atractylodes macrocephala
9–12   grams Poria cocos
1–3   grams Mentha (either spearmint or peppermint)
1–3   grams Fresh ginger
3–6   grams Baked licorice (cooked with honey; I will substitute fennel seed; see information below)

The formula is slowly cooked covered for one hour with six cups of boiling water, then strained and refrigerated until used. Warm to drink. Drink 1/2 cup in the morning before breakfast and 1/2 cup in the late afternoon. Again tea is taken on an empty stomach (1/2 hour before eating or two hours after eating).

Ginseng and friends: Over the years, I have seen many references to the use of Ginseng for hot flashes. I personally have not recommended this herb for several reasons. First, Ginseng (Panax ginseng) is very expensive and the system of herbalism I practice uses the least expensive, most easily available solutions before seeking the rare, expensive, or exotic ones. Second, I don't feel that it is an appropriate herb for most of the women that I have worked with so far. Ginseng is useful to those who suffer from cold and are strongly affected by dampness because it is a warming drying herb. Many menopausal women may need warming but they also usually need more moisture or circulation of the moisture rather than drying. However, Ginseng is a remarkable herb and many women have achieved excellent results from using it. To those women for whom this herb is appropriate, my suggestion is to use it in the more traditional way. Take it only during the fall and winter months and try other herbs in the spring and summer.

Barbara Seaman, in her book *Women and the Crisis in Sex Hormones*, has some excellent information on the use of Ginseng. She states that the benefits of taking Ginseng for hot flashes can be felt in ten days to six weeks, and that frequently better results are obtained when Vitamin E is added to the diet. The dosages given in her book are for capsules: for women weighing 100–130 pounds, 1,000 milligrams; 130–160 pounds, 1,250–1,500 milligrams; over 160 pounds, 2,000 milligrams.

The dosage is divided in half. One half is taken before breakfast and the other before dinner. In my experience, many women will find the dose taken in the evening far too stimulating. My suggestion would be to take the first dose at mid-morning (between 10 and 11 a.m.) and the second dose at mid-afternoon (between 2 and 4 p.m.)

There is a lot of confusion over the use of the word "ginseng" in products. Some products will use the name and have little or no Panax ginseng. This is an area where you will need to educate yourself on the best and most reliable sources. There are several Chinese products that are excellent and can be found in many herb stores. Look for *Renshenwangjiang*, or *Panax Red Ginseng Extractum*. A good substitute for taking ginseng by itself is the Planetary Formula *Tai Chi* which contains not only Panax ginseng, but Siberian ginseng, Tienchi ginseng and Licorice root as well as other herbs that would be very valuable for the kinds of discomforts that menopausal women may be experiencing.

The following herbs are in the same plant family (Araliaceae) as Panax ginseng and have similar uses:

Siberian ginseng (*Eleutherococcus senticosus*). Although the root is the part of this herb that is used for its tonic properties, the Chinese use the leaves as a substitute for black tea and have found that after 2–3 teabags daily for one month, there were fewer problems with insomnia and fatigue. Women who are too stimulated by Panax ginseng may find Siberian ginseng a better choice. The dosage can be as high as 15 grams a day.

American ginseng (*Panax quinquefolium*) offers even another alternative to Panax since it is considered cooler and more moistening than Panax and would not be as stimulating, particularly later in the day. The dosage can be from 3 to 9 grams daily.

Tienchi ginseng (*Panax pseudoginseng*) may be a better choice for some women. While it is only slightly warming, it is also considered a hemostatic (stop bleeding) and may be helpful to women who are having either spotting or profuse bleeding. Dosage 1 to 3 grams a day.

Spikenard (*Aralia racemosa*) is a western warm herb used for gynecological problems. Dosage 3 to 9 grams.

The following herbs are *not* in the same plant family as Panax but have been shown to have similar tonic properties and may be very useful for menopausal women in a similar fashion:

Devil'Club (*Oplopanax horrideum*): a cool herb of the northwest that has been traditionally used for arthritis, rheumatism, and the prevention and treatment of diabetes. Dosage 3 to 9 grams a day.

Suma (*Pfaffia paniculata*): a South American herb with neutral energy that strengthens the immune system and fortifies hormones, especially estrogen. Dosage 3 to 9 grams a day.

Ho Shou Wu—also known as Fo-ti tieng which is a misnomer that keeps being passed from book to book—(*Polygonum multiflorum*): a warm herb that is used to rejuvenate and can be used in the treatment of all health problems where deficiency is a part of the symptoms. A liquid extract of this herb is available as "Shou Wu Chih." Dosage 7–15 grams a day.

Dong Quai—also known as Tang Kuei; there are many different spellings of the Chinese name of this herb—(*Angelica sinesis*): a warm tonic herb that is used for all gynecological problems. It regulates menstruation and therefore is useful for both dysmenorrhea and amenorrhea. Because it promotes blood circulation some women have experienced greater flow using this herb. Due to its moistening properties Dong Quai aids constipation problems caused by dryness in the intestines. Avoid using this herb if there is any bloating or abdominal congestion.

There are many forms for taking Dong Quai. I enjoy occasionally nibbling on a whole root while working in my herb room or adding a whole root to my soup or stew stock. While this herb is quite effectively used by itself, I prefer to give it in formulas that are taken twice a day. It is possible to substitute some local angelicas species (not the common garden one, *Angelica archangelica*) for the Chinese variety. Ask a local herbalist about the species that grow in your area. Dosage is 3 to 15 grams a day.

Vitex —also known as Chaste Berry—(*Vitex-agnus castus*): While this herb is also used in Chinese herbal medicine, its main introduction into the U.S. came from Europe where it has a long history of use. Some recent research from Germany indicates that it is useful for normalizing menstrual flow and the treatment of non-specific breast pains. It seems to have a normalizing effect on the gynecological system and is useful when coming off birth control pills or ERT. It is mostly available in tincture form and I suggest that women add a dropper or two to their teas once or twice a day. Some women have used this herb very successfully as a part of their program to eliminate fibroids.

Motherwort (*Leonurus cardiaca*): A slightly cool herb that is useful for blood circulation, heart problems, arteriosclerosis, nervousness, and insomnia. It is used in most western herb formulas for the relief of menopausal discomforts. The dosage is 10 to 30 grams a day.

Cramp bark (*Viburnum opulus*): This herb used alone or with False Unicorn root (*Chamaelirium luteum*) is used as a general treatment for all gynecological problems. It has a general tonic effect on the uterus and can be used for heart palpitations and rheumatism. The dosage is 3 to 9 grams a day.

Licorice (*Glycirrhiza glabre*) or fennel seed (*Foeniculum vulgare*) are used not only to harmonize formulas but to increase estrogen levels. The main difficulty with licorice is that it can cause people to retain water and increase blood pressure so it needs to be used with caution. The dosage is 1 to 9 grams a day.

Sarsaparilla (*Smilax medica*): The best medicinal variety of this herb is considered the Jamaican variety (*Smilax ornata*). Unfortunately when purchasing this herb there are often inferior substitutions made. Sarsaparilla is included in this list because it stimulates progesterone and some health care practitioners believe that even in menopause maintaining a balance between estrogen and progesterone is very important. The dosage is 6 to 15 grams a day.

Goldenseal (*Hydrastis canadensis*): A very cold herb that is highly useful when there are problems of inflammation. I include it here because Barbara Seaman stated in her book that "goldenseal is a traditional cure for night sweats of any origin." I strongly disagree with this statement. In Chinese medicine those herbs that would be added to almost any formula for night sweats would be either *Cornus officinalis* or *Schizandra sinensis*. Both of these are fruits that have astringent properties (tighten the pores) and are tonifying for the kidneys. Goldenseal is not only an expensive herb but it should be used very sparingly as it disturbs the intestinal flora much like antibiotics do. The dosage is 3 to 6 grams a day.

Herbs to avoid: coffee, tobacco, alcohol. They all put great stress on the adrenal glands and help to age us faster than most of us would wish.

Exercise

For some women exercise sounds like more work and they just don't want to do any more work. Some women enjoy working out and will continue to do so in some fashion for most of their lives. However, for the rest of us something different happens. We may go long periods without doing any type of regular exercise and then when we enter our 40s and 50s become interested in more physical movement and then really take on exercise as a way of life.

A woman of any age can benefit from any type of regular movement (walking, bicycling, dancing, etc.) that lasts from 20 to 30 minutes three to four times a week. Some of the benefits can include having more energy, sleeping better, looking better, having more self-esteem, and not having problems with osteoporosis. If we haven't done anything in a long time then it is best to start slowly. Doing things that we enjoy and that fit comfortably into our lives will help us to succeed. Signing up for a lot of classes or activities that we do a few times and then drop out will give us a feeling of failure and will make it harder in the future to try other activities.

My grandmother walked and danced well into her 80s. She never thought of what she was doing as exercise. I grew up walking with my mother and it is still one of my favorite forms of relaxation and exercise. I always feel "better" after a long walk in the country. Some of the other things I do include yoga which keeps me limber, Tai Chi which keeps my energy flowing and gardening which keeps me in touch with life. Find what suits you and stick with it. My neighbor is in her 80s and has told me many times that she feels that working in her garden keeps her alive.

Kegel Exercise

This exercise was developed by Dr. Arnold Kegel to help women with problems controlling urination. It is designed to strengthen and give you voluntary control of a muscle called the Pubococcygeus (P.C.). This muscle encircles not only the urinary opening, but also the outside of the vagina. Women find that a pleasant side effect of exercising the P.C. muscle is that they have an increased sense of sexual awareness.

To identify the P.C. muscle sit on the toilet and spread your legs apart. See if you can stop and start the flow of urine without moving your legs. The P.C. muscle controls the flow of urine. If you don't find it the first time, don't give up. Try again when you have to urinate. Later after you have learned to identify this muscle you will be able to do this exercise any time you want to without anyone knowing except your sexual partner during love making.

Begin exercising this muscle by contracting hard for a second and then releasing completely. Repeat this ten times in a row to make a set. In a month's time, try to work up to twenty sets a day. From my own experience, even for a woman without a sexual partner, this exercise helps to bring you more in touch with your own body and it reminds you very delightfully that you are indeed a woman, with desire and desirable.

Stress Reduction Techniques

There are many types of stress reduction techniques including Biofeedback, self-hypnosis, meditation, progressive relaxation, etc., that can be learned through books, classes, or videos. These techniques are available throughout the U.S. It was very informative for me to read an article about what the men and women who have been major promoters of stress reduction techniques do for their own health. Not one of them formally used any of the above techniques. Instead they had hobbies; they played with their children; they took time to be with people that they care about; etc. They all did things that were pleasant and changed their daily pace.

The most important thing is to recognize when we are feeling stressed and then find a method that works for us. Personally I enjoy taking a day hike or working in my garden. Once a month, I enjoy a hot tub and sauna at the local spa. I also try to give myself one or two days in the week where I can start the day very slowly and not feel that I have to "do" anything during the day so that the things I do "do" don't feel like work.

Other Therapies

Acupuncture, massage, hydrotherapy, aroma therapy, homeopathy, Bach flowers and flower essences are all techniques that I have used to help women with menopausal discomforts. Acupuncture, massage and hydrotherapy can stimulate the body to have an increased flow of blood and energy. Aroma therapy and homeopathic medicines can be used in a manner similar to herbal therapy. Bach flowers and flower essences are therapies that also can be very helpful for nervousness, stress, and other emotional difficulties.

I can never emphasize enough to myself and to other women that if there are problems in our lives with work, friends, family, or anything else, that for our own health we need to be actively involved in doing whatever is necessary to improve the situation or we will suffer the consequences in the form of poor health and depression.

Natural Healing Therapies vs. Estrogen Replacement Therapy (ERT)

It is interesting to note that of all the numerous menopausal "symptoms" discussed in medical journals and popular magazines, only three are directly related to changes in estrogen production:
1. Changes in menstrual cycle
2. Hot flashes and drenching sweats
3. Vaginal dryness and thinning of the vaginal walls

Some doctors, even those who otherwise use a wholistic approach in all other areas, will recommend that every woman over a certain age (50 plus) take estrogen or a form of estrogen combined with other things. I believe that there is a misconception that has been widely accepted that the only source of estrogen in our bodies is from our ovaries and that upon cessation of our menstrual cycle, in order to prevent health problems, each of us must use ERT. Sadja Greenwood, in *Menopause Naturally*, has one of the best descriptions of the estrogen cycle and the changes that occur as we stop having a menstrual cycle. While she very nicely explodes the myth that our only source of estrogen is from our ovaries, she does not adequately discuss alternatives to ERT.

In the *British Medical Journal* (October 20, 1990), researchers from Melbourne, Australia, describe how they supplemented the normal diets of 25 postmenopausal women with food rich in plant estrogens. After six weeks, those women eating soy flour and linseed showed signs of a modest estrogen response which was accurately assessed by microscopic examination of vaginal cells. While the supplements in the experiment only accounted for about 10% of the calories eaten by the women, plant estrogens account for 50% of the calories eaten in some parts of the world, particularly in Asia. Those levels could possibly diminish the discomforts of menopause as well as the health problems such as heart disease and osteoporosis for which ERT is now being used.

While I am not proposing that we swing the pendulum to the other side and never use ERT, I do feel that each individual woman must be free to decide for herself what is the most effective therapy possible. She must be given the most up-to-date information by her health practitioners and the support to try these therapies or not as she chooses. For a woman who has gone through surgical menopause, perhaps combining therapies could be very effective. She could use ERT for 2–3 months and then taper off as she increased foods in her diet that are rich in plant estrogens and used herbal therapy and acupuncture.

Natural Therapies for Specific Complaints

Hot Flashes: See information on Vitamin E and Herbal Therapy.

Night Sweats: I usually give a Chinese formula in pill form which contains Cornus (see Herbal Therapy) called Lui Wei Di Huang.

Dry Vagina: Vitamin E oil can be applied topically (break open a capsule if necessary). You also can use a salve made with Calendula, olive oil, and beeswax (the only other herbs in the salve I would recommend are comfrey, plantain, chickweed; these are all moisturizing herbs). You can also use coconut oil and K-Y Jelly. *Never use Vaseline.* (Note: oils may damage condoms.)

Osteoporosis: People who are of Black African descent, tall, heavy (here is an advantage for us plump and beautiful women), or big boned or vegetarians tend to have fewer problems with osteoporosis. Heavy meat eaters and thin boned people have the most problems. As we age our bodies seem to have more difficulty in eliminating phosphorus which is found abundantly in meat. Excess phosphorus levels draw calcium from the bones.

To prevent osteoporosis, your calcium intake (after menopause) should be at least 1,500 mg/day balanced with 750 mg/day of magnesium, and of Vitamin D, with the phosphorus level not exceeding the amount of daily calcium. Bone density depends on exercise. Here is a direct case of use it or lose it. It is possible that with a diet rich in calcium, magnesium, and plant estrogens, a body that carries a few extra pounds (10–15), and a daily 20–30 minute walk, no other therapy will be needed.

Long Profuse Periods: See Vitamin A. Also Shepherd's purse tincture is very useful (make sure that it is made from fresh, *not dried*, plants). Take 1–2 droppers twice a day (see Herbal Therapy for how to take a tincture). You can also use your own hair. After cutting your hair, save, burn it to ash, and take one capsule of the ash once or twice a day. Avoid anything that will thin your blood such as aspirin and herbs that are high in coumarins such as Red Clover. Check with your health care practitioner to determine the cause of bleeding.

Insomnia: In Oriental Medicine there are many causes of insomnia, therefore there are also many cures. First find out the reason for your insomnia and work with those problems. Try taking a calcium tea and supplement at bedtime. Or soak in a warm tub before going to bed. Sleepytime tea which is available in most grocery stores also can be helpful. See Herbal Therapy for Siberian ginseng.

Muscle Cramps: Calcium and magnesium can be very helpful for muscle cramps. Also try Vitamin E.

Depression and irritability: While there are many treatments that work including vitamin supplements, herbal therapy, diet, exercise, acupuncture, aroma therapy, etc., it really is necessary to understand where the depression and irritability are coming from and then seek the appropriate help. Begin to help yourself by changing what you can (e.g., cut out sugar, improve your diet, exercise more, take the time that you need for yourself, etc.).

Fatigue: You have to understand if the fatigue is related to physical or emotional problems. Again start by changing what you can change (e.g., your diet, exercise, etc.). See Vitamin Therapy. There are many physical causes of fatigue and it is important to check with your health care practitioner to find out if there is a health problem.

MENOPAUSE MEDICINE

Emma Joy Crone

The final flow that marked the ending of my periods, bloods, or menstrual flow, occurred in France, at a time when I was being a gypsy. I was travelling in Europe with younger women musicians. There were few at this beginning point of my new life—and much of the time thereafter—who could relate to what I was going through. Many older women were not willing to talk about it, or just dismissed me with a remark, "Oh, I had a hysterectomy." The silence was unbearable. I was 49 years old, not ready for the hot flushes, debilitating feelings, pseudoarthritic pains and general depression that hit me.

There were other things happening in my life at the time of my menopause, big changes, new openings, so I realized later that this too had an effect on me. It was 1977 and the darkness of lack of literature on the subject was pretty depressing, most books being by male authors who treated the subject with negativity or disdain. However, there were amusing aspects, one being that whenever I felt a hot flush (and of course providing it wasn't in a public place) I would throw off my clothes and declare to everyone "I'm having a hot flush!" Some women were really embarrassed, others highly amused. I afterwards read that this was a good way of relieving the discomfort and shame which in the past has stopped women from talking, seeking support and generally feeling this was something to be kept in the closet.

Because of all of the above, I decided to retreat to the bush of British Columbia to, as I say to women now, my menopausal hut. I had no car, no neighbors, apart from the farmer and his wife from whom I was renting, and for the first time in years, I grew a garden. This may appear to be typical of one living in the country, but it had a very special feature for me. I decided among other things to grow a special medicine plant to help me through this trying time. I started the little seeds in a tray at the back of my cabin. The farmer from whom I rented would come, and trying to appear casual, would inspect the seedlings which were sprouting. His wife then appeared as they got bigger, bringing one of their goats on a string, ostensibly to graze, and she would peer over the fence.

297

One day she said, "Isn't that marijuana?" I nodded, waiting for the next comment. "What do you use it for?" "Tea," I answered, knowing she drank herb teas. I then proceeded to explain my going through the menopause, how it was affecting me, my fears of aging and how the herb helped to relieve my anxieties, causing me to relax. She accepted this explanation which was in fact true. I had on occasion smoked this herb as well as using it for teas, by soaking the leaves and stems in hot water. As a relaxant I highly recommend this tea.

I was allowed to transplant the seedlings, but to save my landlords any harassment, I planted between sweet peas, around the companion of tomato plants, and between anything that seemed to enjoy its presence. I also kept one in the house to be my friend at this time of aloneness.

This is not written to advocate the use of drugs but simply to describe something I found useful at that time in my life. Many women will find herbal remedies that will personally suit them, and help them get through menopause. Marijuana helped me. I did not abuse it. I gardened, went to bed early, wrote my journal and poetry, and read a lot.

I would sit on a log in the midst of my garden, drinking a cup of my favorite herb tea, feeling a great contentment, surrounded by Mother Earth's bounty. From time to time my sisters visited from the city. I was fortunate to be able to do what I wanted to do.

Because of my hot flushes, I had not had a sexual partner for a while. I found myself throwing off the bedcovers in the middle of the night, and this together with the other emotional changes that menopause brought, did not seem to be conducive to being with another.

Now at the age of 62 I find my body still having hot flushes, much less severe, and only if I don't pay attention to the dietary causes, such as caffeine, alcohol, and sweets. The pseudoarthritic pains have disappeared, and I no longer feel drained if and when I have a hot flush. I fully enjoy life, and am in a relationship after four years of chosen celibacy. There have been many interesting changes in my life. Menopause is now a fading memory, despite the major event it seemed at the time.

THIS MOST IMPORTANT PASSAGE

Elizabeth Gips

It was 1968. I was 47, and too high and holy to ever have trouble with menopause. I meditated every day, did mantra, walked in the woods and lived communally. Weren't all those the requirements for "making it" spiritually? And didn't that guarantee a healthy body?

I had dropped out of a healthy business. I started in the 50s with three thousand borrowed dollars, opened a jewelry counter at Cost Plus Imports. At its height my business had fifty-two employees and grossed $400,000 a year. I had three retail stores, a nationwide wholesale staff and I imported jewelry from countries all over the world. It was fun for a long time. I'd buy antique jewelry and actually tell the "pickers" that I'd pay them more for items than they were asking. Unheard of in the antique jewelry business. Or the import business. The men wanted my business; they treated me with respect or I didn't deal with them at all.

Not knowing what to do with all that money, I ended up buying a mansion in the Haight Ashbury in 1966. Before many weeks had passed, I had taken LSD. My first "trip" was up in my weekend home in Nevada City. Lying on the side of the hill, I listened to the bee humming, to the drone of an airplane, to a chainsaw on the next range over. Eventually they all blended into The One Sound, the great Aum, that which lies beyond god or goddess. Dying to myself, leaving my body and personality comfortable on the hillside, I was given the great and mystical gift of entering the rainbow heart, the molecular world of perfect unity, of love beyond love, of being. Indescribable. This was a classically wondrous mystical experience of union for me. Call it love if you will, call it god; the words are a pale shadow. Whatever it was, it irrevocably changed my life.

Haight Street was blooming when I opened a store there, but I'd drop acid, sit on the floor of my own store and watch people buy jewelry they didn't need.

That did it. Inevitably I dropped out. It was the fashionable thing to do, anyway. One classic afternoon I offered to make a co-op of the business. "If you don't want to take it," I told my employees, "I'm going to drop out."

They turned down the offer a few days later, said they didn't want the responsibility.

How much of my behavior was due to early menopausal discontent, I'll never know. I announced, "I'm going to de-escalate. I'm going to find out what it's like to be poor. That's what spiritual seekers must do."

My mother wrote me out of her will. My husband left for Morningstar Ranch, and I eventually formed The House of the Seventh Angel, a typical hippie commune with an array of typical hippie characters who played music and meditated, that had all the typical hippie problems from dirty dishes to eventually burning down! We hoped we could learn to all love each other equally, discouraged couples, tried sleeping all together in the attic with mattresses all over the floor. It didn't work. There were the same old problems, jealousy, internal angst, and, worst of all, the same sexism. Women were "chicks." I was hurt, confused by my confusion and my anger.

But I was holy, right? I was living communally in the country, just the way we were supposed to do it. This fear, this anxiety, where did it come from? It wasn't the system, so it must be all me, my responsibility. Didn't Gautama Buddha tell us, "We are what we think"?

When those waves of heat started at my toes, sweeping through my body, with their concomitant anxiety, I added fuel to the already hot flames by feeling guilty. This couldn't be happening to me; it was somebody else's body. Finally, I had, as we used to say in those days, to "cop to it." It really was me, damn it. Here I was preaching joy, love, peace, and happiness, and suffering intense pains of apprehension, fear and guilt.

I complained a lot. Something always felt wrong. My lover was much too young for me; my communal family was bickering; my money from years of being a businesswoman was running out, and it was scary. True, my menstrual periods were irregular, but that didn't count. I really *should* have everything under control. But I didn't.

One day someone gave me a Valium. Goddess, it was wonderful! It was a blossoming of peace that began in the heart chakra and spread throughout my body and mind. It was so wonderful that I never took another; I was afraid of getting hooked.

The pain, the pain! I had terrible menstrual cramps that felt like a flame in the female organs. My menstrual periods were only a few days long now, but those few days felt like eternity. I finally remembered that many years ago, when I had had an abortion (illegal in those days) the doctor had told me I had a tumor the size of a baseball inside me.

Finally my belly hurt so much I went to the San Francisco Medical Clinic. Two young doctors examined me. I didn't like the way they looked at each other, eyes sort of slyly sliding past me as though I were some child. They cleared their throats. "I'm afraid you really need to have a hysterectomy," one of them told me. They had an odd sort of look as though this was going to be a great opportunity for them. "Would you like to make an appointment at the hospital?"

"A hysterectomy," I gasped. Whoa! At that point I was unaware of how many unnecessary hysterectomies were performed. I was unaware that a second opinion was certainly a necessity before a decision should be made at all. I also thought that one *ought* to intrinsically trust doctors, and that there was something wrong with me because I didn't. I just knew that I didn't want a hysterectomy. I took a deep breath and looked up. "No," I said, "I'll cure myself. I'm going to start really doing Hatha Yoga every day." They looked at me as though I was crazy as I put on my clothes and walked out.

Hatha Yoga taught me a lot about relaxation. I learned to do it from books, from teachers, from television. Eventually I worked up my own routine, designed for my own body and changing as my body changed. I still do it, not every day but often.

Basically I learned to accept my body much more, to stop fighting it, to relax. I put a lot of attention into my abdominal and genital areas, tightening and relaxing, doing my best to feel what was really happening inside of me.

I knew there was a tumor; I could feel it when I palpated my abdomen. After a year or so, the terrible pain subsided. I still had hot flashes; I still had anxiety. But the pain disappeared and never really returned. I've always wondered if the wonderful yoga stretches and mind calming breathing would work for menstrual cramps as well as it did for my menopausal changes.

As for the tumor, I went through a lot of doctors, most of whom advised me to have a hysterectomy. Finally I found an angel (Howard Salvay in Santa Cruz) who was willing to work with me, examine me regularly and measure the tumor. A few years ago I knew the tumor had suddenly grown large. I went to him, and sure enough, it was enormous. But even when he operated on me, removing a nine-pound, football size, benign tumor, he did not do a hysterectomy! My female organs were clean. *I'm telling you all of this in order to give you courage, the courage to believe your body, listen to your body, and don't get talked into unnecessary operations!!*

As I became closer to my body, and as meditation helped me see my own thought patterns, I understood my anxiety more. I saw that the hot flash came first and that within a second or so my mind would scan my life to pick out a few things about which to feel anxious. There's always something in life to feel anxious about, especially in the middle of the night! So there was this tiny lapse of time between the physical and the emotional reactions. I got pretty good at catching it, saying to myself, "You may feel worried, but don't take it too seriously. It's hormonal, inside you, not really real." That helped.

I found that when I was able to muster the honesty to confide in someone, especially women, about my feelings, that helped. I found if I took hot milk or tryptophan before I went to bed, that I slept better. I used licorice tea (the highest natural source of estrogen) until my pores smelled of it, but it didn't really help me. None of the herbal remedies did.

Most important, for me, has been using estrogen therapy. Until I met Salvay, I couldn't find an M.D. who would give it to me (because of the tumor). It has been a miracle drug for me, ending the hot flashes, helping with anxiety and nighttime trauma. Even now, on the off days when I don't take it, the night sweats often return! I've stayed with estrogen therapy through all of the flap about it: first it was wonderful for post-menopausal women, then it was dangerous and might lead to this and that cancer. Now it's wonderful again and prevents this and that cancer. I know that it has been a miracle for me.

Those days of 1967 seem like another lifetime. Actually, I've been "reincarnated" many times since then. I followed a "spiritual teacher" around the country. Gave that up and lived in a radio commune where I learned how to do real community radio. Gave that up and opened two centers called The Sharing Place where everything was absolutely free. Gave that up and came to Santa Cruz and lived on the streets in a van. Started doing radio again. Decided it was time to have an income; went on SSI for being crazy (since I had given my money away, and that's CRAZY in our society). Went off SSI and had an income coming in. Through it all I had relationships with a series of young men, some of them beautiful, some awesomely terrible. I learned A LOT. What I finally learned was that I didn't want that anymore.

I went through a long period of celibacy during which I learned that I am complete, competent, creative and happy alone. Now, at 67, I have the first sane sexual relationship of my life. I asked to learn to love; I was tired of "falling in love."

I live modestly, but comfortably. I'm busy giving what I've learned to the world through the medium of radio and the written word, and I guess I'm a role model for a lot of younger women. I'm happier than I've ever been. It's some sort of miracle. So never give up envisioning what you really want. You may just get it.

Menopause has been a long and interesting initiation for me. It would be nice if our culture had decent rites and rituals to celebrate this most important passage.

SHEILA AND I WATCH THE SUNSET TURN RED AND GREY

For Sheila

Deena Metzger

A thousand shades of gray
prepare me for old age.
Color fading
as we list toward the poles,
ice carrying us slowly
to the final snow, but

peppers today,
red and burning
against the glacial feet.

UNEXPECTED CHANGES

Chris Karras

Ten years ago, at forty-five, I thought only fleetingly of my approaching menopause. Blissfully ignorant of the facts, I anticipated this rarely discussed "change of life" to complete itself quietly within the space of a few months. I looked forward to no more birth control, no more periodic migraines. The end of my reproductive life would be welcomed. Yes, I admit I had always had a poor attitude toward the monthly mess (Freudians, go away!—I did so "accept my femininity"!)—I had even joked with my same-age women friends about burning my leftover rags and plugs and dancing on the ashes in celebration of the blessed event.

Ten years later, at fifty-five, I am a well-seasoned, somewhat chastened menopausal woman, in menopause proper for 15 months. It's an understatement to say that I am delighted with the outcome of the change but did not always appreciate the process. From the very beginning of my peri-menopause, and for the next five years, it felt as though some strange and powerful force was relentlessly destabilizing and restructuring my body, mind and psyche. No dramatization this! Nothing before in the hormone line had ever shaken me up so much: not puberty, not pregnancy, not childbirth, not lactation. Perpetually stressful, often perplexing and downright crazy-making at times, the process resulted in chronic physical, mental and emotional fatigue for me. As a result, I ran mainly on willpower. What's worse, I no longer had a script! But let me digress briefly:

Early on in the process, I discovered that menopause did not happen in a vacuum but seemed to be profoundly conditioned by the physiological and psychological medium of the particular woman in which it occurred. I could quite easily compare the objective, clinical signs of the menopause transition with my women friends, yet each one of us colored them subjectively and interpreted them within the Gestalt of personal life-style, circumstances, socio-economic and cultural values, even world-view; and, especially, degree of feminist awareness. It's impossible for me, therefore, to isolate my personal experience of menopause from the larger context of my total life-experience or even from the process of aging. I shall have to preface this tale with some relevant, minimum personal history to describe the setting in which my menopause occurred.

We (my husband and I) had moved in and out of the mainstream of society with relative ease ever since coming to Canada from Germany in 1956. Mostly, however, we were "out" with just one of us "in" to make a living. During the years I had stayed at home with our two small daughters, my husband had worked for many years in a respectable engineering position, but couldn't wait to get out. Finally, in our early forties, we were ready to leave the noisy, polluted city for fresh country air, reminiscent of the back-to-the-land movement. By then, we had both shifted gears more than once, had taught yoga and related disciplines, even opened a yoga center, and had participated in some of the saner outcrops of the human potential movement as well as in a few social actions, some of which are still relevant today. During those ten years we had paid little attention to our finances and the situation had become critical. One of us would have to get a *real* job again! We sold what little we owned, built a semi-detached cottage and a cabin on 10 acres, got some sheep, goats and pets and gathered our four-generation family under one roof. We were joined by a friend, a divorced woman with two young teenage daughters. Our total headcount was eleven, ranging in ages from a newborn and a year-old toddler, our grandchildren, to my nearly eighty-year old mother. This experiment in communal living was supported by equal parts of love for family, economic necessity, and a dose of idealism that pre-dated the sixties. However, we hoped that just as soon as everyone else in our household would find a place in society and, with it, economic independence, we would continue our mid-life alone together.

I soon found work as a lay counsellor in a residential service institution for mentally handicapped adults but seemed to be doing little else than dispense an unconscionable array of combination prescription drugs, said to be needed to keep the residents under control. I looked elsewhere for work and landed a full-time office job in the female work ghetto where I am still doing time. My husband picked up odd jobs and did many of the domestic chores, including the cooking.

Five years into our mostly enjoyable new life-style, characterized by organized confusion, the event I had thought of only fleetingly at forty-five was unmistakably upon me. Almost immediately, I wanted nothing more than to live *alone*! The extended family crowd became too much for me; I had little, if any, privacy except in the bathroom or car (sometimes!), and I felt trapped. I needed space, peace and quiet and unfractured blocks of time. My anxiety was compounded by the fact that my now ailing mother, nearly deaf and blind, in her mid-eighties, had to be moved into a chronic care ward of a nearby hospital, which I visited frequently. The images of her in that godforsaken ward haunted me more than I can say. She died there nine months later, in her sleep.

One would have thought that, under these circumstances, a natural event such as my menopause would have passed me by relatively unnoticed. I was certainly distracted and busy enough, healthy enough, and had always adapted well to new situations.

But not *this* time!

So this was menopause! The first two to three years were the worst, given my erratic menstrual pattern with closely spaced and heavy periods, more severe migraines, hot flushes, abdominal bloat, stress-incontinence, heart palpitations, nausea, severe vertigo and, occasionally, even fainting. Add to that irritability, free-floating anxiety, horrific nightmares, insomnia and a rapidly eroding self-confidence and self-esteem. The combined pressures were immense; I still refer to this period in my life as my twilight zone.

Mostly, I worried about my job. I simply could not risk losing it by missing work or goofing off in a client-centered office. And, I worried about driving 46 miles daily when feeling dizzy or being partially blinded by the developing aura of a classic migraine. At home, as the woman in the middle (before my mother's death), I was still the cohesive force; were I to come unglued, a few other things around me would too. I was not in the mood—nor did I have the energy—to pick up the pieces. So I plodded along stubbornly, congratulating myself on still being fully functional.

Then, one day, on my way home from work, I accidentally ran over a rabbit with my car and flipped out. I pulled over and sobbed convulsively. A rabbit for heaven's sake! I cried over a dead rabbit! This must be STRESS, I told myself—or fatigue, or grief, or even depression. In the months to come there were other weeping spells, always in private, usually in the car on my way home. I figured something would have to be done, but what?

I did not feel ill, just wiped out. The last place I intended to look for help was at the friendly neighborhood doctor's office, gynecologist's or psychiatrist's den. The medicalization of menopause (including its psychiatric application) and the medical model of menopause as a deficiency disease did not appeal to me. The unholy alliance of the pharmaceuticals and pro-estrogen physicians did not inspire confidence in me with their aggressive, unsavory campaign, designed to bring the still recalcitrant women in line. All across this land of ours we were steadily assaulted and insulted via the media with promotions about the wonders of estrogen or hormone replacement therapy. This product promotion was blatantly manipulative: first, the fear of wrinkles, loose flesh and sexual rejection and/or abandonment by our male partners said to be in search of younger and firmer flesh ("you wouldn't want to look like a Babushka now, would you, dear?"); next, the fear of disease, especially osteoporosis and heart ailments ("only estrogen will save you, little lady! take it! take it! take it NOW or you'll be sorrrrrry!"); then, the cost-effectiveness calculation with its fear of becoming a burden on the state ("you wouldn't want to become a drag on society when there are so few healthcare dollars!"). What's left? The fear of God, and the fear of death? But give them time.

And, I recalled all too clearly the many misdeeds, to put it mildly, that had been so casually visited upon women everywhere by the practitioners of allopathic medicine and the medical technocrats: Thalidomide, DES, Benedictin, Depo Provera, the Dalkon Shield, and Net-Oen (for women in the third world!); the unnecessary hysterectomies, radical mastectomies, Caesarian sections, episiotomies, and scheduled, induced labor for the sake of the doctor's convenience. The list goes on. There was also that serious attitude problem: have you ever been to a modern medicine man who couldn't hide his underlying assumption that we women are really a lower life-form and rank in intelligence just next to children?

Before I could reach a decision on how to deal with my multiple stressors, I discovered a lump in my left breast. I had lost two dear friends to breast cancer and had instant flashbacks. My husband and I spent a rather miserable weekend. It looked as though I would be seeing a physician after all. I wanted a diagnosis; then I would decide what to do with the lump. As it turned out, the surgeon to whom my G.P. had sent me immediately, declared the lump benign, and we were much relieved. The G.P., however, suggested I have a full check-up with blood tests and a Pap smear. When I showed up for my appointment with him, a substitute physician I didn't know, a solemn-looking elderly Englishman with impeccable manners and who did not condescend, examined me. I was strung up in that ridiculous stirrup position when he asked if I was "on estrogen." I said I was not and didn't wish to be. Surprised, he looked briefly up from the scene of inspection and said: "But *that* tissue looks pretty darn *good!*" Had he been looking for the clinical signs of an atrophic vagina to make the evidence fit the medical assumption, knowing I was over fifty and not "on estrogen"? I wondered. What irony! When I went home I thought of my aging face, wrinkling neck and hands and resented that propriety forbade me to flaunt my vaginal tissue or wear it on my face!

A couple of weeks later I contacted the doctor's office and requested a report on my blood tests from the nurse. All values but one were normal: the TSH (thyroid stimulating hormone) was high. I was not to worry but have it checked again in a year. I concluded, perhaps wrongly, that my thyroid might be low and was being nudged into better action by the TSH. This, I felt, might explain my chronic fatigue and the steady, slow weight gain I had experienced over that last eight years. Given this clue, I had a better handle on my situation. I temporarily reduced my commitments and began a self-management program to deal with the combined impact of menopause, job and home life, such as it was.

I had also begun to get informed. A social scientist, Janine O'Leary Cobb of Montreal, Quebec, had started an educational newsletter in 1984 "for women in the prime of life." She had called it *A Friend Indeed*. The publication contained up-to-date research material pertinent to menopause and related topics. Studying it, as well as her book, *Understanding Menopause*, left me with no doubt that the subject could hardly be exhausted with the usual medical entry of the climacteric: "cessation of menses—hot flushes; dry vagina." The medical model was seriously flawed.

The medical focus, for example, on "dry vagina" as a menopausal symptom, and the pre-occupation with the genital expression of our sexuality by various writers could reach ridiculous proportions, I found. One text suggested that, if sexual intercourse is painful, I am to anaesthetize my vagina with some gucky jelly a half hour before "love-making" (?) but to make sure I wipe my vagina out prior to intercourse so that my partner's "organ" (yes, organ,— I kid you not!) would not be similarly rendered insensate. That ought to give new meaning to the phrase: "Was it good for you too, honey?"—"hm, just wonderful, dear,—I didn't feel a thing!" Needless to say, I was revolted.

My vagina and my sex-life were the least of my problems. I experienced menopause in much less localized, circumscribed ways—predominantly existentially. No medical text covered my concerns.

Over the next two years I watched my nutrition more carefully, added the best B-complex vitamin I could find, took vitamins and minerals (including a calcium substitute) regularly and lost 18 pounds over four months by eating less but better. I walked briskly for an hour each morning before work to promote weight loss and to preserve bonemass. Once I had reached my optimum weight (120 lbs./5' 5 1/2") again, I felt in sync with my body. In the evenings, after work, I practiced yoga regularly for an hour of asanas, pranayama, relaxation and meditation. I felt centered again, as I had been in earlier years. Some of the more distressing physiological signs of menopause gradually lessened (migraines and palpitations) and some even disappeared altogether (vertigo, nausea and fainting).

None of this, however, would have been possible had there not been a spontaneous and gradual exodus of the members of our extended family. Without time, space, and privacy I could not have followed through so well. The urge to live *alone*, however, was still overwhelming even when only my husband and I were left to rattle around in our cottage. I had not expected this and felt profoundly guilty that I wanted and needed distance, at least for a while, from my marriage partner. With my husband's consent and understanding, I settled for the best of two worlds: I claimed the seven hundred square feet of one unit of our semi-detached cottage for myself, furnished it, dragged in my personal belongings, my music, books, plants and pictures and gave my partner "full visiting rights." We continued to keep house together in the other unit. It proved to be a mutually beneficial solution, unusual and intuitive as it was, and this living arrangement did infinitely more for me than hormone replacement therapy, mood-altering drugs or tranquilizers, so often prescribed for "difficult" women like me, could ever have done. Having my own apartment in my own house as well as our shared space was nothing short of therapeutic. Because it worked so well for us, we have kept it that way.

Here in my own space, I could cope much better with my sleep disturbances, the menopausal insomnia that had plagued me for four years. Frequent hot flushes and sudden heart palpitations, usually after a nightmare, interrupted my sleep every night. Now I could get up, do as I pleased without disturbing anyone; I could read, exercise, take a bath, write letters, listen to music, eat or fall asleep on the couch. I began to call those periods my spares. Some of those spares I shall remember forever:

— the night I happened upon Sheldon Kopp's *An End To Innocence, Facing Life Without Illusions*, and read that
> "some forms of madness are no more than failed transitions from one vision of life to the next." (p. 46)
and made a few psychological glitches I had postponed;
—the night I read Gloria Steinem's essay "If Men Could Menstruate" (*Outrageous Acts and Everyday Rebellions)* and laughed myself silly;
—the night I filled out my Living Will and Voluntary Euthanasia forms and really meant it;
—the night I forgave myself for letting my mother die alone in an institution;
—the night I flashed back to my childhood and *re*interpreted it;
—the nights I read Robin Morgan's *The Anatomy of Freedom—Feminism, Physics, and Global Politics*, the book that touched my soul as few others had before;
—the night I drifted in and out of sleep, producing several hypnagogic images, and felt wonderfully relaxed;
—the night I slept six hours and had no spare.

As the quality of my sleep improved steadily, energy returned. I could easily live with the remaining discomforts, mainly hot flushes and much milder migraines. I picked up some of the commitments I had temporarily suspended and saw more of family and friends again. In the meantime, my husband, inspired by my quest for personal space, had laid claim to the now vacant cabin for his own solitude. Friends and family wondered at just whose place we would all gather: his, mine, or ours! But, without exception, they envied us and fantasized about making similar living arrangements.

Friends and family! How very important they are to me! As soon as I felt up to it, I made amends for the times I had been so irritable. I had a vague notion that I might have been the cause of some tensions, conflicts, upsets; I certainly had behaved out of character, at times, during the last few years. It's hard for me to say what prompted me to talk privately to each one of those near and dear to me, especially the two women I had given birth to; was it menopause? The fact I had gotten away with it, as it were, when the breast lump turned out to be benign? Or, perhaps, that I wanted closure? If remaining tensions and conflicts could be resolved, I very much wanted to try. I also wanted my daughters to have a script for their own midlife transition when it came, the script I had to develop as I went along during my, sometimes, critical closing of the reproductive cycle. They will know where to find the newsletters and the books I had found most helpful. My own mother had never discussed menopause with me; it was a taboo subject in 1950, it seemed, when she was fifty and I was sixteen. But I do remember her sometimes strange behavior: taking an over-the-counter bromide potion every night and boozing a little during the day. A few years later, she had settled into chronic melancholia. An artist, intellectual and agnostic, she had been temperamentally manic-depressive all her life. Now she was just sad. When I began my menopause, she was still living; we could have still talked a little, but she was deaf then and we communicated in large letters on scraps of paper and she would nod yes or no.

I do not expect another crisis now until the final one, which even men must face: death! In the meantime, I have work to do. In a world I once heard cultural historian and social critic, Theodore Roszak, define as being on a continuum between the "Calcutta Syndrome" (how to get through the night without starving to death!) and the "Stockholm Syndrome" (how to get through the night without committing suicide!), there is a focus for social action and "the power of one"—as well as for "the power of the collective."

Having traced the physiological and psychological pattern of my climacteric which, I feel, has just about completed itself, I am hard pressed for words that might adequately describe its spiritual impact. More than ever I am convinced that Descartes' "cogito; ergo sum" (I think; therefore, I am) needs reversing to read: "I am; therefore, I think" . . . I am, therefore . . . I AM—YOU ARE—WE ARE.

THERE WILL BE NO BLOOD

Carla Kandinsky

No blood to sing out its warning
each month, the tightness in my
belly, the walking on heavy legs
before it comes. I will sit before
my altar, empty, having nothing to
give the goddess. Full moons will
come and go and not be noted.
Crimson thumbprints on photos once
used for magic spells will become
old blood, turning to simple spots
of rust, useless as junk cars
corroding under a Carolina sun.

I had been warned of this, dire
predictions when I was a girl,
mouthed by rocking chair women seeking
to steal my youth even before the
blood had come. Now are they finally
satisfied, now that no blood touches
my lover's body, my towels, my sheets?
Each morning I still search for the
sign, hopeless as when I was pregnant,
waiting then too for the coming of
that red redemption. Now I am left with
this bloodless life I hold between
clenched teeth like a dog with a bone,
having no use for it as food and
no place to bury it.

THE MYSTIQUE OF AGE
(AN EXCERPT)

Betty Friedan

. . . I looked for patterns beyond the feminine mystique, but there were no patterns, because the women my own age and younger were still in the postwar baby boom and living the feminine mystique, and the few women who were deviating from it were more or less guiltily coping with their own problems, alone. The women who were combining jobs and professions with marriage and motherhood out of choice, not just necessity, were older. They looked different from the frustrated suburban housewives I'd been interviewing. There was vitality in them. Their very skin looked different. I began asking them about their menopause. They hadn't had it. "What do you mean you haven't had the menopause?" I would ask, for they were in their fifties, after all. Their menses had, in fact, stopped; they just didn't remember when. They hadn't had menopause in the traumatic way menopause was supposed to occur. The menopause in America and elsewhere, I think, was considered the end of a woman's life, really. There were just some leftover years to live. In the mental hospitals in the United States, one of the prime diagnostic categories along with *senile dementia* was *involutional melancholia*, a psychosis that had been considered virtually normal for women in menopause and afterwards, a state of extreme depression. But these older women whom I was interviewing didn't have depression; they didn't have the menopause in that sense. I couldn't understand it. I went around talking to some of the experts on menopause, and there were no explanations.

That was my first sense of something new happening with women and age. Does something happen to the aging process when women move beyond that previous biological definition of the female sex role to larger human purposes, a larger definition of personhood?

. . . I had menopause myself somewhere back then in the midst of the women's movement, after *The Feminine Mystique*, but I can't remember when. By now the change that I had seen only in a few women was absolutely epidemic in society. By now millions of women, who were supposed to decline and get ready for death after menopause, were back in colleges, universities, going to work, marching, talking back to male chauvinists, revolutionizing home life, revolutionizing concepts of sexuality, demanding to be preachers and rabbis and priests, moving into space as astronauts. No longer were women three percent of the students in medical school and law school; they were 35 percent. And many of these wonderful, vibrant new women were over 45. The whole picture of aging for women was changing.

UNFORESEEN BLESSINGS

Lea Wood

I first noticed I was on the menopausal slide during a family hike. I stumbled along the trail trying to keep up with my husband and kids, floundered across the stepping stones of the shallow river, and wondered why the collie kept coming back to check on me. I was fifty. My balance was gone, my breath short, my body quickly exhausted.

"This is how it feels to get old," I muttered to myself. "It's going to be downhill all the way now." During most of my life I had engaged in strenuous and frequent physical activity so that the feeling of going down into the valley on my way to death was something of a shock.

I did not consider that I was addicted to cigarettes, and to wine after work; that I got little outdoor exercise, had a demanding job and an even more stressful family life.

I thought menopause was the last degradation of my life as a woman. Society said so in many subliminal as well as obvious ways. I remember a popular cartoon series about middle-aged women who were drawn like pouter-pigeons and made to say trivial and silly things. In ads from hair color to dish soap the message was that to look one's age was horrifying; everything blared "look younger!" I had hoped to age in some beautiful way and felt bleak about this new phase of my life.

Among the first signs were the kind of emotional swings I remembered from adolescence. "Is menopause a teenage re-run?" I wondered. Worst of all were the hot flashes. I had heard about them, but they didn't sound so bad until they flashed through my own body, burning me up in a prolonged body blush that made me want to tear my clothes off. They came and went with a life of their own.

I felt modern going to my doctor for an estrogen program. He put me on Premarin. Not long afterwards, however, heavy and more frequent menstrual bleeding took me back to the doctor who said I might need a hysterectomy, but he would try an additional medication first. It was the birth-control pill, Ortho-Nova, but at the time I didn't realize it had a dual purpose. What it did was to regulate the periods I was still having. They didn't amount to much, but they were so regular I could almost set my watch by them. These medications made me feel more like the self I was used to and the flashes disappeared. I thought the periods would disappear, too.

In two years my life changed. My husband and I parted company on friendly terms, I quit smoking at last, cut down on the wine and lived with my sixteen-year-old daughter. I started hiking for fun and exercise. I still had the demanding job, but other stresses were gone. That was the year that local Sierra Club hikes led to backpacking in the new and wonderful world of wilderness.

At sixty I retired from teaching junior high and asked the doctor how long for heaven's sake was I still going to have periods? He seemed surprised that I was still on the Ortho-Nova, and took me off. The periods ended at last and I still felt fine on Premarin alone.

Then five years later I read a book by a doctor who made a compelling case of estrogens being unnecessary and, worse yet, a cancer risk. He convinced me, and I dropped the Premarin cold. I did not have the sense to taper off and my body went into something of a spin with the sudden withdrawal. By this time my old doctor had gone into the beyond, and I was somewhat on my own. I wondered about going back on Premarin to taper off, but thought that soon my body would adjust.

But adjusting was a long process and during it asthma spasmed my lung sacs and arthritis stiffened my neck. The hot flashes burned again. I hated their random hit, angered at my powerlessness to control them. When an older, wise woman asked why I wasted my energy this way, I decided to think of the flashes as a cleansing fire and waited more patiently for the blissful coolness that followed them. Now, finally, at age 73, I haven't had one for several months. The last reminder of menopause is gone.

During those years between 50 and 65, I weighed fifteen pounds more than I did as a younger person. Uncomfortable and decidedly unagile with this extra tissue, I resigned myself to the thicker shoulders, heavier abdomen and slow-down as one of the crosses of aging.

The asthma and arthritis, however, led to fasts in hope of a cure, and without even aiming for it, I lost my extra pounds. I felt that my own body had returned to me. I love movement, doing things fast, and was delighted to find my agility alive and well. About age 65 I started running and found it exhilarating. It didn't matter that my speed was nil—a run recharged my energy. I never would have believed it possible at that age. I ran alone and in group runs for a couple of years until my body stopped me with a sciatica pain down my leg. I returned to walking.

Menopause should be a *celebrated* change of life. I was surprised that it led to a time of even steadier energy than in the years before. Another triumph besides the cessation of monthly inconvenience, moods, and pain was the freedom from the fear of unwanted pregnancy—even though society thinks older women have little interest in sex.

I was astonished that far from going down into the valley, my sixties turned out to be the most fulfilling decade of my life. Most of the time I had the vitality to enjoy my life, the freedom to pursue what I had not had time for in my years as wife, mother and professional—and wonderful sex in an affair that started when I was 62 and lasted until I was 70 (not because the sex deteriorated).

Dealing with the arthritis, which disappeared, and asthma made me more aware of the desire to live well though aging. In that hope I nourish myself on natural, organic vegetarian food, exercise every day at what I enjoy: T'ai Chi, walking, and gardening; rest when my body asks for rest; and involve myself in the issues of my times. I'm aware of many blessings in my life as I'm living it now, and give thanks for them every day.

INDIAN SUMMER

Ruth Levitan

I carry my climate with me now.
Muggy as a summer storm,
the unsettled weather
of changing seasons
dampens my skin,
reminds me I have survived
the prickly heat of childhood,
flush of first pubescence,
furnaces of passion.
This new heat
tells me that life
with all its hungers, angers, loves,
still glows, radiates,
burns within me.

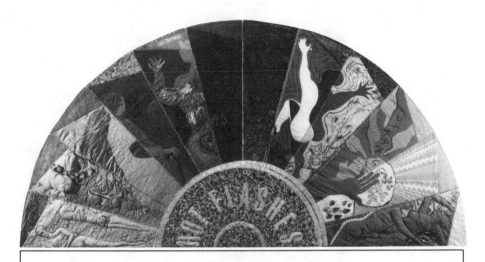

JOURNEY OF TRANSFORMATION

Understanding menopause as primarily a physical experience may block access to its spiritual significance. To understand menopause as a soul-event means attending to it imaginally, regarding its symptoms as symbols, and not being surprised at its close association with underworld experience.

My journey through menopause has brought me to Hestia. She comes bearing none of the usual attributes of the goddess but carrying a book with blank pages, the unwritten volume of the new. I am only beginning to sense what will be written there.

—Christine Downing

BLOOD STOP

Katherine Wells

The moon will abandon me soon,
draw no more blood,
spark no more female alchemy.
My drying pods must turn inward
the way a cut magnolia folds and droops.
Ovarian failure the book says,
as though they'd done something wrong.

Even in my mother's womb
I had my own womb
and a million little possibles
jostling for the signal to travel.
Such overkill. Enough to start a planet.
Only one's been used,
one in a million,
a son nearly grown.
Still hordes remain, landlocked
as chemical valves begin to close,
skin to lose its collagen,
vagina to go slack as a sleeve
when the arm's removed.
Bonfires of the skin,
flames kissing my throat.

It's not the babies I'll regret,
but myself, stuck in an old VW body
concealing a Rolls-Royce engine
with half a million miles left,
dated lines, sagging upholstery.

No one tells you
this is a colossal Non-Event, a doorway to Nowhere,
ice in all directions rather than liberation,
the murder of flowers in a cartel
where young is the only recognized country.

I'm doing a high-tech video fade,
but haven't learned how
to be gratefully invisible,
what to do with age rage,
the urge to hurl bricks through
the slick faces of make-up commercials,
what to do with skin that loses luster
but not its hunger to be touched.

My grandmother's eyes and jaw slide over mine
one frame at a time.
I've got a third of my years left,
thousands of healthy nights most likely alone
with dreams rerunning the one huge love I've had,
a man I'd have jumped into fire for or with.
I try to stretch his warmth to cover me yet.

No decorated cake, no white dress
or cigars passed around,
no sprays of gladiolas as condolence
mark this junction.
No new punctuation when the periods end.
Just questions, calcium and hormones,
a bridge to cross inside a closet,
tampons in the drawer like a stash
of dry, white kindling.

What to do but make a rawhide drum,
search for shrike feathers and hawk talons,
mix ointments from powdered bone
and my last blood,
wrap sleepless nights in stone musk
colluding with darkness
in hard, black sacraments.

Or, can I build a hearth
on the moon's dark side,
silhouette my hands against an evening fire,
learn the music of high, blue desert,
the cadence of solitude.

MENOPAUSAL DREAMS
(AN EXCERPT)

Patricia Garfield

I am startled to see that there are several sinks filled with dirty water. They need to be drained.

—*Author's dream diary, age forty-six and a half, immediately prior to menopause*

The woman whose season of childbearing is complete changes hue like the autumn leaves. Her hair touched with silver, her skin marked with the lines of living, she is nonetheless full of beauty. Much joy may abide in this phase of life. Sad, indeed, that few women are prepared for the process of menopause; few understand what to expect, how to cope with it, or how to make the most of the glory of their autumns—fall can be spectacular.

Menopause is a critical turning point in a woman's life cycle, equal in significance to the menarche, the first intercourse, and the birthing of a baby. For many females it becomes a crisis of major proportions; for some it marks the beginning of self-discovery. We shall see how this process of menopause—its physical manifestations and its psychological responses—is charted in our dreams. . . .

By learning from those who have gone ahead of us in life's dance, by respecting their findings and their essence, we prepare for ourselves a place of value and accumulate a legacy of hope for the daughters who follow. No longer mainly a maiden or a mother, our role now—if we but embrace it—is that of the wise woman. . . .

Estrogen Stimulates Dreaming. Researchers Joan Thomson and Ian Oswald . . . demonstrated (in 1977) that taking estrogen shifts the proportion of sleep time that is spent in rapid eye movement (the characteristic sign of dreaming). When women took estrogen, they dreamed more; when they were estrogen deficient, they dreamed less. Here is the strongest evidence we have for estrogen's connection with dreaming.

When we are deprived of dreaming at night, we suffer during the day. Our whole sense of well-being depends upon sleeping well, especially on our having dreams. Numerous studies have validated the role dreaming plays in making our sleep refreshing. Considering the enormous impact lack of sleep or insomnia has upon people—making them irritable, anxious, under par, and inefficient—the benefits from estrogen therapy for the menopausal woman may outweigh the small risks. Every woman, however, should assess her case with her gynecologist.

Fire and Water: Dreams Depicting Physical Changes
Dreams Associated With Missed Periods

Dirty Water. Each woman's pattern of menopause varies. Some women find that their periods simply stop; others notice their menses growing lighter and lighter until the flow ceases; still others are troubled with excessively heavy periods that require curettage; yet others alternate heavy bleeding with extremely light flows. Most women begin to skip occasional periods a few years prior to menopause itself.

My own pattern, for instance, was mixed. Since this material is generally unfamiliar, especially as related to dream life, I describe it here. My periods ceased completely in 1981 when I was forty-six and a half, but as early as 1975, six years prior to menopause, my extremely regular menses were no longer reliable. Whereas the usual flow was every twenty-six to twenty-eight days, that year it once came at a fifty-day interval, followed by a normal interval, then twice in one month, followed by another normal interval, and then twice in the next month. This erratic bleeding continued for the next year. In 1977 the usually heavy flow concluded with exceptionally light days. Then toward the end of the year there were a couple of months with exceptionally heavy bleeding. In 1978 there was one month with two periods and four months with skipped periods; 1979 was similarly erratic. The last six months of 1980 were marked only by light spotting or no period; this spotting continued for the first two months of 1981, and there the menses stopped completely.

This variation of heavy and light bleeding, as well as missed periods, gave me a chance to observe the physiological process in my dreams. For example, on the occasion when I had nothing but one day of spotting for six months, I had the dream described at the opening of this chapter, about sinks filled to the brim with dirty water. For me, as well as for many women, sinks are frequently a symbol of the womb—corresponding to the womb's capability of being filled and emptied. This dream suggested that there was still a need to release some material. Sure enough, two light but relatively normal periods followed a few weeks later—then, complete cessation.

Later on in the same dream of the dirty water there was another obvious womb symbol:

> I learn that the emblem of a secret order is a vase, an urn, of a deep, almost-maroon red that is set into ceramic tile above the altar. Somehow this understanding entitles

325

me to be initiated into the group. I wear a red velvet gown with a short cape, and a small golden circlet on my head.

Aside from the mystical imagery, the red urn—the container—is of the color of dark menstrual blood. The gown I wear is blood red as well. Vases and urns as well as sinks often serve as symbols for the womb in women's dreams. They, like the womb, function as receptacles for contents. The fact that the water in the sink is dirty suggests accumulated blood; the fullness of the sink indicates the likelihood of another flow. At other times when I have been bleeding heavily, I dreamed of sinks overflowing. The mystical imagery implies a positive attitude toward the natural process of menopause.

Dreams Associated With Heavy Bleeding

Red Doors. At another stage of approaching menopause, when I was bleeding profusely for longer than normal, I dreamed:

> I am climbing up a ramp in a narrow tunnel, on my stomach. At the top I open several layers of red doors to a restaurant.
>
> Then there is a mystery story about some missing jewels. Much searching. One place resembles a home where I once lived that has an all-red meditation room. Later someone asks me if the pearls are pinkish. Yes, they are unusual. A man sets out to hunt.

Narrow tunnels and hallways often represent the vagina, as in this dream; the layers of red doors may have stood for the days of heavy bleeding; the restaurant is the nourishing womb. The missing jewels probably symbolized the lost eggs (the female sexual cells)—there were few ripening in my body at the time of this dream. The pink pearls—ovum-shaped—confirmed this hypothesis. The all-red room of my past waking-life experience relates, no doubt, to the all-red womb.

Sinks, vases, tunnels, hallways, doors, jewels—the woman approaching menopause may well be able to assess the condition of her womb from the condition of these images in her dreams. Because each person has their own individual dream language—in addition to the symbols that are commonly shared because of similar shape and function of the womb—it is important to learn one's personal images. Women can do this most easily by monitoring their dreams carefully, especially during ovulation and premenstrual and menstrual times. She will soon notice what her dreams are saying about her body.

Dreams Associated With Hot Flashes and Night Sweats

Fire Alarm. The chief symptom I experienced was a night-time restlessness—awakening damp, warm, and fidgety—that reduced my usual ample dream recall and left me tired during the daytime.

Daytime hot flashes were, for the most part, exceedingly mild. Since the estrogen level dropped gradually in my case, I rarely mentioned the presence of this symptom in my journal or tied it to specific dream imagery. An exception, however, appears in an entry a couple of years after the menses ceased. It was four days after I noted a hot flash accompanied by heavy perspiration brought on by exceptionally hot weather:

> I am in a house with problems. My husband has just gotten out of his car when a whole pane [pain?] glass window in the house falls forward and hangs at right angles, as though on a hinge. I call to my husband to come help me and he does.

> Later I hear firemen at the door of the house. Now it seems to be a kind of cottage in which an alarm has gone off. Because the firemen get no quick answer, they circle the glass—I hear it ringing—and cut a hole through which they open the door to enter. Inside they spray a preventative liquid. I think there is smoke. A fire person—perhaps a woman—tells me to be careful where I step, that the liquid can burn if it touches the skin. In a later scene we are saying good-bye to a fictional teenage son as he goes off to camp. Much affection among us.

The dream house, which usually represents the dreamer's body, has problems. In fact, later on the same day of the intense hot flash, I had sprained my right ankle (the "right angle" of the dream) on a holiday outing. Like the large window pane, it is a "big pain" that required repair. I am warned in the dream to "watch my step."

Furthermore the dream says that my house is smaller, shrunk to cottage size. This, along with the fire alarm that has sounded, indicates that the change in the body, more specifically the womb—is one that has to do with heat. The positive aspects of the dream include my husband's helpfulness, the appearance of firefighters to control the problem and the preventative liquid that can burn the skin (as hot flashes do). The farewell to a youth may be saying good-bye to the part of myself that began during the teenage years. From another point of view, the teenage boy could be the son we might have had—we have been married for 19 years—but now will not.

A few months after this dream I accepted my physician's urging to take a minimal dosage of estrogen, which resulted in not only elimination of hot flashes and increased sense of well-being but also in greater dream recall. All symptoms vanished.

Fire in women's dreams often represents an emotional heat, as well as a sexual state of feeling "hot." In menopausal women the stimulus for dreaming about fire may be the hot flashes occurring during sleep. Depending upon the woman's experience of menopause and her attitude toward it, the conditions of the fire will vary.

Initiations and Goddesses: Dreams Linked to Self-development
The Dream as Inner Ritual

Women who are able to turn to their dreams for nourishment, understanding, and guidance often find that the menopausal stage brings dreams of staggering impact. In addition to dreams reflecting their physical symptoms and changing conditions, such women discover an inner transformation unfolding at this stage of life.

Deprived of outer rites of passage, women can draw upon the rich inner ritual available in dreams. This nightly panorama sometimes reveals the role models and archetypal patterns that bring a sense of wholeness to life.

Jung has spoken of the value of the second half of life, how this is the time of finding the center of one's being that he called the Self, the whole that was previously hidden or scattered in several directions. He emphasized in particular the affinity women possess for contacting this through dreams.

The woman who communicates with this realm gains wealth beyond compare. She may find herself truly at peace; she may be inspired to strike out courageously in new directions based on guidance from within; she may undertake creative projects; she may discover spiritual joy.

Goddesses, temples, initiations, magical objects, descents and ascents, ritual dances, chants—this sort of imagery is found in the dreams of older women who open themselves to the treasure buried in sleep.

When a woman has struggled to "find herself," when she listens to the words and contemplates the pictures of her dreams long enough, and wrestles to understand their messages well enough, the character of these images undergoes change. A new center emerges. What was buried is reborn. Von Franz tells us that:

> In the dreams of a woman this center is usually personified as a superior female figure—a priestess, sorceress, earth mother, or goddess of nature or love.

This quote did not come to my attention until long after I began to observe such a transformation taking place in my own dreams. I have described my image of the goddess of love elsewhere. Briefly, she was in the form of a large white stone, roughly hewn or natural on the outside with a smooth, flawless hole in the center—a simple, perfect hole. Several more realistic-type goddesses appeared in dreams that I have described in my *Pathway to Ecstasy: The Way of the Dream Mandala*.

The Twin Goddess. At the conclusion of my menopause on the day after Christmas, following six months of no periods or very light spotting, and just prior to the final spotting, I had a remarkable dream of a ritual:

> I am outdoors descending a complex arrangement of circular stairs. It is constructed as though it were around a temple, although no building is there. There are numerous doors and compartments that are waist-high.

> Many people descend with me. A fat woman catches up and crowds me. I feel uncomfortable as she pushes into some small compartment with me as I go through. I try to think why her fatness bothers me so much and I realize I fear that she will smother me. I decide to let her pass, and she does, which pleases me.

As I reach the bottom of the strange descent, I see members of a family of artists I know, particularly noticing the man. They are welcoming some returning voyagers. We greet and embrace.

We speak of a powerful predictive dream I have had that has to do with the breakage or loss of the middle front tooth in the lower jaw of their daughter. . . .

Then the scene shifts and I am seated in a room on a chair, as part of a circle of people belonging to a special group. We discuss the same predictive dream of mine. It emerges that I am being accepted because of my skill in dreams, this one in particular.

The leader, a man with the bizarre code name of Cucumber, proposes a toast to two women who embody the principles of intellect and beauty. I say, "I'll drink to that," and picking up my wineglass set beside me on the floor, I proceed to drink the red wine that fills it. All join the toast.

Then the leader says something like, "Let's do a little 'Loga-Shana.' A little Loga-Shana can't hurt anybody." Everyone rises and, still in the circle, we turn to face his direction. He, with his back to us, demonstrates certain movements and gestures that we follow. The idea is that this secret ritual is safe to communicate to others. Now the women are goddesses. The leader turns partially to the right, at a forty-five-degree angle, and utters, "Loga!" as he spreads his arms open wide at shoulder height and lifts them upward. This is the invocation of Loga. He then withdraws his outspread arms to his body in an embrace, as though to incorporate Loga's essence of intellect; simultaneously he bows his head and dips his body reverently.

Turning to the left, with the same arm-opening gesture, he utters, "Shana!" and then withdraws his arms to his body once more in the identical movement to the left. Doing this incorporates the essence of beauty of spirit. We join the procedure, repeating it over and over.

Ethereal music begins. I know it comes from real singers somewhere in the house because this group does everything with quality. I sense that now at last I can learn some of the things I have yearned to know.

As we continue the repetitive gestures, crying, "Loga! Shana!" I feel myself slipping into trance. I see green fields with people moving over them. At the same time I seem to be writing a description of the ritual, in order to retain it, waking up with the effort.

This complex dream has for me many fascinating dimensions; I will mention only a few. My first impression was awe at the way the dreaming mind can express a partially formed concept. I never heard the word Loga before, but it reminded me of the *Logos*, the word of God that was said to create the universe; perhaps it could be a feminine form of intellect. Shana made me think of the Yiddish-German word for "beauty" (*schön*) that in the dream implied more than physical loveliness. Surely wisdom and beauty of spirit are principles I wish to embody. Awake, it would never have occurred to me to think of them as goddesses who could be invoked and incorporated.

In this dream I find the descent into my depths made more difficult by the presence of the fat woman and my response to her. Not only had I gained a few pounds prior to the dream—later discovered to be a result of a thyroid imbalance that required treatment—but she had negative associations to heavy people I knew, including my mother at a stage when she was physically ill. By "letting her pass" I was able to contact the artist (symbolized by the artist family) within myself. This contact leads to the special knowledge.

From the chalicelike glass I drain the red wine, probably symbolic for the womb being emptied of blood. In the circle of the whole Self, I participate in a ritual that marks my new phase of womanhood.

In addition to all this, I was stunned a few weeks later to learn that the daughter in the artist family mentioned in my dream, just prior to leaving on a trip for Europe, awoke with her mouth and cheeks swollen with infection. She had unexpectedly developed an abscess in a front tooth that required emergency attention. My "predictive dream" was truly predictive. This signal event—Jung would call it synchronous—further marked the dream ritual as significant.

How and why such events happen we do not yet understand. I cherish the content of this telling dream and the many of like nature that succeeded it. Surely there is more in dreams than we can fully comprehend.

The Value of Menopausal Dreams

We have seen that dreams of the menopausal years often indicate the physiological changes that are taking place within the dreamer's body. They may also dramatize her sense of barrenness and emptiness, not so much of the loss of capacity to have children—the woman may have had as many as she wished—but rather a feeling of uselessness in life. If the woman who feels this way searches sincerely, either with or without the assistance of a therapist, she may find new fertile ground—a purpose—for the years ahead.

Some women can find their internalized menopausal rite of passage in a dream. Awake, they may seek an unexplored direction, a way to revitalize their energy for abundant and luxuriant new growth. With the freedom from birth control, from the nuisance of equipment for menstrual periods, from the emotional swings of the reproductive years, and from heavy commitments to home and children, the menopausal woman finds she can pursue interests that formerly eluded her.

We shall see how undertaking new activities not only stimulates us momentarily, it literally adds growth to our brains. What we have regarded as old age is, in large part, ill health or boredom. As physical activity and good nutrition strengthen the body, intriguing mental activity strengthens the mind.

In addition to travel, to pleasurable hobbies, to time with loved ones, to creative pursuits in pottery, jewelry design, painting, language study, charitable or other projects they have always wanted to try without previously having the time to do so, women of menopausal years may find new self-development and spiritual direction. Who knows, perhaps this preparation will serve us well in the unknown beyond?

LAST EGGS

Dena Taylor

Tiny bottles of colored powders
stand on shelves along the walls
A sweet cinnamon smell wafts
through rosy light
Smiling fetuses float in glass bowls
waiting to be lifted and held

Wise and ancient women are busy
measuring, mixing, weighing, feeding
You can have a baby too, they tell me
Oh no, I've hardly any eggs left
and those that are, well, they're old
The women laugh gently: it's very easy
These herbs will bring everything back
Oh no, I say again, I've already had
my children, they're nearly grown and gone
We will take care of you, they chant
We will take care of the baby

And then my body remembers the wonder
Remembers how precious
the births and babies were
Yes, I say to the women, yes

Awake, the next morning
the once-familiar
sticky mucus of ovulation
stretches between my fingers

OVULATION ON THE SUMMER SOLSTICE

Christina Pacosz

Fireflies are blinking,
many bright eyes opening
and closing in the deepening night.
Deep inside my body
an egg is letting go,
a difficult lesson
I am still learning.

Pain just below the solar
plexus, rhythmic, miming labor,
but less intense. No sweat,
no screams except one,
where, where did youth go,
old egg on your finite journey,
do you know?

The last light of the first day
of summer fluoresces the sky,
blue, becoming bluer, then bluest
night. I sit and stare, feeling
a fist clench, then relinquish
my flesh, a small sacrifice
on the standing stone of my body.

All is possible, but not this
wrenched red life, soon to die
in a gush, the stench of iron, sharp,
rising like the odor of water at dusk,
or a newly-forged knife of hot steel.

Just once, just once,
do you hear? little half-life,

little lost one, *just one child.*

A JOURNEY OF TRANSFORMATION

Louise Thornton

When my first symptom of menopause, sudden attacks of dizziness, began two years ago at the age of 47, I became terrified for my life. Brain tumor! was my first response. I had always been afraid that I would die from one and here it was. Fortunately a friend who is a nurse assured me that I was probably suffering from no more than the onset of menopause.

I didn't entirely believe her, but she proved to be right. One day after one of these attacks I went home, my body cramping as it had at the age of thirteen when menstruation began, and slept, thinking I was coming down with the flu. When I awoke there was blood on the sheet. While I was greatly relieved that I was not dying of a tumor I was also aware of my mortality in a way I had not been before. I looked out into the redwoods across the canyon from my studio and felt great sadness, remembering that young girl of thirteen who was pale and trembling as her body writhed with cramps. I knew she was leaving me forever. She had been through so much, but I did not want to let her go.

At this point in my life I had already grieved for more deaths than I thought I should have to endure. Four years earlier I had lost a mentor who died long before I was ready to let her go. A year later I ended a painful 21-year marriage, leaving the only life I had ever known as well as my adolescent children who chose to remain in their home. The following year my oldest child was diagnosed with paranoid schizophrenia, and I lost him as I had known and loved him. A year later a new relationship ended, and my father began succumbing to Alzheimer's disease. I did not want another ending but it was breaking upon my body whether I was ready for it or not.

As I began to experience more symptoms of menopause—a dark heaviness in my muscles, lead in my bones, ropes wound around my chest that tied me to the earth as my body held on and held on and did not bleed for 34, 38, 42 days— I would slip out of bed at five in the morning, gaze at the moon in the quiet dark and begin to weep. Sometimes I wept out of loneliness. Sometimes I wept for my son. Sometimes it was for my daughters who felt distant from me. Most often it was for the passing of time itself. The rich moist place inside me that had grown three babies was shrinking. The primary way I had of identifying my Self, as a mother, was being taken from me.

Often I would think of that young girl who had stood ashen before the mirror, the color drained from her face, as her body began its mysterious journey. What was particularly startling to me as I thought back over my life was that, despite the passing of time and the assumption of many responsibilities, I never entirely ceased being that girl. I became a girl-woman who tried desperately to please everyone but her Self.

As a child I knew deep abandonment, my father seriously mentally ill and my mother lost to me again and again with each new baby sister. As I came to be mother not only to my five sisters but to my mother as well, and as I was told by my father that girls were dishrags (to his credit he did send me to college so I could support my Self if I became a widow), I tried very hard to be good. If I were perfectly good, I believed, someone would love me enough not to abandon me. I did not yet know that someone could love me but not be able to remain in an emotionally intimate relationship because of unresolved childhood pain.

I grew older, married, quickly gave birth to three children and poured myself into being a perfect wife and mother. It did not work. My husband abandoned me for his job and his computer. My daughters grew from sweet children into angry adolescents who told me I was laying guilt trips on them when I asked to see them more often. And most of my son's childhood was a long nightmare for both of us as the early but unrecognized symptoms of his illness (obsessive compulsive behavior, paranoia, thoughts of suicide) manifested. Finally he left me completely and entered a psychiatric hospital.

After I took it upon my Self to find a cure for him and failed, I was catapulted into a feeling of powerlessness. The dreams I had had for many years of being unable to control my car became more frequent. Sometimes one of my children (small again) was in the driver's seat while I froze, helpless, in the back. At other times I was driving but the car insisted on going backwards down steep, precarious hills. Once my two cats drove the car while I watched in horror from the back seat. In one dream I was again in the back seat, the car was running smoothly through the quiet desert and the space behind the wheel was empty. The car traveled on a stretch of unmarked sand, moving on and on through lavender and soft brown shades of silence.

I woke from these dreams in the middle of the night, heart pounding, even though my car never crashed. And so I began to ask the question: why am I so terrified of being out of control? I could not tell whether it was because my wounded inner child was dominant in my life or because this inner child felt she and she alone was responsible for everyone and everything, and it was overwhelming. In the desert dream, I realized, the car was perfectly under control, guided by a spirit or power certainly present although I could not see it. I wanted to know this power and whether it was inside or outside of me. And this was the beginning of my passage into adulthood.

Until this point I was not aware that I had very few models of women who had successfully evolved into autonomous, fully adult beings. Until recently many women, hundreds of thousands, died tragically young from the complications of childbirth or from illness and exhaustion, and this was true in my family: the mother of my mother's mother died at 42, her daughter at 46 while pregnant with her fourteenth child, my paternal grandmother and most of my aunts in their fifties. Those female relatives who did survive into old age cared for their declining husbands until their husbands died and then they also sank into illness.

When I turned to books on women's spirituality, thinking I might find in them representatives of the woman who is no longer fertile but is far from aged and is vital and strong, I could find no direct acknowledgement of her existence. Primarily I found references to woman's value as mother, the source of life, and as nurturer. While there were also numerous references to other rites of passage (first menstruation, marriage, birth), there was no mention of menopause. It is as if once we can no longer create life we become invisible and are not valued.

Is this because until the last fifty years or so more women than not died before reaching menopause? Or they were made to bear children until their bodies rescued them by becoming infertile and then they fell into exhaustion and old age? Perhaps mine is one of the first generations of women who are able to view menopause not as the signal that life is over but as another, vital cycle in our evolution towards wholeness.

The search for wholeness is a spiritual quest, and as we enter menopause we are given an opportunity to deepen and strengthen the bonds we as women have always had with the essential elements of life: birth, death and transformation. As we enter this important transition in our lives we can call upon the aspect of the feminine known as the goddess, symbol of our innate beauty and capacity for empowerment and the source of meaning and purpose in our lives. This goddess, who was once revered in the entire civilized and uncivilized world, continues to manifest her Self in the Life Force and in each of us as we participate in balance and harmony for our Selves and for the earth as a whole.

What is particularly exciting about the goddess is her constantly transforming nature. In *Lost Goddesses of Early Greece* (Beacon Press, 1978), Charlene Spretnak explains how the three phases of a woman's life—maiden, mother and crone—were linked with the three phases of the moon. The new moon represented the pure maiden, growing in strength and magic. The full moon symbolized the mother, fully empowered. The waning moon was the crone, filled with wisdom and ready to die and be reborn as the waxing moon.

In Native American spirituality the counterpoint of the goddess is Mother Earth: she who gives birth to us, sustains us, teaches us with her sometimes harsh lessons, comforts us, renews us, welcomes us back into her body at our deaths. Sometimes she has other names: among the Navajo the highest place in the pantheon is held by Estsanathehi, The Woman Who Changes, and who has the gift of renewing herself whenever she grows old.

Among the Nootka people of the village of Ahousat on Vancouver Island are the stories of Copper Woman, her daughter Mowita, and Mowita's grandmother, Old Woman, who are all aspects of the same being. In her book, *Copper Woman* (Press Gang Publishers, 1981), Anne Cameron tells the story of how when Old Woman became bent with advanced age her spirit left her body. Not knowing if she could survive without her, Mowita lay on a bed of skins and asked Old Woman to enter her. Old Woman heard her and impregnated Mowita with her spirit; Mowita became Old Woman and Old Woman became Mowita.

The journey in which Old Woman is participating is not only the one I shall make at death but a continuation of the spiral of transformation I began at birth and continued to move through as I began menstruation, developed into a full sexual being, bore children, raised them, severed from them as the center of my existence, returned to my original Self. Each time I complete another cycle of the spiral I die and am reborn. Menopause is simply another cycle, another part of the journey.

This journey, like all other journeys, can be divided into three stages: severance, threshold and emergence. These stages are not always clearly differentiated; often they overlap. One stage may be begun before the previous one has been completed. This often necessitates going back to the preceding stage to tend to unfinished business. At other times we may find that we do indeed complete the cycle but that life plunges us again into the same journey only at a more intense, deeper level. What is essential is movement along the spiral.

Severance

While the changes required to obtain transformation are essential, for there is no rebirth unless there has been a death, they are often accompanied by great resistance. We fear what we do not know and cling to what we do know. In our culture menopause is often called The Change, as if it embodied the essence of change for women, or it is called The Change of Life. These names are powerful for they suggest that this is a time when our lives are undergoing profound transitions which in themselves release bursts of energy and growth.

However, in our culture menopause is not regarded as a time of power for women. When I say the word to a woman she often grimaces and speaks only of hot flashes and extreme discomfort or of migraine headaches that leave her incapacitated or of the increased dangers of osteoporosis or other frailties accompanying age. These physical discomforts are exacerbated by our culture's beliefs that aging is not a natural phenomenon but a failure to remain young. Who am I if I am no longer considered beautiful, a woman may ask herself.

What am I to do with this body that is betraying me? And what will I do with myself now that I am no longer wanted?

These are almost impossible questions to answer if one accepts the belief that a woman not only loses her femininity but her very reason for existence once she is no longer fertile and begins to age. Even if one does not accept this belief, however, severance is difficult for we are called to separate from the way we have perceived ourselves for the last thirty-five to forty years: young, fertile, almost invincible, needed, needed, and again, needed by our children, spouses/lovers, and other family members, by our employer or by an organization or group, finding our identities by immersing our Selves in other people's lives.

In my own instance letting go of these aspects of my Self created a profound sense of loss. I grieved not only for the loss of my youth and my strong, vigorous body but for the loss of the dreams of my youth which had been broken or radically altered and which could not be entirely mended because there was not enough time; I had already begun the descent into darkness.

And when I thought I had finally come to the end of them and could settle into a permanent state, life crashed down around me once more. Just recently my oldest, precious daughter moved away, began using hard drugs, was jailed three times, and was finally brutally assaulted. As I drove alone to the city where she lay in a hospital, her chances of survival only five percent, I screamed "This can't be happening!" But it was, and I calmed my Self, calling on all the sources of strength I have acquired during the last few years. She survived and is now in physical and emotional recovery and will be entering a drug rehabilitation program very soon.

However, several months after she was injured the relationship I had with someone who talked of being together for the rest of our lives ended abruptly, not by my choice. For four more months while I struggled with finding the best physical rehabilitation program for my daughter I held my Self together because it seemed required of me. The day after my daughter left my house for a treatment facility, however, I spiraled into despair. I now had two disabled children, I realized. I was completely depleted. I could not imagine going to work. I would never find happiness. I wanted to die.

Fortunately I have learned how crucial it is to have a support system intact, so I used this and was able to crawl through this time, which lasted for only a few days instead of the months it would have taken me at an earlier time in my life. When my daughter at one point secretly made plans to return to the city where she was injured so she could buy drugs again, I finally got it: if I was going to survive I had to sever from her. I can not lose my Self in desperate attempts to keep her alive. Whether she lives or dies is in the domain of the Spirit, and I have learned to surrender to this law of the universe, enabling me to return one more time to my Self.

Being able to return to the Self necessitates this severance, but it is often difficult in a culture where women are overwhelmingly assigned the role of caretaker. I am speaking not only of those women who have children at home but of those who have other kinds of all-consuming responsibilities. A friend who is childless and works in the mental health field said to me recently, "We find our children." Every night she tries to avoid taking her "children" home with her but they come nonetheless. I did the same when I taught in an elementary school and would still be doing this with my college students had I not worked extensively on detachment. Very often I see this double mothering: children at home and children at work.

If women do not have primary responsibilities at home they often expend even more energy at work, assuming responsibilities far greater than they can comfortably manage. I am not speaking of women who have found their life work and pour themselves into it with a passionate intensity or of women who must work long hours to provide for themselves or their families; I am speaking of women like Elizabeth, an office manager for whom I once worked.

She arrived at 7:00 in the morning, often stayed until 7:00 at night and joked about "running the company" which she did (for low pay). She never left her desk . . . not for coffee breaks, not for lunch. She and only she knew every aspect of the small company; she was needed to the extent that almost all business was put on hold if she became ill, so she came in while sick.

At the core of such over-responsibility is a desire to escape the Self, very likely because of childhood abuse; I have engaged in this willing slavery repeatedly, finding false refuge in overmothering and caretaking, rather than feel the excruciating pain of abandonment. Thus letting go of these escapes can be terrifying, as illustrated in the next section, but they are crucial. The death of the Self under such circumstances is inevitable.

Ultimately severance is exhilarating and life-affirming for everyone. Children, mates, other family members, friends and associates are finally allowed to fly free to follow their own rightful longings. And in each of us who are journeying through menopause, the Self, buried for so long under responsibilities for others, can finally begin to emerge, trembling, exquisitely beautiful and new.

Threshold

The task of the threshold stage of menopause is to learn to know and love this new but mortal Self. Now that it is clearly evident that one does not live forever, each of us may realize, perhaps for the first time, exactly what it is she really wants to do or become or accomplish before she dies, and what greater gift could there be than this knowledge? However, while the treasure that each of us eventually obtains is great, the search itself is often difficult.

In any transition this stage is the time of chaos. A death has occurred but there is not yet a rebirth. For those of us who have severed from deadly over-responsibility or control, a blank horizon may stretch before us colorless and void. As we look at this horizon stretching endlessly into the distance we may realize for perhaps the first time that each of us is alone.

My early experiences with the threshold were of this nature. I felt as if I had suddenly landed in an alien land where no one desperately needed me, and I did not know how to live in this world. I wandered around lost, wondering if I had not made an overwhelming mistake in separating my Self from the only life I had ever known.

Not only was I alone in a strange land with no clear direction for my life but my body was presenting clear evidence that I was growing older, every muscle in my body aching, the blood in my womb stagnant and dark. At other times exhaustion was so deep and profound I felt that surely I was dying and if not, I wanted to die and as soon as possible.

In my cyclic, ongoing experiences with this stage of menopause, exhaustion continues to challenge me, but I am learning to acknowledge and honor the need for long hours of solitude and sleep. In this surrender to the dark I often find healing both of my body and of my spirit. In my dreams I return to the womb of the Earth Mother, to the Underworld, and dream of urns and coffins, tombstones and graves, of bodies of water which are in continual flux and in which I sometimes plunge, terrified, but never drown.

The spirits of my ancestors and of inner and outer guides come to me in various forms: hawk, eagle, owl, swan, deer, elk, coyote, wolf, bear, innocent child, Old Woman, Old Man. My unconscious, an integral part of the psyche and most often identified with the feminine, has become a strong ally. My dreams not only illustrate exactly where I am in the chaos and the nature of the fears that may be preventing me from moving through to the other side but what aspects of the Self I may call upon to help me make this transition.

This does not mean that I am not lonely. Sometimes my loneliness is so profound that I fear it is my permanent state. Despite this fear I have been able to develop several treasured friendships and one of the things I hold to me when I again feel abandoned are the words of my friend Rose who is 57 and has created a rich life for her Self in the past few years. One morning when I was crying again she told me: "The gift of loneliness is Self." These words, which I think she borrowed from May Sarton, have repeatedly proved true for me.

At other times I am frightened. What if I look deep inside my Self and there is no one there? Or what if I find that I can not stand the person that I find, that she is rotten to the core and does not deserve to live for her Self?

This stage, like the one before it, requires great courage. As I let go of all the previous ways of defining my Self, and as I accept the fact that I am indeed aging and must seek wholeness now while I still have time, I risk everything. I may find that indeed there is no longer any meaning to my life and I must create it in order to live. And although I may find a Self when I look within, however frightened and small it may seem, I may discover that this Self has been brutally wounded and is in dire need of healing.

The other side of these fears is the excitement and joy of healing my Self and creating meaning for my life. Primary in this stage of the journey has been my work with my compassionate and highly skilled therapist who continues to remind me that I have strong internal allies: anger, strength, humor, love, tears. In addition, I attend several twelve-step meetings every week which invariably remove my feelings of isolation and connect me with my spiritual center. I also see my acupuncturist/herbalist often. She has enabled me to live relatively free from the pain that, once I began menopause, permeated every muscle in my body from the time of ovulation until I began to bleed. Through regular visits to her and drinking specific herbal teas she prescribes this pain is greatly alleviated.

Perhaps most significant in this transition has been my relationship to Mother Earth. When I have been in deep physical pain I have lain down on my back, my arms and legs outstretched against her body, and asked her to heal me. And when I have felt that I could not endure yet another loss, that the pain was more than I could bear, I have flung my body against her and wept until there were no more tears and I felt drained of everything. Then, quietly, she has seeped into the newly-created space inside my Self and filled me with love and serenity. I have looked at the mountains solid and strong against the horizon and watched the shadows of clouds drift across the escarpments or heard the sweet song of a bird call to me from across a canyon and felt at peace. In comforting and caring for me she has taught me to comfort and care for my Self.

The paradox of existence is that the one thing we can count on is change. This time of chaos does end. In the meantime the suffering we may endure gives us the opportunity to develop courage and strength and to create parts of the Self that never before existed. Each of us can emerge as a survivor who has found her strength in the wounding and in the healing of those wounds.

Emergence

At emergence each of us comes out of the time of chaos as a woman who is actively seeking autonomy. She realizes that at this time of her life her strength lies not in her youth or in her ability to bear children but in her own personal power, and she embraces this power like a warrior. She is an adult woman who has endured and has learned that the gift of this endurance is wisdom. And so she continues her transformation, and while she is ever evolving she is at the same time fully complete. She is whole.

Sometimes this autonomy begins in a very simple manner. One of the things I immensely enjoy is walking alone in a large redwood forest near Santa Cruz. When a woman was murdered in this forest by a man who had previously killed many other women, and murdered while I was in another part of the same woods, my horror quickly turned to outrage because the police closed the forest. I knew walking there had become dangerous, but I was angry that one person had robbed me of a place sacred to me.

After several months the man was caught, and the forest was reopened. At first I could go no further than a hundred yards without turning back in sudden fear, imagining a man, his penis jutting out, hidden behind a tree. Each time I returned I focused again on my spiritual center, and each time I was able to go further. Finally on a particular walk, a medicine walk, I was able to journey through the entire forest, climbing up through the quiet, wind-lulled slopes to the highest point where I could see the ocean, brilliant with light, in the distance. The forest was again mine.

Autonomy in one part of my life, however small, often leads to autonomy in other, greater spheres. At one point I was working for an abusive employer and while I felt I was terribly needed by the children whom I taught, I became ill from the working conditions. Once I resigned I was astonished that not only could my life begin again but the job, which I had allowed to dominate my life, fell into nothingness. The institution where I had worked spun off into its own universe on the other side of the galaxy and ceased existing for me.

That experience gave me the courage to let go of lovers with whom I was obsessed but who were skitterish, like birds, always ready to fly away. When each left for the final time I wept, long and hard, but I did not beg. I let go, gathering my Self together once more.

I have been able to do this because of a major shift in my thinking. The girl-woman believed that:

A woman only finds happiness through marriage and children. The marriage model I knew, that of my parents, was composed of loneliness, control, and denial. Thus I will find happiness based on these things.

The autonomous woman who is emerging believes that:

I find happiness in loving and nurturing my Self, balancing all of my needs and desires and honoring all of my powers. This marriage of my needs and powers has a spiritual basis and is composed of trust, self love and the courage to be an adult woman who takes responsibility for her own healing and growth. I find happiness based on these things.

Sometimes I imagine I am on an open road in Alaska illuminated by brilliant light. At other times I am attracted to someone with an open, kind face, and I imagine my Self with this person. Then I remember: I cannot be with anyone now. I am being called to the openness in my Self.

Each woman who is journeying through menopause is being called to this openness. In her arms she cradles her Self which she is now free to nurture and protect. And if she becomes afraid she has but to look to her mother, the Earth, who is constantly transforming and being transformed, changing from young maiden to woman to crone in the course of a single day, and she will find both comfort and strength.

> Behold, I go forth to move around the earth.
> Behold, I go forth to move around the earth.
> I go forth as the great black bear that is great in courage.
> To move onward I go forth.

> —Osage warrior song

OPENING TO THE WISDOM OF MY HEART

Kathleen Sims

First Week

At last the pain of my dis-ease Endometriosis is gone. For twenty-nine years I bit my hands and cursed my fate to be a woman with every cycle of the moon. So I decided to have this hysterectomy. I decided to be wounded to heal myself. Demerol, my friend, sent me visions and I have lived through the pain of the great cut.

> You see, I am alive.
> You see,
> I stand in good relation
> to the earth.
>
> —Kiowa song

Second Week

Today I returned to the hospital to reclaim my uterus. She is the size of my fist, my strong woman muscle. Her spasm brought me in desperation to meditation and gave me red to color the rocks of Mother Earth.

My womb will not be burned in an incinerator. She will be buried with good honors this fall.

Fifth Week

I am waking at all hours, sweating, feeling, thinking . . . becoming a wise woman as I throw off covers and tear off my clothes.

Soon I will have to rise at dawn and return to work. My gynecologist says take estrogen, the magic drug of this decade. Take it until you are seventy. It stops hot flushes and osteoporosis. It will keep your vagina moist. Best of all it will keep you young.

I shall take this Premarin drug but I wonder, do I really need a gynecologist when my female organs are now in the freezer?

Tenth Week

Another horrid migraine today. I told my gynecologist that the estrogen gives me headaches. Take it one more month she says. I screamed over the phone lines. No. No. No.

I don't want anymore pain. That's why I had the hysterectomy.

I went instead to my family doctor. She is the honest one. She looks me in the eye and says I am the guinea pig. We all are. Our whole generation of women.

First they put us on birth control pills and now we are the recipients of Estrogen Replacement Therapy.

She too feels that I should not flirt with the possibility of osteoporosis. But I will swim. I will study Tai Chi. I will make my bones strong. I will have no more pain.

And I am beginning to glimmer deep feelings inside the flushes. They are heat. Heat is energy. I will not take Premarin. I will have stronger energy!

Sixteenth Week

I am a woman who will never bear children. I will never know the pain of my cervix opening for their passageway. I will not know the pain of their growing up and leaving me. My energies will flow into my songs, my dances, my paintings and my love. I will be mother to my dreams.

BODY METAPHORS
(AN EXCERPT)

Genia Pauli Haddon

Women today reaching menopause at around age fifty can expect to live twenty-five to forty more years—one-third or more of their lives. These are the years that correspond to the mythological figure of the Crone. They are marked by the emergence of yang-femininity physiologically, emotionally, sexually, behaviorally. Conceptualizing menopause as a point of cessation rather than as a phase of development reflects the natural patriarchal bias against honoring the Crone. . . .

Without the Crone dimension neither woman nor God-Feminine is complete. The "change of life" is a universal and normal process for all women, not an aberration or disease. Yet the predominant medical attitude is that the bodily changes accompanying the perimenopausal period are pathological, to be treated as a hormone-deficiency disease. The treatment of choice is "estrogen replacement therapy," or ERT. The goal is to artificially elevate estrogen levels to premenopausal levels, thereby preventing the bodily and behavioral changes that naturally reduced estrogen levels would bring about. . . .

Women who become comfortable with the qualities represented by the Crone, perhaps within a therapy group, sometimes even report finding hot flashes pleasurable. A woman whose sense of God-Feminine is developing may spontaneously begin thinking to herself as she feels a flash starting, "The Goddess is touching me." Perhaps the hot flash is a physiological experience corresponding to the "fiery darkness" attributed to Lilith and the dark moon, as symbols of yang-femininity.

During the years of "the Change," many women experience unaccountable blue feelings, irritability, anxiety. The severity of emotional distress may be influenced by nonphysical factors as well as by hormonal variations. Some studies suggest that women who have invested themselves very intensely in mothering have the greatest difficulty adjusting when their bodies bring them to the point of initiation into the final third of life, where nonmaternal modes of fulfillment are to take precedence. Cultural prejudice against the Crone may make the transition difficult and forbidding. The face of the young maiden

347

represents ideal femininity; the face of the Crone is considered ugly, evil, disgusting. As lines and wrinkles inevitably appear, and perhaps moles, liver spots, warts, and facial hair as well, women may feel shame, grief, anger, disgust with themselves. At the same time, new resources of yang energy are becoming available. Anthropologist Margaret Mead is reported to have said that the greatest creative force in the world is a menopausal woman with zest. If environmental circumstances or the woman's own habitual attitudes block the flowing forth of this zestful creativity, the thwarted potential curdles within. . . .

Decrease of estrogen level has been construed to mean a corresponding decrease in both femininity and sexuality. It is true that those feminine attributes that coordinate with peaking of estrogen become less central with the climacteric: vaginal sexuality, sexual receptivity, ovulation, impregnation, gestation, nurturance, mothering. These are expressive of yin-femininity, matching the full moon and the Mother or Virgin-Mother images of God-Feminine. If that were femininity in its entirety, it would be accurate to say that decreased estrogen levels result in loss of femininity. However, as these yin expressions of femininity are declining, expressions of yang-femininity are coming to the fore. Furthermore, although fertility and vaginal sexuality decrease through the menopausal period, the sex drive tends to increase. As with perimenstrual sexuality, post-menopausal sexuality is more clitoral than vaginal, more assertive than receptive; probably due to relative preponderance of prolibidone (libido-promoting hormone) in both circumstances. As the clitoral (yang) style of sexuality takes precedence over the vaginal (yin) mode, the woman may experience a parallel shift in other areas of her life. She may find herself generally less nurturant and more assertive in both her relationships with others and her style of creativity. Ideally she will discover how to be a pushy woman in the positive sense as she grows into the Crone dimension of her feminine identity. . . .

For the most part, menopause has been considered an illness rather than the normal closure of menstrual and reproductive life; it has been defined medically in terms of symptoms, as degeneration, and as deficiency disease; its normalcy as a natural physiological event remains undocumented by the scientific community. I believe this is due in part to patriarchy's built-in fear of the Crone and yang-femininity. If it is true that as the Patriarchal Age is founded upon cultural expression of phallic physiology and experiences, so the coming Cultural Age is to reflect yang-feminine values, then perhaps symbolic importance attaches to the fact that a greater than ever portion of the population consists of postmenopausal women, or Crones. This is due to repeated increases in average life span, while the average age at which menopause occurs has remained constant. Therefore, long ago few women lived much beyond menopause at age fifty; now the average life expectancy is some twenty-five years beyond menopause. Thus most women can expect to experience being the Crone physically and emotionally—with concomitant opportunity to explore and integrate the spiritual meanings of that aspect of God-Feminine. As there come to be more and more Crones around, the spiritual values of yang-femininity may gradually become commonplace as well.

Menopause is a time for confronting death while there is still time to live. It is a true initiation, a doorway through death to a new phase of life. Fear of natural menopause, fear of the Crone, translates also into dread of death. Through bodily experiences of yang-femininity, in both menstruation and menopause, women (and men who relate sensitively to them) have opportunities to encounter the dark death side of the Divine.

THE METAPHYSICS OF MENOPAUSE

Suzanne Laberge

the sacred does not cease to manifest itself . . .

—*M. Eliade*

I am a woman of a certain age
becoming invisible.
I walk the streets unseen.

the mirror knows me not; shows me my mother, sometimes,
sometimes a stranger, turning gray

I am losing identity

Losing red tides
losing my familiar red ties
my rhythm
bonds to matter
to mater
to ma terra

loosening

I have headaches, I am irritable, impatient.
Blood seeps from me; I am a swamp; I am becoming dry
and barren; a husk, crisp under heedless foot.

summer is ending, harvest in, winter wind waits
over the hill

it seems the Change is more cursed than the Curse
oh squandered years! fertility ran rampant within me

a waning moon sets

no more tampax or kotex or folded toilet paper wadded
kleenex or little cups or sponges or moss or pills or
swelling or cream or gel or condoms or loops or coils or
diaphragm; no more fearful reckoning of dates; no more
attending to the moon

liberation!

who welcomes me to this new country?
what are the boundaries? the landmarks?
who is here to know me?
who do I know? who am I
here?

Cleansing tears, deep grieving, blood thinning to water;
my face swollen for two days; never, for mother, lovers, or
children, have I wept so profoundly as for this end of 40
years of self, of possibility, of position

In a quieter time of reflection, I wait, I rest
I simply am aware of a humming
a kind of whirlwind, a kind of vortex

shift center of focus from
PROCREATIVE TO PURE CREATIVE

unrequired love flows
the largest flower, yes

Just before it died my backyard plum tree, previously
unremarkable, produced a glorious crop, a multiplicity of
plums; I marvelled and made jam. I offer my blossoming;
soon, plums for all; soon enough, winter.

A DIFFERENT PERSPECTIVE

Patricia Mathes Cane

"Hotflashes, pain, blood, the crazies, a time to dread." I grew up with these images of menopause thinking that this would be my lot in life. Even worse than the "curse," this would be a time to grit my teeth and suffer what my mother and grandmother and generations of women had endured before me, with the hope that eventually my life would return to "normal."

In my late forties, as the time of menopause neared, I was determined to try to do it differently. I talked with a woman at our local health food store who encouraged me to prepare myself by practicing meditation for relaxation and stress reduction and by taking chinese herbs (a formula which consisted of ten different herbs including dong quai) to strengthen and harmonize the cycles and systems of my body. I found all this to be very helpful in regulating my more erratic periods and heavy cramping, my more frequent feelings of edginess and my emotional swings from elation to depression, all of which were new for me.

I had gotten to the point of thinking, "Hey, I can handle this!" when suddenly the larger context of my life changed abruptly, throwing me out of control into soul-stretching directions, bringing a much deeper meaning to this menopause of body and spirit.

An earthquake of 7.1 magnitude hit Northern California, badly damaging my home and possessions, destroying the homes and businesses of neighbors and friends, deeply scarring my local community for years to come. My basic sense of security which I had taken for granted over the years, was lost in a matter of fifteen seconds. Illusions of all sorts were shaken loose from secure inner moorings. Much of the familiar around me was broken or destroyed.

During this same period of time, the slaughter and repression of innocent people in Central America increased. The cousin of my Salvadoran friend Victoria was disappeared, along with her infant son, in one of many raids which claimed hundred of lives. Six Jesuit priests, their housekeeper and her daughter were massacred by the Salvadoran military which receives over a million dollars a day from my own country. Two Catholic nuns, colleagues of a dear friend, were killed in a Contra ambush in Nicaragua, murdered by "freedom fighters" supported by my country. And in other parts of Latin America, friends were being threatened as they worked for justice and truth on behalf of the Families of the Disappeared.

At the same time in another part of the world, changes in Eastern Europe and the Soviet Union were taking place, changes I never dreamt I would see in my lifetime—a new order, a perestroika—opening these countries to freedom and possibilities for life.

For several months I felt stunned by all these larger and smaller events—vulnerable, out of control, numbed, powerless, shaken to the core, wanting just to return to my own comfort and security, to get back to "normal." It was enough for me just to be going through menopause. I didn't deserve to have everything else come crashing in on me, too!

The inner image I had of myself at this time was that of a frightened child hanging onto the window ledge of a tall building. I had just barely enough energy to hang on each day. There were times when I just needed to stop and cry and mourn, but I didn't have the privacy or the time to do this. My patience was stretched to the limits as my husband and I painstakingly picked up and repaired our home. I felt irritable with friends who called to see how we were doing or to give advice, but who couldn't understand the shattering depths of what we were experiencing. Often I felt like screaming or running away, but I would somehow manage to pull myself together and face the next day of reordering my home and life. I wasn't sure what I could blame on menopause and what on physical and emotional stress!

About a month after the quake in the midst of our personal trauma, my husband and I were invited to be delegates to the international Congress of FEDEFAM—the Federation of Families of the Disappeared of Latin America. In the last two decades it has been documented that over 100,000 people have been disappeared by death squads or military regimes. When we arrived at the Congress in Lima, Peru, the delegation of 200 representatives (mostly women) from 15 different countries had to be sequestered in a hotel compound with armed guard protection. Just to be present at such a meeting brought death threats to some of the Peruvian delegates.

The stories of these women were incredible. Sylvia, a Peruvian teacher, told of her sister's disappearance three weeks previous. Unlike most of the families of the disappeared, she did find her sister's body three days before the Congress—gang-raped by the military and badly mutilated. She had never been involved in human rights work before but was present at the Congress to gain courage and strength from those who have experienced similar tragedies. And she was determined to help organize the people in her area who were being victimized. I remember looking into her eyes and wondering how long it would be before she, too, would be disappeared because of what she believed in.

One of the women who touched me most deeply was Antonia, a member of the Mothers and Grandmothers of the Plaza de Mayo of Argentina, one of "las locas," the crazy women, as they had been disparagingly called by the officials. During the military regime six members of her family were disappeared—two sons, their pregnant wives, and two unborn children. She never had the joy of seeing her grandchildren, but has since been made an honorary grandmother for the love and life she has given to so many others. Often I was in tears as she shared with me her experiences. During what would have been her years of menopause, when the needs of most women become more personal and self-directed, Antonia was out in the streets protesting the return of her six disappeared family members, facing the anger and hostility of a murderous military, or she was in the home of a victim's family giving aid or comfort or advice. On one occasion I overheard her talking with Sylvia, the Peruvian teacher, who was having to deal with fears of returning to her small town after the Congress. Antonia, with great pain and with great love, described how it is never easy. But by facing each moment, one at a time, with faith and with the support and solidarity of the other women, she has been able to find the courage to keep on going and to overcome her own fears. And from this she has received the energy and inspiration to commit her life to working for justice for others around her.

Shortly after we had arrived at the Congress, a Bolivian delegate had asked us, "How many people have been disappeared from your family?" . . . Yes, we had indeed lost quite a few personal possessions in an earthquake and had suffered some stress and discomfort, but in no way have we ever experienced what it must be like to be torn apart by the sudden disappearance of someone we love dearly. We have never felt the constant agonizing questions: Where are they? Are they still alive? Are they being tortured at this moment? How are they being murdered? Where are their bodies?

Returning home after the Congress, I had a very different perspective. I struggled to listen to both the reality within me and without me, and to face some of my feelings and delusions. I began to see some connections between these world events and what was being called forth in my own life and spirit at this time of menopause: a perestroika, a reordering of my body and spirit.

It was important to honor the pain and the discomfort of my own processes in menopause. But I also desired not just to get stuck in that. My life experience had been different from many of my friends who were going through menopause and needed time for themselves to be and to develop their own lives. I had married late in life after years in the convent and a career as an educator and counselor, and had never had children. So my needs at this time of life were different. Antonia of Argentina had been a real inspiration to me. Here was a woman who had taken her own physical and emotional pain at the most difficult period of her life and had channeled her energies into helping create something beyond herself based on justice, truth and love. I somehow wanted to do that, too.

Some other realizations came to me one day when I was cleaning up the mess in my home. I had repaired a broken painting, a favorite of mine, and was in the process of hanging it back up on the wall where it had hung for many years, when all of a sudden I had the thought, "I don't have to hang this here, why not try someplace else?" Then as I looked around at other treasures, I started thinking, "What would be a better, happier, more creative way of doing this? My home reflects myself and my own process. How do I want to creatively reorder my life and spirit for the remaining years I have to live?"

Shortly after the quake I had looked in the mirror and had seen an earthquake victim going through menopause, with skin beginning to wrinkle, hair turning gray, energy waning, a woman vulnerable to life's vicissitudes, to history's grinding movement.

But now I again looked in the mirror and found a woman, vulnerable, yes, and closer to death, but also a woman softer, more filled with life, with compassion, with wisdom, with light. How to honor all these parts of me? How to enable what has been buried deep within me to surface? How to recommit to that subtle life-giving process learned only by listening in silence to my heart?

All those years of illusion about menopause. I often think of how the rose gives forth the brightest and most beautiful flowers as summer is nearing its end. As a plant has certain requirements for growth and flowering, so too, my life and spirit. At this point I wanted to reclaim and recommit myself to whatever would help encourage this deeper mystery of my unfolding spirit. For some years I had been a nun in a religious order, but after leaving the community I needed to let go of the piety, ritual and regimen to regain a sense of my own life. Now I somehow needed to reclaim some practices of the spirit to live more fully the life/death/life cycles I was experiencing.

Over the last few years I have found several practices very helpful in honoring this deepening process and have tried to make time for these in my daily life. A year ago I went to a Buddhist retreat and learned something about the practice of Mindfulness. Participating in the retreat were 75 peace activists, all of whom had the desire to learn this practice to further their peace-making. Mindfulness is essentially very simple and yet very profound. It consists of breathing slowly and fully to calm the mind and spirit and being joyfully present in the moment. Mindfulness can be practiced washing the dishes, driving the car, being with friends. Many things change when the mind is quieted of its incessant chatter and the spirit is joyful and present.

As I reflected on the life and commitment of my friend from Argentina, I realized that her life and pain and commitment to justice were being lived out with a sense of mindfulness. Touching the moment, whether it is very difficult or ecstatic, I feel grounded in the reality of what simply is. Breathing deeply and fully, being simply present to myself and to God, I am slowly able to shed the pretensions and images I have built up around myself over the years as my armor and defenses in life.

Some body movement, too, has become important. I have found Tai Chi a wonderful way to express and heal and connect with myself and with nature. During a visit to China some years ago, I became fascinated with this kind of movement. Early in the morning thousands of people were out in the parks starting their days with this ancient form of movement. When I first started learning, I felt clumsy and awkward, but then I remembered the Chinese. This was no new-age fad for them, but young and old, master and novice, graceful and clumsy were all doing this together—a movement of the people. This thought brought ease and grace and enjoyment to my own attempts at doing Tai Chi. One of my favorite movements is called Passing Clouds. I stay peacefully centered in the moment while moving my arms in circles around me—a point of peace and being and wisdom amidst the passing clouds of life.

Prayer has become essential for me, but has greatly changed since my years of religious practice. I now sit quietly, breathe deeply, and relax in the presence of God/Goddess. From this silent being present I learn much and am filled. At times I ask for deepening wisdom, to be a person of love, compassion and light, to be most fully who I am called to be. And I unite myself in oneness and solidarity with those who are suffering injustice in Latin America, Africa, throughout the world.

I am simply one person on this planet, but somehow I feel that I, along with every other person, have a part to play in the large historical drama. Several years ago during a trip to Central America to areas my country has tried to destroy and control, I decided that I would like to help rebuild and repair what my tax dollars have destroyed. With a friend I started working with women's groups in Guatemala and Nicaragua teaching methods of stress management and relaxation, and in turn learning many things about compassion and life from the women. From these experiences we developed Project CAPACITAR and in the spirit of the Nicaraguan word "capacitar" try to enable, self-empower and encourage the gifts of women in different worlds. Our work focuses on connecting first world women with third world women in mutual understanding and healing and we have been invited to share with women in different countries in Central and Latin America and in South Africa.

As I now go through this period of my life, this time of menopause, I am learning that there are no roadmaps or patterns to rely on. The territory is open and new at each moment. I have come to trust the deep down listening process of the heart which keeps revealing and unfolding and surprising, connecting me with Gaia, Mother Earth, the greater cycles of spirit as my own body changes and ages. I am part of the Whole!

INQUIRY

Dona Luongo Stein

You no longer leak
your sorrow
each month
over my legs, through my slacks
into the sheets

You no longer prepare
your thick nest
for my lost daughters
no longer swell
then shrink
as the moon crosses
the salty waters of heaven

How are you? Now that you
no longer squeeze the little stars
I once looked for
as if newts, toads, tadpoles
would swim from your space
into my hands for rocking and song

I don't know what humming
goes on behind closed lips
when I feel you flutter, rock
in the rowing of love
your dimension, unpeopled,
full of moons
silent, calm.

CELEBRATING THE VIRAGO: THIRD STAGE OF WOMANHOOD

Maureen Williams

When I first considered writing this piece, I searched through my extensive personal library for material dealing specifically with the menopausal woman in pre-patriarchal societies, but found such to be virtually non-existent. This puzzled me since in those ancient Goddess-oriented times the older woman was respected and valued. Then I realized that the reason for the dearth of information is a familiar one to someone in my field of studies: Any writing that might have existed on this subject has been expunged from the record. Since this aspect of womanhood is the one which men understand least, find most difficult to deal with, or indeed, to acknowledge at all, there is even less on record than one normally expects to find. It is as if a woman who has reached menopause ceases to exist because she is considered to be beyond sexuality and fecundity, therefore beyond womanliness. Thus she is relegated to the ranks of gender neuter, along with the senile and the eunuch, and as such, of not much use or interest to anyone. So, in order to write this piece, I am left with supposition based on my knowledge of matriarchal times, presented here in order to encourage the older woman to see herself in a different light, one that might still be shining today if those ancient matriarchies had not been overthrown.

The modern attitude to menopausal woman seems to continue the dismissal indicated above. As pointed out in *The Menopause Book*, Freud warns she is "quarrelsome and obstinate, petty and stingy . . . sadistic and anal-erotic." Sadly, how we see ourselves as women approaching menopause is often based upon such prejudiced but popularly held views, and the confusing attitude that our society has towards women in general. While older men tend to be thought of as wise, older women are branded as irrational, even mad, certainly "past it"—it of course being sex and childbearing—or at best, of little use, harmless and easily dismissed. Yet it was not always so. If we women knew our hidden history, ancient truths that are as veritable today, surely we would take heart and look forward to the third stage in our lives. Virago: the very word has lost its original meaning of a strong, experienced and wise older woman. Together, let us celebrate the Virago.

Although the historical record would seem to have been drastically altered, there are societies today where this ancient knowledge has not slipped entirely from race memory, where women eagerly anticipate menopause. Among the Mohave Indians, women view menopause as a sign of achievement, the point in their lives when women become free to do as they please. In China, the older woman is greatly respected; she, not her male counterpart, becomes the community's counsellor. The Chinese grandmothers, as they are called even if they have no grandchildren of their own, are loved and needed to help with child-raising while the younger women go to work. In a study done by the International Health Foundation of attitudes towards menopause, British women were asked whether menopause means the end of their attractiveness to men; 85 percent replied: Certainly not! As a Brit myself, I like to think that this attitude stems from a strong self-image, culturally-based knowledge that women are valued as individuals, are more than sex objects and child-bearers. I believe this British female sense of self-worth is derived from our matriarchal heritage.

The pre-patriarchal culture I'm most familiar with is that of the Kelts who once roamed the whole of the European continent, then about 400 B.C., migrated westward, to settle in the British Isles. Successive invaders of Britain pushed the Keltic clans into the fringes of the islands, where their descendants still reside in Scotland, Ireland, the Isle of Mann, Wales, Cornwall and Brittany. From their myths and artwork, we know that early Keltic society was quite remarkable, with women and men co-existing in mutual respect and equality. A Keltic woman could fulfill any role she pleased: tribal leader, head of the family, warrior, spiritual leader, healer, artist, educator or enchanter. As with most early agrarian societies dependent upon the earth to put forth her bounty, the creating deity of Pagan Kelts was Female. Mortal men regarded women as living images of their Goddess, a creature mystical and magical, the fountain of life, revered throughout the three stages of womanhood. Virgin, Mother, Virago: each stage was valued in ways rarely seen in modern societies.

The Virgin: To the Pagan Kelts, this first stage of womanhood was essentially a time of choices, with the virgin free to choose her own role in life, her sexual partners (homosexuality was entirely accepted), whether she wished to be a wife or remain single, and a mother, with or without marriage. This was a time when love between sexual partners was given freely, without guilt; children born out of wedlock were considered gifts to the entire community, to be cared for and loved by all. The Keltic virgin was a lively young woman, bold, free, strong and pure of mind and spirit, and innocent though sexually wise.

The Mother: Since Keltic tribes were matrilinear, motherhood was the foundation of clan loyalty, just as their supreme deity was the Mother of All Living. Presumably women who had chosen to be lesbians could fulfill their desire to have children by taking a male partner simply to become pregnant. Though some women, of course, would choose to remain childless. It is known that there was a class of reclusive warrior women among the Kelts who led their clan into battle, and trained the young male warriors, and the women who would succeed them, in this sense fulfilling the motherhood role.

The Virago: With younger women to take care of hard physical work, the wives child-bearing and running the home, the Keltic woman came into her own as the virago. Finally she was freed to live for herself, to offer her experience and knowledge to the community, helping others while gaining self-fulfillment. The water that flowed through her as the fountain of life was menstrual blood, "wise blood" as it was termed in some cultures. Even after a woman ceased to bleed monthly, she continued to be revered because now she retained this special blood within her veins, keeping it for herself, as it were. Thus she became the wisest of women, mature enough to lay claim to those once proud titles of the older woman: virago, crone, hag, and witch.

Among the Kelts, the witch was one of the most important roles for the virago: usually an older woman, past menopause, who had studied throughout her life, learning to be in touch with nature, her own, and that of the world around her, to qualify as the tribal herbalist, healer, midwife, counselor, magician and sexual instructor. When she was ready to hang out her shingle, both female and male virgins came to her cottage for advice and love-potions. Wives and husbands also came, separate or together, for counselling and herbal help when the body seemed to be faltering, as well as the sick and ailing of all ages, nobles and peasants, anyone in need of charms and spells.

There were many other tribal roles in which the Keltic virago eagerly anticipated fulfilling herself. She was now eligible to become leader of the sacred dancing that played a major part in religious ceremonies; or tribal storyteller, for without a written language, Kelts depended upon her for their history and entire litany of learning; or the teacher of all manner of crafts and arts, which had taken years of practice until a woman, in the third stage of her life, could attain the perfection of her artifacts and pass on her skill to apprentices.

The Keltic virago woman was also considered to be a very skilled lover, an art to which she could dedicate herself after menopause with little fear of pregnancy. She could now join the enclave of sacred harlots whose assignment it was to give and take pleasure in the sexual magic ceremonies that ensured the future well-being of the tribe. Because of their great power, sacred harlots were protected by tribal taboo from unwanted attention; one gained access to their much desired beds by invitation only.

So it seems that in a matriarchal society, there were many roles waiting for the older woman. Yet, peering into our distant past is surely only of value if it serves to enhance our present and give hope to our future. Knowing about the old way, about a time when woman in all three stages of her life was respected and valued, should help to allay some of the fears of menopausal women and repair some of the damage to our self-esteem that modern society inflicts. While we cannot entirely change our society's attitude to us, we can change our attitude toward ourselves. We can use this heritage. By taking heart in the knowledge of our matriarchal past, we begin to view ourselves for ourselves, and refuse to allow these strong self-images formed out of race memory to be shattered.

My personal experience as a woman entering menopause gives credence to the notion that knowledge of our matriarchal past benefits both our present and future. I began delving into the culture of my own Keltic forebears in my late thirties. The discovery of the startling female heritage that I have just recounted was a revelation that gave me spiritual strength. Once I came to know my ancient sisters by gaining knowledge of their position in society, I realized that within my ethnic memory existed the kind of positive self-image I needed to carry me into menopause and beyond. I thought: What does it matter how the world today treats or views me; I possess this original strength, this gift from the past. I came to see deity as essentially female, myself as goddess, soon to become virago, soon to enter the stage of greatest wisdom and freedom in my life.

Going beyond my own culture, I found that women the world over have this common matriarchal heritage. The ancient virago, that wise crone, is in all of us. The witch, nature's healer, born naturopath with knowledge of her own body, follower of the eco-feminist way, she is there within every one of us, her sacred knowledge waiting to be discerned and appreciated.

I am presently in the early stages of menopause since my monthly bleeding has tapered off almost to nothing. And whilst I have suffered none of the discomforts we are warned to expect, certain physical changes have occurred: an increase in weight, though I've not changed my lifestyle of sensible eating and regular strenuous exercise; more grey hairs among the auburn; more lines on my face. None of this dismays me. On the contrary, since I know my essential self to be undiminished, I accept these marks of aging with pride. Within, I am as I was born: Keltic goddess, virgin, mother, and now virago, my entire being enriched by the landscape of the two ages through which I've journeyed to reach this third stage of womanhood. My erotic self is enhanced by the experience of my nearly 50 years—no one can tell me I'm passed it! I feel I'm on the brink of all manner of exciting innovations in lovemaking; my childbearing days being over, this will be pure erotic love for its own sake. Perhaps I am one of the lucky women who will go through menopause without anguish or physical hardship. What I believe is that because I learned to emulate my Keltic forebears, I resurrected within myself that strong wise woman, the virago who knows how to celebrate herself no matter what may transpire.

BODY AS SACRED

Joan Borton

Women have not experienced their own experience.
Stories give shape to experience, experience gives rise to stories.

—Carol Christ, *Diving Deep and Surfacing*

Remembering our experience before menstruation is important for women approaching menopause. Menarche (the onset of menstruation) and menopause (the actual cessation of the menses) are two balancing movements in our body's natural rhythm. There is a deep connection between the times of beginning and ending our fertility. There is much to learn and gain from re-membering our experience as young girls. Many of us have negative memories about our preparation for menstruation, or sadness about what we gave up as childhood seemed to end. Our experience, negative or positive, is part of our story. It is what was so. Sharing these experiences with other women, telling our stories, gives us the opportunity to include and not forget. Accepting what was so and learning from that experience, we actually become freer to make choices about this time of life as we approach our menopause. As we give ourselves permission to experience our own experience and then share that with others, we do shape our experience.

My mother's message about menstruation was: being a woman is becoming like me.
So I became my mother. It was *her* menses not mine. Maybe that is why I want to really experience myself in this passage.

—woman in her late forties

We who are going through the life passage of menopause can rename our experience, choosing to discover our bodies as life-giving and thus sacred, connecting us with the divine. Many of us now in mid-life were not aware of this potential for spiritual learning in our early years. We had no "waiting house" in which to receive this knowledge. Various different cultures have prepared young women in such a natural way with their "waiting house" or moon hut. The older women, who no more had the bleeding, tended there the women in "moon time" while young girls assisted them, learning from these old wise women. In our culture few menstruating thirteen-year-olds on their own would have recognized the spiritual movement of being acted upon by nature, becoming one with nature as we let go into the rhythm of shedding and replenishing. Nor would we have been aware of nature's amazing balancing process. Winnifred Cutler, a reproductive biologist, and her associates note that "it takes about seven years from the first menstrual period until a woman is fully fertile, and it takes about seven years for the reverse process (total infertility) to be complete." The number seven has long been a symbol of creative fullness. That fullness is experienced when we choose to be conscious and become one with our bodies. The seven-year span ending our fertility gives women the opportunity to trust our bodies and learn from them, and then to cooperate with their process: thus holding our bodies as sacred.

This was Christine Downing's intention as she went on her *Journey Through Menopause*. In her preparation research she had read both male and female medical and psychological accounts of the climacteric period which were written from the perspective of medical pathology, seeing the event of menopause as a deficiency disease. This view is based on the equation that femininity equals motherhood; menstruation and menopause refer only to reproduction processes, and the womb is solely an organ for making babies. Many of us have been affected by this focus. The extreme sense of loss and ending which some women feel as they approach menopause is closely related to this medical interpretation. In contrast, Downing presents her intention regarding her own experience:

> To learn ever more deeply that the body-event is soul-event, that the two belong together, lies for me at the very heart of what this transition signifies. Most of what I have read about menopause disappoints precisely because it does not recognize that, speaks only of body or only of soul. I want to speak of the soul of the body, its withinness, and to go into the bodily events, the changes, the "symptoms," and discover their inherent symbolic meaning. I am persuaded that the soul meaning is not added on, not found through some movement of transcendence, but within the physical experience itself.

Experiencing menopause as a "soul event" as well as a body event opens us to a more inclusive way of journeying through this passage. For there is surely grief and darkness in the letting go of our fruit-bearing years. But there is also a release in letting go of the old which makes way for the new—truly the journey of change; that too involves risk and venturing into the unknown.

Jean Bolen, author of *The Goddesses in Every Woman*, suggested a mythic way of viewing our uterus and the transformation in our body. She sees the process as a pilgrimage, the purpose of which is to "quicken the divine" in the pilgrim. At a workshop on "Women's Spirituality," she spoke of woman's spiritual pilgrimage as an inward one led by a new symbol for the Holy Grail, the womb. Like the chalice, it holds life-giving blood that is sacred. The object of the quest becomes no longer something out there, sought after in the fashion of the medieval knights on pilgrimage. We ourselves bear the chalice within. Journeying to our own experience within our body, we can meet the divine. As we open ourselves to the changes taking place in our womb, as we reflect, remember, grieve, rejoice and live the changes, we engage the divine, we become one with the divine as we become one with our own experience.

Our womb can be a place of meeting the divine through grief. The process of letting go of the childbearing years for some women involves all the stages of grief, as Elizabeth Kubler-Ross outlined them. For example, a woman who had loved being a wife and mother stopped menstruating quite suddenly at 40. She kept "putting a pad on each month." It was too soon for her. She hadn't had time to prepare herself. She held on. She did not want what was so to be. This kind of denial is often followed by the other stages of grief: anger, bargaining, depression and finally acceptance. There is a lot to letting go and acceptance, this is a bodily lesson that the womb has been teaching us since we became young women. Each month we have been reminded that we are not in control, that we are part of a rhythm that goes beyond us and connects us with the moon rhythms of the universe.

Many of us meet the divine through our womb's dis-ease, or potential disease. The experiences of having gynecological checkups which raise questions and propose solutions having to do with a D&C, hormone therapy, a hysterectomy and/or treatment for uterine cancer force us to face our mortality. There is great grief in that and it is often experienced in all of its stages. Any woman who has dealt with these concerns can recall becoming enraged at a medical secretary, lab technician, doctor, friend, relative or perfect stranger; after the fact realizing that the intensity of anger was not proportionate to the situation. The outburst may have been carrying the heavy freight of looking at death perhaps for the first time. Our womb often gives us the opportunity to walk with our fears through "the valley of the shadow of death" and encounter more deeply than ever before the divine in our life.

During the passage through menopause when women choose to become one with their bodies, some women find that this choice opens memories of physical and/or sexual abuse. The grief involved in this remembering needs tender healing support and therapy (therapaeia), as defined by Downing, meaning attention of the kind one devotes to the sacred. Through this kind of therapy and healing even in that violent darkness, there is the potential for meeting the divine. There is a darkness for many women at this time which has been called depression, and is often treated as such medically. Sometimes that is appropriate. Sometimes the experience of darkness is part of the spiritual journey into the unknown. Our dreams and nightmares bear out our fears of leaving the familiar and moving into the new. This darkness is often experienced as being without a sense of purpose. There is an emptiness that previously we have been able to fill. Staying with that emptiness, like staying with the emptying process of our womb, can be a deeply spiritual time. It is not easy, but there are many pilgrims along the way who encourage this as the way to "the place of break-though into abundance," in Joseph Campbell's words.

For women who have not borne children this is often a time of acknowl-edging grief that they have been dealing with for years. It is helpful to share this grief with others who have not given birth, as it is a different experience. For some women there is a feeling of relief. One woman expressed her feeling this way: "At last my friends will be learning what I have been coming to accept during the time that they were bearing and raising children and becoming grandmothers." Women who have not borne children have come to know the meaning of being a woman that others of us will come to through the passage of menopause. We will be given the opportunity then to say "yes" to being a creator in a new and different way. Our Native American sisters have always celebrated the experience of woman that goes beyond procreation. The spirit which pervades all creation has many names but, according to Paula Gunn Allen in *The Sacred Hoop*, "at the center of all that is created is Woman, and no thing is sacred (cooked, ripe, as the Keres Indians of Laguna Pueblo say it) without her blessing, her thinking."

Far beyond a fertility goddess "she is a true creatrix for she is thought itself, from which all else is born." One of the Keres ceremonial prayers refers to "Woman" as "mother of us all, after Her, mother earth follows, in fertility, in holding and in taking again us back to her breast." Allen speaks for her people seeing "the power of woman as the center of the universe" . . . which "is both heart (womb) and thought (creativity)." This creative power is often dis-covered by women as they journey through menopause.

Each of us traveling our particular road at this time of life has the opportunity to own our experience of this creative power. We may need to walk through times of grief and darkness to come through to this place of new life. Our sister pilgrims encourage us on the way. It is a solitary journey at times, as each of us is unique. But when we choose to stop at the Women's Well and draw on the life-replenishing water, we know our oneness with each other and with the underground stream of life-giving energy that feeds all creation.

BIOGRAPHIES

Ann Stewart Anderson is a visual artist who lives in Kentucky, where she was born. Her work, which often combines painting and needlework, depicts images of women, not as traditional objects of veneration or beauty, but subjectively, as females dealing with their lives as women. Her work has been exhibited internationally, and is included in the Atlantic Richfield and Alabama Power and Light collections. She has taught at the School of the Art Institute of Chicago.

Dori Appel has been published in *Beloit Poetry Journal, Calyx,* and *Sojourner,* among others and in the anthology *When I Am An Old Woman I Shall Wear Purple.* Her plays include *Female Troubles, Fun House Mirror* and *Girl Talk* (co-authored with Carolyn Myers), a "serious comedy" about friendships between women throughout the life cycle.

Connie Batten is trying to remain as conscious as possible of the unfolding process of menopause. Through talking with other women about their experiences during this powerful life passage she is deepening her understanding. Currently she is working on a book in which her own story weaves together with the stories of these other women.

Henrietta Bensussen grew up in Los Angeles, moved to the San Francisco Bay Area in the sixties and plans eventually to live in a forest in Oregon. She works as a secretary to a publisher and spends much of her free time helping to put out the lesbian newsletter, *Entre Nous.*

Doris Bircham ranches with her husband in southwest Saskatchewan. She is a nurse with two grown children who are involved in the business of cattle ranching. Her poetry and non-fiction have been published in periodicals, anthologies and aired on CBC radio.

Audrey Borenstein has published thirty works of fiction in literary journals, as well as essays and poetry, and four books of nonfiction. She is co-author of a chronicle of local history published in 1989. Her awards include an NEA Fellowship and a Rockefeller Foundation Humanities Fellowship.

Joan Borton is presently writing a book on menopause based on her workshops and individual work with women in Massachusetts. The mother of three grown children, she is a play therapist and an early childhood clinical consultant to parents, schools and day care centers.

Sandy Boucher has published four books: *Turning the Wheel: American Women Creating the New Buddhism, Heartwomen: An Urban Feminist's Odyssey Home, The Notebooks of Leni Clare,* and *Assaults & Rituals.* She has a masters degree in the history and phenomenology of religion and lives, teaches and writes in Oakland, CA.

Claire Braz-Valentine is a widely published poet, fiction writer, journalist and playwright. Her play, *This One Thing I Do,* about the suffrage movement, was published by Samuel French and her latest play on Frida Kahlo is being produced in theatres across the country. She works with men in prisons, is a Spectra Artist in The Schools and facilitates writing workshops in Santa Cruz, CA.

Patricia Mathes Cane is a teacher, counselor and artist. She is the director of Project Capacitar, which focuses on connecting First World and Third World women. She facilitates stress management workshops with women's groups in Nicaragua and Guatemala as well as South Africa. Her work involves enabling, self-empowering and encouraging the resources of women in many different worlds.

Mary Dominick Chivers, born in 1938, grew up in Wyoming and returns every summer. She lives with her husband and son in Andover, Massachusetts, and has recently completed a book of short stories about her father's life as a Wyoming doctor. She is at work on her first book of poems.

Erica Lann Clark has been writing and telling stories since she was seven. Her first career as a promising playwright was brought to an untimely conclusion by a divorce that left her the single parent of two baby boys. A progression of jobs—teaching, fundraising and massage—followed, and now, 25 years later, the boys have become men, mom's gone menopausal, and hence, this essay.

Elayne Clift is a writer and health communication specialist. Her monthly column "Through the Looking Glass" appears in *New Jersey Woman,* and a collection of her essays, *Telling It Like It Is: Reflections of a Not So Radical Feminist,* was published by KIT Publications. She is married and has two teenage children.

Lucille Clifton teaches at the University of California at Santa Cruz and in Maryland. She is a former Poet Laureate of Maryland and has been nominated for the Pulitzer Prize in poetry. Her books of poetry include *Quilting, Next, An Ordinary Woman, Two-Headed Woman* and *Good Woman.* She has also published several children's books.

Janine O'Leary Cobb is the founder and publisher of *A Friend Indeed,* the international newsletter for women in menopause and midlife. Her book, *Understanding Menopause,* was published in 1988 by Key Porter Press in Toronto. She is a sociologist, teacher, wife and mother of five, as well as a lecturer and consultant on menopause.

Emma Joy Crone is a writer and networker who continues to disseminate words to increase the visibility of aging women. She published the newsletter, "A Web of Crones," for four years and now, at 63, is aging dis-gracefully on an island in British Columbia.

Geeta Dardick is a writer and photographer, specializing in non-fiction articles on parenting, farming, business, travel, disability and health. She has been published in *The Christian Science Monitor, East-West Journal,* and *Mothering,* among others. She is the author of *Home Butchering and Meat Preservation.*

ellen is associate editor of *Sculpture Gardens Review.* Her work has appeared in *Earth's Daughters, New Los Angeles Poets Anthology,* and *Poetry LA,* among others. She has received writing awards from *Z Miscellaneous* and New York Poetry Society.

Clara Felix was born in 1921 in Bronx, New York, of Russian-Jewish immigrants. Her three children are living proof that even an imperfect marriage can bring undeserved rewards. Her work as a late-blooming nutrition writer and consultant proves that life can begin (again) at 60. She plans to spend the rest of her life in the San Francisco Bay Area.

Marigold Fine is a video artist and producer living in Santa Cruz, CA. She has done freelance writing for several publications and for her own therapy and amusement. Women's lives and stories are of vital interest to her.

Linda Nemec Foster received her M.F.A. from Goddard College in Vermont; she currently lives in Michigan. Her poems have appeared in *Nimrod, Negative Capability, Passages North,* and other journals. A collection of prose poems, *A History of the Body,* was published by Coffee House Press in Minneapolis.

Betty Friedan is the author of *The Feminine Mystique.* She founded the National Organization for Women (NOW) in 1966 and served as its president for many years. She is a Distinguished Visiting Professor at the University of Southern California and in 1989 taught a course on Women, Men and the Media. She has three grown children.

Patricia Garfield is an international authority on dreams. A clinical psychologist who graduated summa cum laude from Temple University, she has been studying dreams professionally for 20 years. She is the author of *Creative Dreaming.* Her diary of over 39 years contains more than 20,000 dreams.

Sally Miller Gearhart is a San Francisco lesbian-feminist professor, activist, and writer. She is a product of the ten-cent picture show and the penny postcard, and lives her life on a mountain of contradictions. She believes fervently in the rights and dignity of non-human animals. She also believes in the healing power of aikido and barbershop harmony.

Elaine Goldman Gill owns The Crossing Press with John Gill. She's particularly proud of several things: her two sons, who seem to be growing up OK; the defeat of a nuclear reactor in Ithaca, N.Y. in 1973, engineered by her and John Gill; and the existence of the press, a politically open institution.

Jill Jeffery Ginghofer lives in Santa Cruz, CA, with her husband and three children. She works with and for women. Her poetry and prose have appeared in *Touching Fire: Erotic Writings by Women, Cosmopolitan, Feeding the Hungry Heart* and in other publications.

Elizabeth Gips has had many incarnations in one lifetime: housewife, mother, grandmother, big-businesswoman, hippie, poet, scholar, lover of spirit. She has had a radio program, "Changes," for the last 15 years in Santa Cruz, CA, which is a celebration of evolution and consciousness. Her life gets better the older she gets.

Marylou Hadditt, 62, is a crone who writes about her various roles as newspaper woman, mother, wife, recovering mental patient, lesbian, and social worker. She writes to heal and discover. She is now revising her play, *Rights of Passage, A Celebration for Midlife and Menopause* and is editor emeritus of *Sonoma County Women's Voices.*

Genia Pauli Haddon is the author of *Body Metaphors: Releasing God-Feminine In Us All*. She operates Haelix Plus, Inc. in Connecticut, where she provides individual and group resources for spiritual transformation, including depth psychotherapy, Kripalu yoga, shamanic techniques, and whole-brain audio technology developed at the Monroe Institute. She is working on a new book, *Spiritual Emergence at Menopause: The Teachings of Red Ridinghood's Grandmother*.

Joan Joffe Hall is a Professor of English and Women's Studies at the University of Connecticut. She has published four books of poetry, most recently *Romance And Capitalism At The Movies*, as well as a chapbook of fiction, *Summer Heat*. Her work appears in *Word of Mouth*, a collection of short-short fiction from The Crossing Press.

Heather is an ex-New Yorker who considers herself bi-coastal, dividing her time between California and Vermont. She's a lesbian feminist, a cat person, and a therapist working with severely disabled kids. She's published two books of poetry.

Carla Kandinsky has self-published eleven chapbooks, including the "Nekkid Ladies" series. She has been a San Francisco Bay Area Artist's model for 30 years. Berkeley Poet's Cooperative published her book *Instead of a Camera* in 1985. She is coordinator of the poetry series at Oakland's Coffee Mill, where she is known as Mama Kandinsky.

Chris Karras, 56, lives in rural Ontario with her husband of 37 years. Originally from Germany, they emigrated to Canada in 1956. She taught yoga for a decade and is presently employed as a licensed registered insurance broker. She is a committed letter-writer and a member of Amnesty International.

Maura Kelsea, RN, FNP, practices in Santa Cruz, CA, at the Santa Cruz Women's Health Center and in her private practice, Wellcare Associates. She provides health counseling and body-process work. She enjoys oceanside walks, back-packing and cross-country skiing. She is married and mother of two.

Gail M. Koplow is a past fiction editor of *Sojourner*, presently working on a collection of poems about love entitled *Fear on the Weekends*. She is the mother of several grown children.

Suzanne Laberge is a nominal grandmother who has been a housewife, hippie, social rebel and business woman. Presently she is a graduate student at Lesley College studying Expressive Therapy.

Candida Lawrence lives in Santa Cruz, CA. She writes stories and non-fiction. She has published in *Passages North, Ohio Journal, Missouri Review* and other literary journals. She teaches pre-schoolers and has taught 3–5 year olds for 25 years.

Ursula K. Le Guin is the author of the *Earthsea Quartet* series, *The Beginning Place, Buffalo Gals and Other Animal Presences* and *Dancing at the Edge of the World: Thoughts on Words, Women, Places.* She was born in Berkeley, CA, in 1929, educated at Radcliffe, and is the mother of three children. She is a member of the National Organization of Women and Women's International League for Peace and Freedom.

Ruth Levitan is a retired Oakland, CA, elementary school teacher who writes poetry and short stories. She has received awards for her poetry from the Bay Area Poet's Coalition, and the Villa Montalvo Literary Arts Competition, among others.

Mary Lou Logothetis has been an associate professor of Parent-Child Nursing and Women's Health in the College of Nursing at Valparaiso University, Indiana, for 11 years. She has over 20 years experience in a variety of roles related to the health care of women, with special interest in the menstrual cycle and its effect on women's lives.

Janet McCann has been teaching writing at Texas A&M for 22 years. Her poetry has appeared in several literary journals including *Southern Poetry Review.* Her most recent chapbook, *Afterword,* was published in 1990 by Franciscan University Press. She received a Creative Writing Award from the NEA in 1989.

Frances Ruhlen McConnel teaches Creative Writing at the University of California, Riverside. Her first book of poetry, *Gathering Light,* came out in 1979 and her second, *What the Bear Ate,* is seeking a publisher. She has almost completed a short story collection, *Sins of the Mothers.* Her family includes an academic husband, two creative daughters and two bewitching grandchildren.

Ginny MacKenzie teaches creative writing at the School of Visual Arts and C.U.N.Y. in New York City. Her poems have appeared in many literary magazines including *The Iowa Review, The Nation,* and *Ploughshares.* She is the author of a poetry chapbook, *By Morning,* and the editor and co-translator of the American and Chinese poetry anthologies, *New York/Beijing* and *Beijing/New York.*

Louise Mancuso is an Italian-American woman and writer, who, after 25 years, is just beginning to find her own voice. Her work has appeared in *Feminist*

Voices, Broomstick and *The Phoenix*. She is grateful to have made it through menopause without suffering, or causing, too much damage. She is presently editing an anthology on lesbian relationships.

Ann Mankowitz is a Jungian Analyst practicing in Santa Fe, New Mexico. She has an M.A. from Cambridge and a Ph.D. in psychology from the National University of Ireland. *Change Of Life: A Psychological Study of Dreams and the Menopause* was published in 1984 by Inner City Books in Toronto, Canada.

Nancy Mathews is a third generation Californian and is writing *Growing Up In California*. Her women's writing group provides much needed support. She is active with peace and environmental groups and tutors Learning Disabled adults at Santa Rosa College.

Brooke Medicine Eagle, an intertribal Indian metis, raised on a Crow reservation in Montana, is an Earthkeeper, artist, teacher, healer, performer, and songwriter dedicated to learning from Mother Earth/Father Spirit. Her vision and work have been documented in *Shaman's Drum, East-West Journal, Woman of Power* and other publications. An autobiography, *Buffalo Woman Comes Singing* (Ballantine, 1991) is her first book.

Maude Meehan, author of *Chipping Bone* and *Letting Go,* is a writer, editor, wife, mother, grandmother and political activist in movable order. She is a frequent lecturer in fields related to Women's Studies and for several years has led writing workshops in Santa Cruz, CA.

Ann Menebroker is the author of eleven books of poetry; her most recent is *Routines That Will Kill You.* She has co-edited two poetry anthologies and edited and published two poetry magazines. She is a board member of the Sacramento Poetry Center.

Deena Metzger is a poet, novelist, playwright and psychotherapist. Her books include *Looking For The Faces Of God, What Dinah Thought, The Woman Who Slept with Men to Take the War out of Them,* and the diary/novel *Tree* about healing from breast cancer. She is married to poet Michael Ortiz Hill, has two grown sons and lives at the end of a dirt road with the wolves, Owl and Isis.

Jane L. Mickelson is a voiceover narrator and freelance author who lives in Northern California with her family. She is deeply involved in the women's spirituality movement. Her other interests include music, reading, travel, herb gardening and textile arts.

Pat Miller, born in 1928, did what was considered desirable for women in the fifties: she married and raised children. As a "homemaker" her interests center around population dynamics, ecological issues, the creation of a humane sustainable planetary society, the worldwide establishment of basic human rights and international conflict resolution.

Constance Mortenson lives in Powell River, British Columbia and writes for *Women's Weekly* in London. Her work has appeared in numerous small magazines including *Alberta Poetry Yearbook*. She presently has three novels looking for a publisher and is working on a trilogy about a Logging Clan.

Jean Mountaingrove, 65, lives and gardens on a southern Oregon mountainside while exploring her experience of aging from a feminist perspective. She helped start the Old Lesbian Organizing Committee to give national voice to concerns of old lesbians, and is active in the Southern Oregon Country Lesbian Archival Project.

Marjory Nelson at 61 is exploring how to be an old woman who is also fat, lesbian, a writer, gardener, swimmer, emerging poet and artist, new grandmother, single at last, who supports herself as a hypnotherapist, and dreams of old women rising: crusty on the outside and soft in the middle.

Greta Hofmann Nemiroff is co-director of The New School of Dawson College in Montreal where she teaches Women's Studies, Humanities, and English. She is the author of *Reconstructing Education: Towards a Pedagogy of Critical Humanism* and *Interesting Times: Women in Canada: 1970-1990*. She is married and mother to three adult children.

Miki Nilan stumbles into each era of her life with a sense of surprise at the tables spread before her. Barren or bountiful, each has nourished her spirit. She has had short stories published in *The Bridge* and *Expression*. Her essay, "Tell Me Where I've Been," appeared in *Anna's House*, Fall '89.

Karen Ohm is a retired classical musician and former teacher of music. She works in Boulder, Colorado, as a computer assistant for the National Institute for Standards and Technology. She is now dealing with the effects of Post-Polio Syndrome, a disabling condition, but overcomes most obstacles with regular hydrotherapy and massage as well as a positive attitude.

Christina Pacosz has been an artist-in-the-schools for the Washington State and South Carolina Arts Commissions and a North Carolina Visiting Artist for the last four years. She has published four books of poetry including *This Is Not*

A Place To Sing (West End, 1987).

Evelyn M. Parke is a Communications Specialist for Bank of America. In the seventies she produced a full-length vampire film and in the eighties finally settled down to write. She is an obsessive needlepointer and ardent baseball fan. She writes essays for fun when it is not baseball season. She is 54, divorced, and has no children, by choice.

Carol Pascoe writes humor for periodicals and, under another name, is a poet and author in the mental health field, specializing in bereavement. "The relationship between grief and humor is not as dubious as it may sound," she says. "I've found that people who are afraid to throw back their heads and laugh are also afraid to let go and love. And, of course, people who cannot fully love will never truly grieve." Her poetry has appeared in *The New York Quarterly, Five Fingers Review,* and *The American Writer,* among others.

Fionna Perkins lives with husband, ponies, cats, and a large poodle among the trees of the Mendocino Coast. Her recently published work includes a fable, "Lady-Queen of the Night," in *Mendocino Review.* Readings of her stories and poetry have been aired on the "Women's Voices" program on KZYX.

Eleanor J. Piazza lives in the redwoods of Northern California. She earned a Master's degree in French and World Literature from San Francisco State University. For three years she lived in a Native American community where she learned a deep respect for ancient visions. Also known as Sumahsil, she is an activist in her community and exalts the Spirit of Woman.

Marge Piercy has a new novel forthcoming from Knopf in 1991. Her most recent novel, *Summer People,* is in Ballantine/Fawcett paperback. She has published eleven volumes of poetry of which *Available Light* is the most recent. She and her husband live in Wellfleet, Massachusetts.

Vickie C. Posey survived early menopause, but not without a struggle, one that led her to make some decisions about her life. One decision was to do some writing. She lives in Raleigh, North Carolina, where she works with an innovative literacy program called *Motheread.* She is married and is the mother of a daughter and son.

Pat Rhoda moved to an acre of land in Stockton, California, two years ago where she lives with her husband of 26 years and three lively adolescent cats. Writing does not come easy, this being her first and perhaps only attempt, but she wanted to share her experiences on the subject, it being close to heart and all.

Trudy Riley has been a social worker for 30 years and a feminist for 20. She began writing five years ago, at age 54, after taking a lesbian writers workshop. She lives in the Los Angeles area. "Commercial Messages" is her first published work.

Elisavietta Ritchie is editor of *The Dolphin's Arc: Poems on Endangered Creatures of the Sea*. Her book, *Flying Time: Stories and Half-Stories*, was recently published. She has read at the Library of Congress, and, under USIA auspices, in Brazil, the Far East, and the Balkans.

Pela Sander, a native Californian, is a mother and grandmother. She lives in Santa Cruz, CA, and is a practitioner of traditional medicine. She is a licensed Acupuncturist, Massage Therapist, and Herbalist. She has a private practice and works at the Santa Cruz Westside Community Health Center. She also gives classes across the U.S. and Canada.

Pat Schneider has published widely in literary journals including *The Minnesota Review*. Her libretto has been recorded by the Louisville Symphony, and performed by Robert Shaw and the Atlanta Symphony in Carnegie Hall, New York City. Fourteen of her plays have been produced, nine published. She lives in Amherst, MA, where she is the Director of Amherst Writers & Artists.

Penelope Scambly Schott is a poet and essayist. Her work has appeared in *The American Voice, Lear's, The Georgia Review*, and elsewhere. Her most recent collection of poetry is *These are My Same Hands*. Currently she is collaborating with her mother and daughter to explore the lives of three generations of women.

Marcia Seligson has written for virtually every major magazine in America, primarily on the subjects of female/male relationships, sexuality, health, entertainment, and all issues concerning women. She is the author of eight published books, including *The Eternal Bliss Machine: America's Way of Wedding and Options*. She has written two children's books.

Joanne Seltzer has published over three hundred poems in literary journals, anthologies and newspapers including *The Village Voice* and *Blueline*. Her essays, book reviews and short fiction have appeared in *The Small Press Review* and *Studia Mystica*. In 1989 Bard Press published her latest chapbook of poems, *Inside Invisible Walls*.

Gretchen Sentry is a former fashion model, designer, coordinator and artisan who was introduced to writing through the Women's Re-Entry Program at

Cabrillo College in Santa Cruz. Her work has been published in *Coydog Review, Good Times,* and *Porter Gulch Review.*

Kathleen Sims is a teacher, poet, practitioner of T'ai Chi Ch'uan and a rainbow warrior in service to the children of Mother Earth.

Dona Luongo Stein has been widely published in magazines, journals, anthologies, texts, and in the collection, *Children of the Mafiosi* (West End Press). Currently she teaches and writes in the Monterey Bay area of California. She is poetry editor for *Matrix.*

Amber Coverdale Sumrall is a lapsed Catholic, Wife and Teacher. She is co-editor of *Touching Fire: Erotic Writings By Women* (Carroll & Graf, 1989) and the forthcoming *Catholic Girls.* Her poetry and prose have most recently appeared in *New Voices From The Longhouse, The Women's Review of Books, Mid-America Review, Pearl, My Father's Daughter,* and *Word of Mouth.* She is addicted to the written word, LP's, the cinema, and her two teenage cats.

Dena Taylor was born in San Francisco in 1941. She has published in *Mothering* and is the author of *Red Flower: Rethinking Menstruation* (Crossing Press, 1988). She lives by the ocean with her two nearly adult daughters, where she works as a paralegal and free-lance writer. Part political activist, part hedonist, she is currently working on the proverbial novel and is looking forward to the feisty fifties and beyond.

Louise Loots Thornton is the co-editor of *I Never Told Anyone: Writings By Women Survivors of Child Sexual Abuse* (Harper and Row, 1983) and *Touching Fire: Erotic Writings By Women* (Carroll & Graf, 1990). She teaches writing and literature at Gavilan College in Gilroy, California, and lives near Santa Cruz amid dolphins and falling stars.

zimyá a. toms-trend of *mother courage productions* is an educator, whether employed as a therapist/counsellor, consultant, radio programmer, writer or filmmaker. Because she is an eclectic and eccentric anarchist activist she derives inspiration from Marshall McLuhan's quote: "If you're not part of the solution, then you're part of the problem."

Ellen Treen grew up in Michigan, went East to be educated, then bounced from coast to coast while raising four children. She now lives alone in Santa Cruz, CA, knitting, reading, and writing short fiction. Her work has been published in *Coydog Review, Porter Gulch Review,* and *In Celebration of the Muse.*

Gloria Vando is founding editor of *Helicon Nine* and a Poet-in-the-Schools in Missouri and Kansas. Her poems have appeared in *New Letters, Poets On,* and *Seattle Review,* among others. Her manuscript was a finalist in the Poetry Society of America's 1990 Alice Fay Di Castagnola Contest. In 1989 she was awarded the first Kansas Arts Commission Fellowship in Poetry.

Patrice Vecchione is the editor of three collections of poetry, including *Faultlines: Children's Earthquake Poetry.* Her poetry has most recently appeared in *Touching Fire: Erotic Writings By Women, Ikon, Quarry West,* and *Puerto del Sol.* She teaches poetry in Monterey Bay Area schools.

Katherine Wells is a mixed-media sculptor, poet, and performance artist. Her poetry has appeared in *Kayak, The Southern California Anthology,* and *Saturday's Women.* She has had numerous solo exhibitions of her visual work and was recently featured in *The Georgia Review.*

Kathy M. White works as a Rehabilitation Counselor for disabled youth in Berkeley. She has been writing and publishing poetry for nine years and is presently working on a chapbook of her haiku. She lives in Oakland with her husband and two children, who constantly provide many rich images for her writing.

Maureen Williams is a Kelt from Kernow presently living in the mountains of northeastern Pennsylvania. Britain's mystical past is the major influence in her writing. *Thirteen Keltic Moons,* her celebration of the Old Religion, was published in 1990 by Kittatinny Press. Her collection of stories, *Time Belongs To The Moon,* is forthcoming.

Clara E. Wood is the founder and director of Women In Midlife and Menopause (WMM), a support group in Washington, D.C. She has written short stories and poetry for over 30 years and has several publications to her credit. She lives in Greenbelt, Maryland.

Lea Wood is a 73-year-old feminist and peace and environmental activist who has lived in California since 1950. She has been an office secretary, conference and court reporter, housewife and mother of one, junior high teacher, environmental columnist, as well as a writer of plays, one filmscript, and numerous family chronicles.

RESOURCES

Informational Books

Brewi, Janice and Anne Brennan, *Mid-Life: Psychological and Spiritual Perspectives*. N.Y.: Crossroad Publishing Co., 1982

Brown, Judith K., et al., *In Her Prime: A New View of Middle-Aged Women*. Massachusetts: Bergin & Garvey Publishers, Inc., 1985

Cobb, Janine O'Leary, *Understanding Menopause*. Toronto, Canada: Key Porter Books, 1988.

Costlow, Judy et al., *Menopause: A Self-Care Manual*. Santa Fe, NM: Santa Fe Health Education Project, 1989 (Can be ordered from P.O. Box 577, Santa Fe NM 87501)

Cutler, Winifred Berg, M.D. and David A. Edward, Ph.D., *Menopause: A Guide for Women and the Men Who Love Them*. N.Y.: W.W. Norton & Company, 1983

Dickson, Anne and Nikki Henriques, *Women on Menopause*. Rochester, Vermont: Healing Arts Press, 1988

Doress, Paula Brown, Diana Laskin Siegal and the Midlife and Older Women Book Project, *Our Selves Growing Older: Women Aging with Knowledge and Power*. N.Y.: Touchstone Books, 1987

Downing, Christine, *Journey Through Menopause: A Personal Rite of Passage*. N.Y.: Crossroad Publishing Company, 1987

Garfield, Patricia, Ph.D., *Women's Bodies, Women's Dreams*. N.Y.: Ballantine Books, 1988

Gillespie, Larrian, M.D., *You Don't Have to Live with Cystitis*. New York: Avcon Books, 1986. See chapter on "How Menopause and Aging Affect Your Urologic Health"

Greenwood, Sadja, *Menopause Naturally: Preparing for the Second Half of Life*. San Francisco CA: Volcano Press, 1989

Haddon, Genia Pauli, *Body Metaphors*. N.Y.: Crossroad Publishing Company, 1988

Hufnagel, Vickie, M.D., *No More Hysterectomies*. N.Y.: Susan K. Golant, 1989

Lark, Susan, M.D., *The Menopause Self-Help Book*. Berkeley: Celestial Arts, 1990

Mankowitz, Ann, *Change of Life*. Toronto, Canada: Inner City Books, 1984.

Martin, Emily, *The Woman in the Body: A Cultural Analysis of Reproduction*. Boston: Beacon Press, 1987.

Parvati, Jeannine, *Hygieia: A Woman's Herbal*. Monroe, Utah: Freestone Publishing Co., 1978.

Reitz, Rosetta, *Menopause: A Positive Approach*. New York: Penguin Books, 1977.

Rogers, Natalie, *Emerging Woman: A Decade of Midlife Transitions*. CA: Personal Press, 1980

Scarf, Maggie, *Unfinished Business: Pressure Points in the Lives of Women*. N.Y.: Ballantine Books, 1988

Taylor, Dena, *Red Flower: Rethinking Menstruation*. Freedom CA: The Crossing Press, 1988

Walker, Barbara, *The Crone: Women of Age, Wisdom, and Power*. San Francisco CA: Harper & Row, 1985

Weideger, Paula, *Menstruation & Menopause*. N.Y.: Alfred A. Knopf, Inc. 1975.

Wilson, J., *Women, Your Body, Your Health*. N.Y.: Harcourt, Brace, Jovanovich, 1990

Publications

A Book About Menopause by Miryam Gerson and Rosemary Byrne-Hunter. To order, send $4.00 to Montreal Health Press, P.O. Box 1000, Station Place du Parc, Montreal, Canada H2W 2N1; tel: 514/272-5441

A Friend Indeed, a monthly newsletter whose "intention is to explore menopause as mythology, as biology, as feelings; to offer moral support to those who need it; to offer an exchange of information from woman to woman; and to gather together in one place relevant information so that women can make knowledgeable decisions." Box 515, Place du Parc Station, Montreal, Canada H2W 2P1, tel: 514/843-5730

Healthsharing: A Canadian Women's Health Quarterly, issue on menopause, Winter 1990. 14 Skey Lane, Toronto, Ontario, M6J 3S4

Hot Flash, the official publication of The National Action Forum for Midlife and Older Women, Box 816, Stony Brook, NY 11790

Woman of Power, issue #14

Articles

"Estrogen replacement: What are the risks?" in *Consumer Reports Health Letter,* November 1989, Vol. 1, No. 3

"On menopause and the toll that loss of estrogens can take on a woman's sexuality," by Jane Brody, *The New York Times,* May 10, 1990

"The Estrogen Fix," by Andrea Boroff Eagan, *Ms.*, April, 1989
"The Menopausal Years" by Beth Reimer, M.D. Daly City, CA: PAS Publishing, 1980

Miscellaneous
Stanford University Study on Menopause
Dr. Marcia Stefanick, Project Director

Organizations
Santa Cruz Women's Health Center
Santa Cruz, CA
Maura Kelsea, N.P.

North American Menopause Society
c/o Dr. Wulf Utian
Dept. of Obstetrics and Gynecology
The Mt. Sinai Medical Center
One Mt. Sinai Drive
Cleveland, Ohio 44106

The Institute for Reproductive Health
Vicki Hufnagel, M.D.
8721 Beverly Blvd.
Los Angeles, CA 90048
tel: 213/854-6483

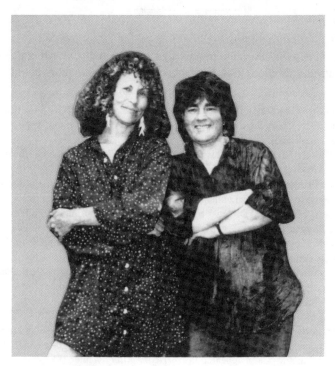

Photo by Heather Treen

Amber Coverdale Sumrall is co-editor of *Touching Fire: Erotic Writings By Women* (Carroll & Graf, 1989), *Catholic Girls* (Penguin/New American Library, 1992), and is editor of *Lovers* (The Crossing Press, 1992). She is a widely published poet and writer and lives in Santa Cruz, CA.

Dena Taylor is a freelance writer and researcher. She is the author of *Red Flower: Rethinking Menstruation* (The Crossing Press, 1988) and has published work in *Mothering*, *Matrix* and local newspapers. She lives with her two teenage daughters in Capitola, CA.

The editors are currently at work on an anthology about women's sexuality in midlife and beyond, to be published by The Crossing Press.

Some of the work in this book has previously appeared in the following publications to which authors and publisher gratefully acknowledge permission to reprint:

"A Journey Homeward" by Connie Batten appeared in *Woman of Power*, #14.

"Meeting The Tiger" by Sandy Boucher appeared in *Snake Power*, Vol. 1, #1, 10/89.

"Sweet Insanity" by Claire Braz-Valentine appeared in *In Celebration Of The Muse: Writings by Santa Cruz Women* (M Press, 1987).

"Giving Up The Rag" by Elayne Clift is reprinted from *Telling It Like It Is: Reflections of a Not So Radical Feminist* (KIT, 1991).

"The Mystique of Age" by Betty Friedan is reprinted in part by permission of the author from *Productive Aging* (Springer Publishing Co., 1985).

An excerpt from "Menopausal Dreams" by Patricia Garfield is reprinted from *Women's Bodies, Women's Dreams* (Ballantine, copyright 1988) by permission of the publisher.

"Flossie's Flashes" by Sally Gearhart is reprinted by permission of the author from *Lesbian Love Stories* (Crossing Press, 1989).

An excerpt from *Body Metaphors: Releasing God-Feminine in Us All* by Genia Pauli Haddon (copyright 1988 by Genia Pauli Haddon) is reprinted by permission of the author and The Crossroad Publishing Company.

"Eggs" by Gail M. Koplow appeared in *Sing Heavenly Muse*, #18, 1990.

"Space Crone" copyright 1976 by Ursula K. Le Guin; first appeared in *Co-Evolution Quarterly*; reprinted by permission of the author and the author's agent, Virginia Kidd.

"Forty-Five" by Janet McCann appeared in *Hurricane Alice*, Winter 1989.

"Aunt Lena Is Committed To Bellefonte State Hospital" by Ginny MacKenzie appeared in *Ploughshares*, Vol. 13, #4, 1988.

"The Neglected Crisis" by Ann Mankowitz is reprinted from *Change of Life: A Psychological Study of Dreams and the Menopause* (Inner City Books, 1984) by permission of the publisher.

"Grandmother Lodge" by Brooke Medicine Eagle is reprinted by permission of the author from *Red Flower: Rethinking Menstruation* (Crossing Press, 1988).

"Sheila and I Watch the Sunset Turn Red and Gray" by Deena Metzger is reprinted by permission of the author from *Looking For The Faces Of God* (Parallax Press, 1989).

"Changing Woman" by Jane L. Mickelson appeared in *Mothering*, Spring, 1986, in a slightly different version.

"Migraine" by Greta Hofmann Nemiroff appeared in *A Friend Indeed*, Vol. III, #6.

"The Changes," copyright 1981 by Fionna Perkins, reprinted by permission of the author from *When I Am An Old Woman I Shall Wear Purple* (Papier Maché Press, 1987).

"Something to look forward to" by Marge Piercy, is reprinted from *Available Light* by permission of Middlemarch, Inc. (copyright 1988 by Alfred A. Knopf, Inc.).

"Annunciations, October" by Elisavietta Ritchie appeared in *Visions*, 1989.

"The women we have become" by Penelope Scambly Schott appeared in *The American Voice*, #16, Fall 1989.

"Body Briefing" by Marcia Seligson appeared in *Lear's*, March 1990.

"In The Crevices Of Night" by Gloria Vando appeared in *Rampike: The First Anthology of Missouri Women Poets.*